CW00429856

Guidebook on

Enteral Medication Administration

Joseph I. Boullata,
PharmD, RPh, BCNSP, FASPEN, FACN
Editor

American Society for Parenteral and Enteral Nutrition

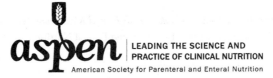

LEADING THE SCIENCE AND
PRACTICE OF CLINICAL NUTRITION
American Society for Parenteral and Enteral Nutrition

The American Society for Parenteral and Enteral Nutrition (ASPEN) is a scientific society whose members are healthcare professionals—physicians, dietitians, nurses, pharmacists, other allied health professionals, and researchers—dedicated to ensuring that every patient receives safe, efficacious, and high-quality patient care.

ASPEN's mission is to improve patient care by advancing the science and practice of clinical nutrition and metabolism.

NOTE: This publication is designed to provide accurate authoritative information with regard to the subject matter covered. It is sold with the understanding that the publisher is not engaged in rendering medical or other professional advice. Trademarked commercial product names are used only for education purposes and do not constitute endorsement by ASPEN.

This publication does not constitute medical or professional advice, and should not be taken as such. To the extent the information published herein may be used to assist in the care of patients, this is the result of the sole professional judgment of the attending health professional whose judgment is the primary component of quality medical care. The information presented herein is not a substitute for the exercise of such judgment by the health professional.

2 3 4 5 6 7 8 9 10
Copyright © 2019. American Society for Parenteral and Enteral Nutrition.

Print ISBN: 978-1-889622-36-1
eBook ISBN: 978-1-889622-37-8

Suggested citation: Boullata JI. *Guidebook on Enteral Medication Administration*. Silver Spring, MD: American Society for Parenteral and Enteral Nutrition; 2019.

Printed in the United States.

Dedication
To the mother who kept her son alive,
When others said he shouldn't survive

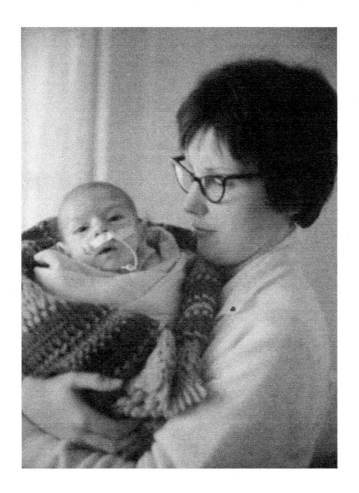

Contents

Preface

Far too often, the administration of an oral medication to a patient with an enteral feeding tube is an afterthought left to the discretion of the patient at home, a caregiver, or an inpatient nurse. At that point, the two basic options are either to improvise or to seek suggestions. With the former approach, the thought given to the preparation and administration methods is less than what is deserved for such complex pharmaceutical formulations. The potential for both obvious and unrecognized medication errors is always present. For the latter option, the person administering the medication may be guided, at best, by a knowledgeable pharmacist with a strong appreciation of clinical pharmaceutics or, at worst, by someone whose advice lacks an adequate evidence base. In either case, until now, there has been no single reference source available that is dedicated to this clinically important topic.

The purpose of this *Guidebook on Enteral Medication Administration* is to pull together the available information from multiple disparate sources into one easily accessible resource. The result is a book that provides the requisite background as well as specific recommendations for individual medications. The first part of the book contains chapters covering enteral access devices, drug interactions with nutrition, foundational principles of drug solubility and bioavailability, and the most current recommendations for drug preparation and administration. The second part of the book contains individual drug monographs, which summarize pharmaceutical and pharmacokinetic data, review enteral administration and nutrition considerations, and conclude with specific recommendations on how to prepare and administer the drug. References to the relevant literature are included.

The book is intended for use by healthcare providers including pharmacists, nurses, dietitians, and physicians involved in managing patients with an enteral access device, regardless of patient care setting. The book attempts to capture all the information that an individual provider may need—whether that is the simple recommendation at the end of a monograph, the available supporting data for that recommendation, or the foundational science that underpins the approach to enteral medication administration in general. For many years, the response by drug manufacturers to queries about how to prepare and administer a drug through an enteral feeding tube would be, "Why would you want to do that?" or "Our drug product is only approved for oral administration," or "We cannot be liable for the product if you destroy it for an unapproved method of delivery." As the industry has become more aware of the hundreds of thousands of patients requiring enteral medication administration, I expect that more information will be forthcoming.

This inaugural work has been limited to the most commonly prescribed oral drugs, to include most of the top 200 medications. Of note, the terms drug and medication are used interchangeably throughout this book. Additionally, this book is not intended to serve as an all-inclusive pharmacotherapeutic reflection of all populations (eg, pediatrics, geriatrics, pregnancy, lactation) or morbidities (eg, organ dysfunction, drug interactions). Within these limitations I hope that users will find this *Guidebook on Enteral Medication Administration* valuable as they provide the best care for their patients.

—JBoullata, PharmD (2018)

Acknowledgments

I would like to acknowledge a number of people without whom this work would not have been possible. My initial concept for the book was quickly appreciated by Peggi Guenter, PhD, RN, FAAN, FASPEN, who encouraged further development, including fruitful discussions with Jennifer Kuhn, MPS, former director of publications at the American Society for Parenteral and Enteral Nutrition (ASPEN), which eventually led to this interdisciplinary organization agreeing to serve as publisher of my *Guidebook*. The project has since been overseen by Catherine Wattenberg, director of publications at ASPEN, with the invaluable guidance of Elizabeth Nishiura, MA, who painstakingly copyedited all the work you find in these pages. I thank each of the authors who contributed a chapter and offer a special note of appreciation to Kayla Kotch, PharmD, who assisted with compiling some of the monographs, which included seeking input from manufacturers. My thanks also to the reviewers who took the time to provide constructive feedback on the content. Additional thanks to Lauren M. Hudson, MS, RD, LDN, my department director at the University of Pennsylvania Health System, for her support of the time and effort necessary to stay on top of this project. Thanks also to Stella L. Volpe, PhD, my department chair at Drexel University, Juan Muniz, PhD, and William Lane, RPh, for their support of my ongoing work in the pharmaceutical nutrition laboratory. Lastly, I would be remiss not to thank my loving wife, Laurel, who put up with many, many days and nights of me working on this project.

Contributors

Christel A.S. Bergström, PhD
Associate Professor in Pharmaceutics
Department of Pharmacy, Uppsala University
Uppsala, Sweden

Joseph I. Boullata, PharmD, RPh, BCNSP, FASPEN, FACN
Clinical Professor, Department of Nutrition Sciences, Drexel University
Pharmacy Specialist in Clinical Nutrition, Hospital of the University
    of Pennsylvania
Philadelphia, Pennsylvania, USA

Peggi Guenter, PhD, RN, FAAN, FASPEN
Senior Director of Clinical Practice, Quality, and Advocacy
American Society for Parenteral and Enteral Nutrition
Silver Spring, Maryland, USA

Hans Lennernäs, PhD
Professor
Department of Pharmacy, Uppsala University
Uppsala, Sweden

Reviewers

Hassan Almoazen, PhD
Assistant Professor and PhD Program Director
University of Tennessee, College of Pharmacy, Department
    of Pharmaceutical Sciences
Memphis, Tennessee, USA

Lingtak-Neander Chan, PharmD, BCNSP, FACN
Professor of Pharmacy and Nutritional Sciences
University of Washington, School of Pharmacy and Graduate Program
    in Nutritional Sciences
Seattle, Washington, USA

Michael L. Christensen, PharmD, BCNSP
Professor
University of Tennessee Health Science Center
Memphis, Tennessee

Mark G. Klang, MS, PhD, RPh, BCNSP
Core Manager, Research Pharmacy
Memorial Sloan Kettering Cancer Center
New York, NY

Andrew Mays, PharmD, CNSC
Clinical Pharmacy Specialist Nutrition Support
University of Mississippi Medical Center
Clinical Assistant Professor
University of Mississippi School of Pharmacy
Jackson, Mississippi, USA

Mary S. McCarthy, PhD, RN, CNSC, FAAN

Senior Nurse Scientist, Center for Nursing Science & Clinical Inquiry
Madigan Army Medical Center
Tacoma, Washington, USA

Carol McGinnis, DNP, APRN-CNS, CNSC

Clinical Nurse Specialist: Nutrition Support
Sanford USD Medical Center
Sioux Falls, South Dakota, USA

Fundamentals of Enteral
Medication Administration

Enteral Access Devices and Connectors

Peggi Guenter, PhD

Introduction

When oral feedings are not an option or do not adequately meet nutrient needs, enteral nutrition (EN), also known as *tube feeding,* can be used to support patients' nutrition requirements. Generally, patients who require nutrition via feeding tube also need medications delivered by this route. Patients receiving EN can be found in a variety of healthcare settings, ranging from the intensive care unit to long-term care and the home care setting. To best provide optimal medication delivery, clinicians must understand enteral feeding devices; the methods and sites of EN delivery; new enteral connector standards and products; and nursing, pharmacist, and caregiver medication delivery procedures. This chapter provides a thorough and timely discussion of a variety of enteral access devices (EADs) in the US market, including short- and long-term feeding tubes, as well as the administration sets and syringes with the new EN connectors. It also explains medication delivery processes using the latest equipment for patients in institutional care as well as home care and across the age-spectrum as appropriate.

Enteral Delivery System

Enteral Nutrition Access Devices

When a patient requires EN, the optimal device and location (gastric vs small bowel) for its delivery must be selected. Multiple factors, including the patient's age, lifestyle, gastric motility, risk of aspirating refluxed gastric contents, alterations in gastrointestinal (GI) anatomy, preexisting medical conditions, and anticipated length of therapy, affect the choice

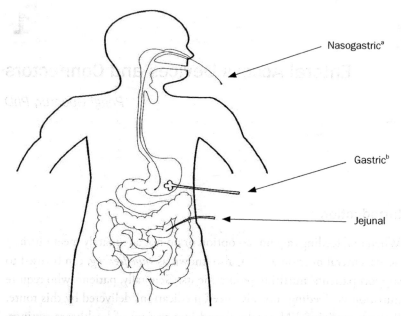

Nasogastric[a]

Gastric[b]

Jejunal

Figure 1-1. Enteral access devices. [a]The tube can also be advanced to become nasoduodenal or nasojejunal. [b]There are also combination gastrojejunal tubes. © American Society for Parenteral and Enteral Nutrition.

of EAD. Use of the stomach for gastric feedings is generally reserved for patients with normal gastric emptying and a low risk of pulmonary aspiration.[1] Small bowel feedings are the preferred choice in the presence of conditions such as gastric outlet obstruction, gastroparesis, increased risk of aspiration, and pancreatitis.[2,3] The use of gastrojejunal (GJ) tubes, which allow for simultaneous gastric decompression and small bowel feedings, may be indicated for gastric outlet obstruction, severe gastro-esophageal reflux, gastroesophageal regurgitation, and gastroparesis.[2–4] The decision to place long-term access depends on the estimated length of therapy, the patient's care setting and clinical conditions, and the special needs of the patient and caregivers. Figure 1-1 is a general illustration of EN device access into the GI tract.

Short-Term Enteral Nutrition Access Devices

EADs inserted via the nasal and oral routes are usually placed for short-term use in the hospitalized patient. However, in some situations, a

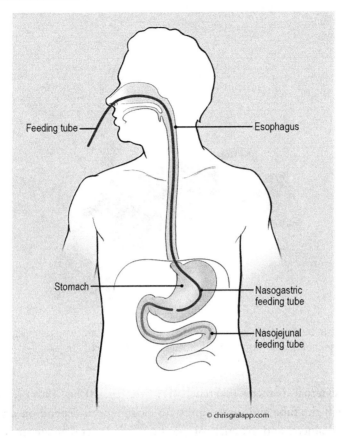

Figure 1-2. Nasogastric and nasojejunal feeding tube position. Illustration © Christine Gralapp. Reprinted with permission.

nasogastric access in the outpatient setting is appropriate. Some patients or caregivers are able to place an EAD in the home setting. Clinicians consider the estimated duration of enteral therapy when determining nasal tube placement vs tube enterostomy. Generally, tubes used for short-term therapy (less than 4 weeks) are placed nasally or, in some cases, orally, at the bedside blindly, endoscopically, or in interventional radiology under fluoroscopic guidance.[1] These tubes include nasogastric (NG), nasoduodenal (ND), nasojejunal (NJ), and nasogastric-jejunal tubes (NG-J). See Figure 1-2.

Nasoenteric feeding tubes come in a wide array of diameters and lengths, with multiple options such as stylets, feeding and medication ports, weights, and various tips. EADs are conventionally measured by

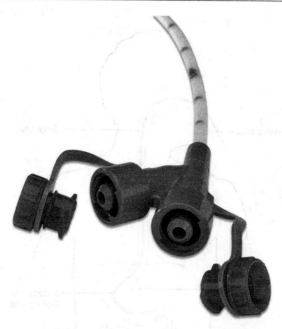

Figure 1-3. Dual ports on an enteral access device. Reprinted with permission from Cardinal Health (http://www.cardinalhealth.com).

their external diameter in French (Fr) Size (eg, 10 Fr). However, flow through the tube and susceptibility to clogging can depend on a tube's inner diameter and material composition. The inner diameter may vary depending on the specific material used to construct the tube. In general, polyurethane tubes have a larger internal diameter than silicone tubes of the same outer diameter.[5] Most nasoenteric feeding tubes have a single lumen with either one port for feeding or two ports in a "Y" configuration, one for feeding and the other for medication administration and/or flushing (Figure 1-3). These ports can accommodate a feeding administration set, an enteral syringe, or both. Dual ports into a single lumen can allow for both feeding and medication administration and/or irrigation. However, to maintain tube patency, medications should be administered through the EAD only after the enteral formula is temporarily stopped and the feeding tube is flushed with water (see Chapter 5).

NG and nasoenteric feeding tubes are inserted when short-term access is indicated. If longer-term access is required, they can also provide an opportunity to assess tolerance of enteral feedings prior to placement of an enterostomy tube. These types of EADs are passed transorally or transnasally, although the nasal approach is better tolerated in the conscious patient. NG or nasoenteric feeding tube placement is contraindicated in the presence of obstructing head, neck, and esophageal pathology or injury preventing safe insertion. Once placed, these feeding tubes should not be used until proper distal position is confirmed. EADs can also be placed with electromagnetic or direct camera visualization tools to confirm tube placement within the GI tract; however, without those tools, radiography remains the gold standard for confirming placement.[6,7]

Although NG tubes are the easiest EAD to insert, no procedure is without risk. Tube placement should be performed by clinicians with familiarity and competency in this skill. Larger, stiffer tubes used for gastric decompression should be converted to a smaller-bore EAD as soon as possible for patient comfort and to decrease the risk of associated complications. The length of the tube necessary for gastric placement can be estimated by measuring the distance from the tip of the nose over to the earlobe and then down to the xiphoid process plus 10 cm.[8] Aspiration of gastric contents, auscultation of insufflated air over the stomach, and absence of patient coughing or choking suggest but cannot ensure correct tube placement.[7] Figure 1-2 shows a properly placed nasoenteric tube. Confirmation of correct position of a newly inserted EAD is mandatory before EN or medications are administered.

Long-Term Enteral Access Devices

For long-term use (greater than 4 weeks), feeding tubes are placed into the stomach or small bowel via enterostomy (ie, opening in abdominal wall). A variety of techniques (ie, endoscopy, fluoroscopy, open laparotomy, and laparoscopic surgical methods) are used for enterostomy. Long-term percutaneous EADs (eg, gastrostomy, jejunostomy, and gastrojejunostomy tubes) may be placed with local anesthesia of the abdominal wall and intravenous conscious sedation, which may be a better option than general anesthesia in some patients. Gastrostomy tube placement using fluoroscopic techniques in interventional radiology suites is also a safe method. Figure 1-4 shows a placement of a commonly used gastrostomy tube.

Long-term EADs are available in a variety of diameters and lengths. The internal retention bolster of the gastrostomy tube keeps the tube

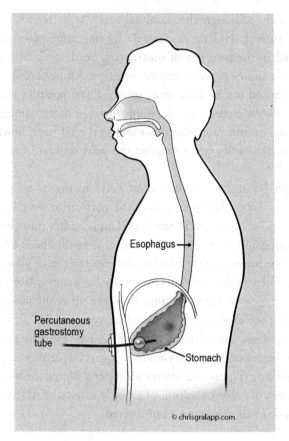

Figure 1-4. Percutaneous gastrostomy tube. Illustration © Christine Gralapp. Reprinted with permission.

from slipping out of the stomach. Solid internal bolsters, which are constructed of silicone or polyurethane, are more commonly used with initial percutaneous enterostomy tube placement. Balloon-type internal bolsters made of silicone are inserted more commonly with open or laparoscopic surgical tube placement, with fluoroscopically placed tubes, and as replacement devices. These balloons generally only have a lifespan of 3 to 4 months, but some may last longer (see manufacturers' descriptions for more information on balloon longevity).[9] Enterostomy feeding tubes may have multiple ports. Typically, separate ports are included for feeding and medication and/or flushing, similar to the short-term tubes (see Figure 1-3). If the internal bolster is of the balloon type, an additional third port is present for balloon inflation or deflation.

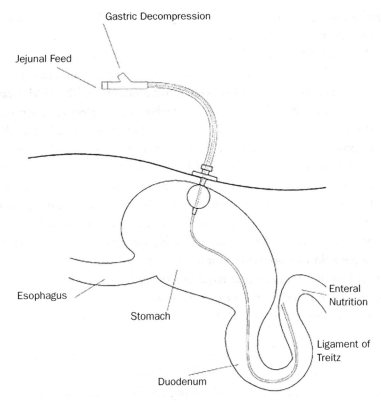

Figure 1-5. Gastrojejunal feeding and decompression tube. Reprinted from reference 3: Vanek VW. Ins and outs of enteral access. Part 3: long term access—jejunostomy. *Nutr Clin Pract.* 2003;18:201–220.

A postpyloric tube should be placed when a patient has impaired gastric motility, pancreatitis, or pancreatic surgery, or any time that enteral feeding into the small bowel is required. Some tubes are dual lumen, with a postpyloric distal end for feeding and another lumen terminating in the gastric pouch to allow for simultaneous stomach decompression. Gastrojejunal tube placement may be performed initially or at an appropriate time after gastrostomy tube placement. A gastrojejunal tube (Figure 1-5) can be placed during laparotomy or by endoscopic or fluoroscopic technique, using any of the methods described previously.[3] With these types of EADs, the patient benefits from gastric decompression while receiving EN into the small bowel.[3] It is important to note that the jejunal lumen of this type of tube can be easily clogged when medications are not prepared or administered appropriately. Also, the distal jejunal portion may flip back into the stomach, leading to unexpected adverse consequences.

Skin-level EADs, also known as *low-profile EADs,* are an excellent option for the patient who is concerned about cosmetic appearance and does not wish to have a visible feeding tube extension. This device can also be more comfortable for the patient who is active, sleeps in the prone position, or only needs intermittent therapy. Low-profile EADs may also be helpful for children or those likely to pull on conventional tubes. To attach a feeding extension set to the skin-level EAD, the patient must have good eye-hand coordination or caregiver assistance. Low-profile EADs are usually placed as an exchange tube for a pre-existing gastrostomy tube; however, they can be placed at the time of initial tube placement.[10] Skin-level devices are also available for jejunal access. Skin-level tubes are held in place with an inflated internal balloon or a distensible internal retention device that requires a trocar for placement. See Figure 1-6 to view the device and the extension set.

Jejunostomy tubes have their distal tip in the jejunum. These tubes can be useful in patients with a nonfunctioning or resected stomach and can be used as short-term or long-term EADs. These devices can be inserted surgically, endoscopically, radiologically, or laparoscopically. They are often surgically placed during another procedure.[3] See Figure 1-1 for an illustration of a jejunostomy feeding tube.

Enteral Nutrition Delivery Methods

To plan the appropriate medication delivery schedule for a patient receiving EN, clinicians and caregivers must be cognizant of the formula delivery method and feeding schedule. Administration of EN should be guided by the patient's age, lifestyle, underlying disease, nutrition status and nutrient requirements, type of EAD, and condition of the GI tract. Formula may be administered using bolus, intermittent, or continuous techniques, or a combination of these methods. *Bolus feedings* are defined as formula delivered to the EAD via a syringe over a short period of time. Usually, the bolus and gravity methods are well tolerated when EN is administered into the stomach. The feedings may be initiated with full-strength formula 3 to 8 times per day, with volume increased every 4 hours in adults as tolerated up to the goal volume.[7] The goal volume equals the amount of formula that closely meets the patient's

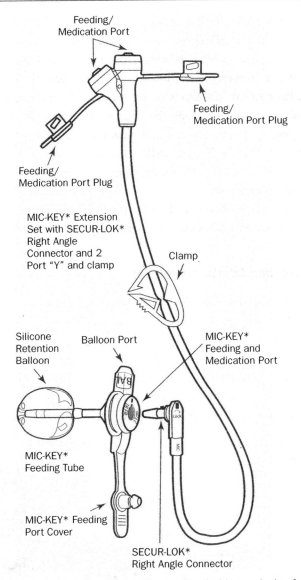

Figure 1-6. Skin-level device and extension set. Used with permission from Halyard Health. (https://www.halyardhealth.com).

predicted nutrient needs. *Intermittent feedings* are delivered to the EAD via a feeding container or bag over 30 to 45 minutes, with or without an enteral feeding pump. In a *continuous feeding,* an hourly rate of EN is administered using a feeding pump. A continuous feeding can be given in the stomach or small bowel, but a pump is required for small bowel feedings and is preferred for gastric feedings in critically ill patients, as a controlled administration rate of continuous feedings often enhances tolerance.[7] Formulas usually are started at 10 to 40 mL/h and advanced to the goal rate in increments of 10 to 20 mL/h every 4 to 8 hours as tolerated. Patients can also receive continuous feedings over a portion of the day only, such as during nighttime hours, and that method is referred to as *cyclic feeding*. For example, an adult patient might receive formula at 100 mL/h from 7 PM to 7 AM so that he or she can be mobile during the day. EN delivery may be improved by using a daily feeding volume target over 24 hours that prompts makeup of missing feedings within set guidelines.[11] These volume-based feeding protocols have been recommended to provide the patient adequate nutrition in a given 24-hour period.

Enteral Nutrition Administration Sets

A patient who requires intermittent or continuous feedings may have that formula delivered via gravity or a feeding pump. To easily deliver the formula, it is aseptically poured into an administration container (open system), connected with an administration set and then attached directly to the EAD. In a closed system, the ready-to-hang container is attached to the administration set and then attached directly to the EAD. See Figure 1-7 for an illustration of an administration set. These administration sets now

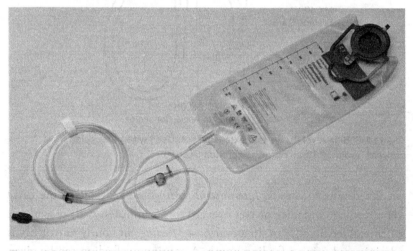

Figure 1-7. Enteral nutrition administration set for an open system. Reprinted with permission from Cardinal Health (http://www.cardinalhealth.com).

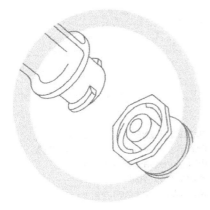

Figure 1-8. ENFit® connector. Reprinted with permission from Global Enteral Device Supply Association (http://gedsa .org). For more information, visit: www .stayconnected.org.

have the ENFit connector (Figure 1-8) at their distal end, which meets the ISO 80369-3 standard to prevent connecting an enteral administration set to an intravenous line or any small-bore connector not intended for enteral nutrient delivery.[12]

Enteral Nutrition Pumps

Enteral feeding pumps have advanced as the needs of patients receiving EN have evolved. These pumps are used routinely in every patient care setting and with every patient population. Some pumps are small and lightweight, making them particularly appropriate for ambulatory patients in a home care environment. All pumps are designed to be accurate to within 10% of the programmed EN delivery volume unless specifically documented to be more stringent.[7] Pediatric and infant enteral pumps require even more accuracy, delivering EN within 5% of the set volume. In a child or infant who requires full enteral support, a pump that delivers a volume that is off by 10% is problematic, given the risk for compromising growth and development. Some infants require use of a syringe pump to provide small volumes of EN with more accuracy.[7]

Enteral Syringes

When delivering bolus feedings, particularly in the home care setting, patients will often use a large syringe to administer their formula via the gravity bolus method. They may remove the plunger from the syringe after attaching the syringe to the feeding tube, then pour the formula into the

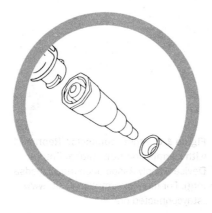

Figure 1-9. ENFit® transition set.
Reprinted with permission of GEDSA
(http://gedsa.org). For more
information, visit:
www.stayconnected.org.

syringe, and quickly administer the feeding. This approach should only be done as tolerated. Enteral syringes, whether large enough to administer formula or smaller to administer medication, now have the ENFit connector.

In patients who currently have long-term EADs without the ENFit connector, a transition connector, a type of interim adapter, will be needed to attach the ENFit syringe or ENFit administration set to the EAD. See Figure 1-9 for an illustration of that transition set.

Enteral Medication Administration

Patients receiving EN often require administration of medications through that same EAD. Understanding the complexity of drug delivery through a feeding tube and maintaining appropriate techniques to prepare and administer medications may help avoid an obstructed tube, reduced drug efficacy, or increased drug toxicity. Safe delivery of medications in patients receiving EN is optimized when preparation and administration techniques ensure bioavailability without further complicating the patient's overall care. Guidelines for administering medication via EADs are available,[13-21] as are multiple surveys of enteral drug administration practices and techniques.[20,21] The survey results suggest that practice differs significantly from guidelines, and several common practices could interfere with appropriate medication delivery.[20,21] According to the surveys, 38% to 98% of practitioners flush tubes before, between, or after medications are administered.[20,21] Only 32% to 38% of practitioners always administer drugs separately from one another; 52% to 60% dilute liquid medication; and 75% to 89% avoid crushing modified-release dosage forms.[20,21] Not following these best practices may contribute to adverse outcomes—tube obstruction, reduced drug efficacy, and increased drug toxicity in particular. See Chapter 5 for further details.

Enteral syringes have been recently developed in a variety of sizes with the ENFit connector to allow for medication and formula delivery into the newer EADs manufactured with ENFit connectors. Because of concerns around syringes with the reverse orientation (compared to Luer Lock or Cath-Tip syringes) and problems with low-dose medication accuracy due to additional syringe dead space, a new syringe (called the *low-dose tip syringe*) was developed, successfully tested, and received expedited US Food and Drug Administration review and approval. These syringes need to be filled using a specific process, which is outlined later in this chapter.

EADs are prone to clogging for a variety of reasons. One is accumulation of formula sediment in the lower segment of the tube, especially during slow administration rates of energy-dense formulas or those containing fiber.[22] Clogging is also more likely in small-diameter tubes and occurs more frequently in silicone tubes than polyurethane tubes.[7] Another common cause of tube clogging is the improper administration of medications via the tube.[7] Gastric tubes are reported to clog more frequently than small bowel tubes, presumably because of contact between enteral formula and acidic gastric fluid.[23] Because the feeding tube is often the lifeline to the patient and can be difficult and costly to replace, it is essential that the tube is flushed appropriately with water to maintain patency. For adults, a flush volume of 15 mL is usually adequate. To limit excessive free water administration, flush volumes for NG tubes should be limited to 1 to 3 mL in neonatal patients, and 3 to 5 mL in pediatric patients. Excess free water is particularly concerning for a child who is fluid-restricted, and, for this reason, small air flushes may be used. Purified water should be used for tube flushes, especially in immunocompromised or critically ill patients, and when the safety of tap water cannot be reasonably determined.[7]

Documented procedures and guidelines for medication administration through an EAD with clear step-by-step instructions can assist caregivers in optimizing the therapeutic response of the medication and preventing complications such as tube occlusion. Before enterally delivering any medications, it is important to assess tube size and tube tip location and note which medications can be crushed or dispersed and which ones can be switched to liquids or suspensions. It is also important to note that flushing is required between each medication administered. These flushes could amount to a large volume of water and must be taken into consideration when assessing the patient's hydration status and providing the daily water prescription. Accounting for the volume of water from flushes is particularly important if the patient is using a pump that intermittently delivers water.

Before administering medications via the enteral route, it is also crucial to verify tube placement using current guidelines.[7] Be sure to use clean technique, including hand hygiene, placing a clean cloth under connection, and ensuring that syringes are clean and dry and water is fresh and clean (or purified as appropriate). See Appendix 1-A for practice recommendations and medication administration techniques for inpatient settings using the ENFit connector. An instructional video of these processes is available at http://stayconnected.org/enfit-medical-guidelines.

Home Care Considerations

Patients and caregivers in the home care setting are most often responsible for EN and medication administration through the EAD. Now, with EADs with ENFit connectors, it is even more important that needs of the home patient be addressed. Childproof caps need to be in place, when appropriate, and the pharmacies and infusion companies that supply medications must provide the proper equipment so that the patients or caregivers can prepare and administer the medications safely through the feeding tube. Appendix 1-B describes options for a medication preparation and administration procedure that can be customized for your patient and caregiver at home. This appendix can be printed and used for caregiver or patient education.

In the home care setting, patients often reuse syringes and other equipment, even when they are labeled for one-time use only. Therefore, patients and caregivers need to be taught how to properly clean these devices. An instructional video of these processes at home is available at http://stayconnected.org/enfit-medical-guidelines.

Conclusion

To best schedule and deliver medications through a feeding tube, it is essential to understand where the EADs are placed anatomically, where the tube tip lies, and how the EN is delivered. The introduction of the

ENFit enteral connector and ENFit-compatible EN delivery system, best practices, and definitive procedures for both inpatient and home settings are keys to prevent complications and optimize therapy.

References

1. Vanek VW. Ins and outs of enteral access. Part 1: short-term enteral access. *Nutr Clin Pract.* 2002;17:275–283.
2. Vanek VW. Ins and outs of enteral access. Part 2: long-term access—esophagostomy and gastrostomy. *Nutr Clin Pract.* 2003;18:50–74.
3. Vanek VW. Ins and outs of enteral access. Part 3: long term access—jejunostomy. *Nutr Clin Pract.* 2003;18:201–220.
4. Lord LM. Enteral access devices: types, function, care, and challenges. *Nutr Clin Pract.*2018;33(1):16–38.
5. Fang JC, Kinikini M. Enteral access devices. In: Mueller CM, ed. *The ASPEN Adult Nutrition Support Core Curriculum.* 3rd ed. Silver Spring, MD: American Society for Parenteral and Enteral Nutrition; 2017: 251–264.
6. Smithard D, Barrett NA, Hargroves D, Elliot S. Electromagnetic sensor-guided enteral access systems: a literature review. *Dysphagia.* 2015;30(3): 275–285.
7. Boullata JI, Carrera AL, Banchik LH, et al. A.S.P.E.N. safe practices for enteral nutrition therapy. *JPEN J Parenter Enteral Nutr.* 2017;41:15–103.
8. Taylor SJ, Allan K, McWilliam H, Toher D. Nasogastric tube depth: the "NEX" guideline is incorrect. *Br J Nurs.* 2014;23(12):641–644.
9. Heiser M, Malaty H. Balloon-type versus non-balloon-type replacement percutaneous endoscopic gastrostomy: which is better? *Gastroenterol Nurs.* 2001;24:58–63.
10. Yarze JC, Herlihy KJ, Fritz HP, et al. Prospective trial evaluating early initiation of feeding in patients with newly placed one-step button gastrostomy devices. *Dig Dis Sci.* 2001;46:854–858.
11. Heyland DK, Cahill NE, Dhaliwal R, et al. Impact of enteral feeding protocols on enteral nutrition delivery: results of a multicenter observational study. *JPEN J Parenter Enteral Nutr.* 2010;34(6):675–684.
12. Guenter P, Lyman B. ENFit enteral nutrition connectors: benefits and challenges. *Nutr Clin Pract.* 2016;31(6):769–772.
13. Kurien M, Penny H, Sander DS. Impact of direct drug delivery via gastric access devices. *Exp Opin Drug Deliv.* 2015;12(3):455–463.
14. Wohlt PD, Zheng L, Gunderson S, et al. Recommendations for the use of medications with continuous enteral nutrition. *Am J Health-Syst Pharm.* 2009;66:1458–1467.

15. Williams NG. Medication administration through enteral feeding tubes. *Am J Health-Syst Pharm.* 2008;65:2347–2357.

16. Beckwith MC, Feddema SS, Barton RG, Graves C. A guide to drug therapy in patients with enteral feeding tubes: dosage form selection and administration methods. *Hosp Pharm.* 2004;39:225–237.

17. Dickerson RN. Medication administration considerations for patients receiving enteral tube feedings. *Hosp Pharm.* 2004;39:84–89,96.

18. Magnuson BL, Clifford TM, Hoskins LA, Bernard AC. Enteral nutrition and drug administration, interactions, and complications. *Nutr Clin Pract.* 2005;20:618–624.

19. White R, Bradnam V. *Handbook of Drug Administration via Enteral Feeding Tubes.* London, UK: Pharmaceutical Press; 2007.

20. Guenter P, Boullata J. Nursing2013 survey results: drug administration by enteral feeding tube. *Nursing.* 2013;43(12):26–35.

21. Boullata JI. Drug administration through an enteral feeding tube. *Am J Nurs.* 2009;109(10):39–42.

22. Lord LM. Restoring and maintaining patency of enteral feeding tubes. *Nutr Clin Pract.* 2003;18:422–426.

23. Powell KS, Marcuard SP, Farrior ES, Gallagher ML. Aspirating gastric residuals causes occlusion of small-bore feeding tubes. *JPEN J Parenter Enteral Nutr.* 1993;17:243–246.

APPENDIX 1-A

Procedure for Inpatient Settings:
Preparing and Administering Medications Using ENFit®

Purpose: Outline the preparation and administration of medication doses using the ENFit system. This procedure will be applicable to patients of all age groups in inpatient settings.

Background: The ENFit® system is the new ISO standard for enteral connectors. It promotes patient safety by reducing the risk of misconnection between unrelated systems by implementing a unique mechanical design. The syringes are available in 2 tip versions: low dose and standard dose.

The standard ENFit tip is used on most syringe sizes. The low dose tip (available in smaller sizes as defined by the manufacturer) was developed to address clinicians' concerns about dosing accuracy when delivering small medication volumes. For syringe performance information on the low dose tip and other currently available products, see GEDSA's ENFit Low Dose Tip presentation (www.stayconnected.org).

ENFit Standard Tip Syringe

ENFit Low Dose Tip Syringe

MEDICATION PREPARATION: FILLING A SYRINGE USING A BOTTLE FILL CAP

Always consult the syringe manufacturer on instructions for use. These are guidelines for general filling practices and do not supersede the manufacturer recommendations.

Current fill caps will NOT work directly with the new ENFit syringes. This procedure will demonstrate different ways to to fill ENFit syringes.

Liquid medication bottle with open top

Liquid medication bottle with press-in oral syringe adapter

CURRENT

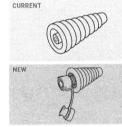

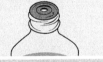

NEW

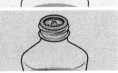

Step 1. Make sure that the medciation bottle has an ENFit compatible fill cap such as the ones shown above.

Step 2. Attach the syringe to the bottle adapter.

Step 3. Turn medication bottle upside down.

Step 4. Quickly pull and push syringe to cycle (eliminates air bubbles).

Step 5. Pull plunger back to desired dose.

Step 6. Turn bottle right side up and remove syringe.

APPENDIX 1-B

Procedure for Home Care Settings:
Preparing and Administering Medications Using ENFit®

Purpose: Outline the preparation and administration of medication doses using the ENFit system. This procedure will be applicable to patients of all age groups in home care settings.

Background: The ENFit® system is the new ISO standard for enteral connectors. It promotes patient safety by reducing the risk of misconnection between unrelated systems by implementing a unique mechanical design. The syringes are available in 2 tip versions: low dose and standard dose.

ENFit Standard Tip Syringe   ENFit Low Dose Tip Syringe

FILLING THE SYRINGE WITH A MEDICATION STRAW

When an ENFit bottle cap will not fit the medication bottle or it is impossible to remove the current bottle adapter, fill the syringe using a medication straw.

Example of a Medication Straw

| Step 1. Connect the ENFit medication straw to the syringe. | Step 2. Insert straw through existing adapter or directly into bottle. | Step 3. Cycle the syringe to help eliminate air bubbles and then draw up medication to desired dose. | Step 4. Disconnect straw from syringe and gently tap to remove any remaining medication. | Step 5. Make sure there are no air bubbles at the lower end of the syringe. | Step 6. Carefully tap or flick the syringe to remove air bubbles or excess fluid in the moat. |

FILLING THE SYRINGE USING A MEDICATION CUP

If the medication is delivered in a dose cup and needs to be transferred to an enteral syringe, the syringe can be prepared in two ways. NOTE: Filling the syringe via a dose cup is not the preferred method for filling the syringe.

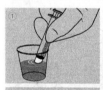

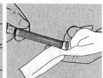

| Step 1. Submerge tip of syringe into medication cup after priming syringe. | Step 2. Cycle the syringe and then gently pull up on the plunger to fill syringe to desired dose. | Step 3. Tap/flick the syringe to remove air bubbles. | Step 4. Wipe off end of syringe to remove excess medication in tip. |

Drug Interactions with Nutrition

Joseph Boullata, PharmD

Introduction

Regardless of the route of administration, the effects and bioavailability of medications are influenced by a wide array of factors, including interactions. The most commonly appreciated interactions are those between one drug and another. Mechanistically, they can be described as *pharmaceutical, pharmacokinetic,* or *pharmacodynamic* in nature. The number of potential interactions is very large, and, despite significantly improved predictive models used in drug development, some clinically relevant interactions are only recognized after the medication is widely available in the marketplace.[1,2] Drug interactions with nutrition are no less important than drug-drug interactions.[3] Unfortunately, clinicians' degree of familiarity with drug-nutrition interactions is far less than their knowledge of drug-drug interactions and may be limited to a few more frequently identified types, including some common food-drug interactions. In the context of administering medication through an enteral access device (EAD) (ie, feeding tube), this chapter offers an overview of drug-nutrition interactions and then discusses interactions between drugs and enteral nutrition (EN) specifically.

Drug-Nutrition Interactions

Definitions and Classifications

Drug-nutrition interactions reflect a physical, chemical, physiological, or pathophysiological relationship between a medication and (a) one (or multiple) nutrient(s); (b) food in general; (c) specific foods or food components; (d) nutrition status; or (e) metabolic status.[3-5] As with any drug

Table 2-1. Examples of Drug-Nutrition Interactions

Precipitating Factor	Object	Examples
Drug	Nutrient	• Carbamazepine lowers biotin status. • Isoniazid impairs vitamin B_6 status.
Drug	Nutrition status	• Quetiapine increases weight gain. • Sorafenib is associated with sarcopenia.
Drug	Metabolic status	• Capecitabine may cause hypertriglyceridemia. • Olanzapine may cause hyperglycemia.
Nutrition status	Drug	• Obesity results in lower ertapenem levels. • Vitamin C deficiency prolongs pentobarbital action.
Specific nutrient	Drug	• Vitamin D reduces atorvastatin concentrations. • Iron supplements reduce doxycycline concentrations.
Food component	Drug	• Calcium reduces ciprofloxacin absorption. • Protein interferes with levodopa absorption.
Food	Drug	• Grapefruit juice increases simvastatin toxicity. • Enteral nutrition impairs ciprofloxacin absorption.

Source: Data are from references 3 and 4.

interaction, one element of the relationship is considered the precipitating factor (the "perpetrator") while the other is the object (the "victim") of the interaction. The precipitating factor may be any of the listed components (eg, drug, nutrient, food, or nutrition status), with any other component as the object of the interaction. As a result, several subtypes of drug-nutrition interaction exist, and they could be individually described as "food-drug" interactions or "drug–nutrition status" interactions, among others. Table 2-1 describes each category of drug-nutrition interaction with examples. For a drug-nutrition interaction to be considered clinically significant, there is an expectation that therapeutic drug response is altered and/or nutrition status is compromised. Altered drug response or nutrition status may be represented by a 20% or greater change in biomarkers or kinetic parameters from a baseline or anticipated effect. The time frame over which this change occurs varies with the precipitating factor and object. The severity of consequences may vary, with some individuals at higher risk based on their age, genetic variants, organ function, or disease state. As a result, the clinical significance or severity of the drug-nutrition interaction (like that of the drug-drug interaction) may be difficult to predict. The classification depicted in Table 2-1 provides a systematic approach to identifying, recognizing, and understanding drug-nutrition interactions.[3,4] Identified drug-nutrition interactions can each fit into one of the classification subtypes as new data become available. Ideally, clinicians would like to be able to *predict* all possible drug-nutrition interactions, or assess their clinical relevance, even when published data are unavailable. This type of analysis requires a keen clinical eye and an appreciation for the mechanisms of interactions.

Mechanisms of Interaction

A model that links drug-nutrition interactions with their physiologic effects and clinical outcomes helps differentiate interactions by mechanism.[4] Such a model runs parallel to mechanisms involved in drug-drug interactions. Some interactions are based on physicochemical reactions that take place in a nutrition delivery device or the lumen of the gastrointestinal (GI) tract (ie, pharmaceutical interactions). These interactions have the distinct potential to alter the bioavailability of one or more substances. Other interactions are the result of actions at cell membrane transporters or metabolizing enzymes (pharmacokinetic) or yield an antagonistic, additive, or synergistic effect on physiologic function (pharmacodynamic). The potential consequences of these interactions are altered bioavailability, distribution, clearance (ie, elimination from the body), and clinical effect of the drug (or nutrient). When the interaction is sufficient enough to alter a drug's (or nutrient's) effect or disposition, including altered biomarkers (direct or functional), it has the potential to be clinically significant. For example, taking a drug with a meal may significantly alter the drug's bioavailability compared to administration in the fasted state, based on the ratio of area under the concentration-time curves (AUCs) under each condition falling outside of 80% to 125%.

In drug development, techniques such as quantitative structure-activity relationship (QSAR) modeling and physiologically based pharmacokinetic (PBPK) modeling, or approaches through the Biopharmaceutics Classification system (BCS) or Biopharmaceutics Drug Disposition Classification system (BDDCS), are used to predict the likelihood of interactions. Additionally, our colleagues in computational biology are using an integrative-systems approach to better predict interactions based on known properties of drugs, foods, nutrients, and physiologic proteins.[6] This emerging approach even incorporates gene targets to further refine outcome prediction. However, we still need methods to account for differences between patients that are much less granular than genetic characteristics. For example, interindividual variability in GI function (eg, motility) and differences in intestinal permeability between gut regions can influence bioavailability.[7,8] The clinically relevant drug transporters (both the respective gene and protein expression) vary by segment along the GI tract, including the small and large intestines.[9] The low-solubility/ permeability medications (BCS Class 1) that also have high affinity to CYP3A (an enzyme with its own inter-/intrasubject variability) are risk factors for high intrasubject variability in absorption.[10] Additionally, although studies using physiologically based computer modeling to examine the effects of fed vs fasted states on drug bioavailability are helping to improve predictions, they also expose the interpatient variability.[11] Therefore, what follows is a brief description of drug-nutrition interaction subtypes, which takes into account both the newer approaches to prediction and the limitations of those models. Although some representative data are cited, the ability of the clinician to make predictions based on class effect, potential mechanisms, or unexpected clinical outcome observations remains indispensable.

Medications

The influence of medications on nutrition status in general or on the status of specific nutrients or metabolic biomarkers can be significant and is important to consider during patient care.[12] Many different mechanisms are at play that can influence global status (ie, body weight, volume status), individual nutrient stores (eg, hypokalemia, hypozincemia), or metabolism (eg, dyslipidemia, dysglycemia). Drugs can influence food intake, digestion, and absorption. The effect on intake may occur through the central nervous system, more local GI mechanisms, or both. Clinical manifestations can be as much patient-specific as drug-specific. These unintended drug effects can include changes in appetite, body weight, and composition, as well as GI effects (eg, taste disorders, mucositis, nausea, vomiting, abdominal pain, constipation, and diarrhea). Sometimes, nutrition status is influenced by a less-common or less-obvious adverse drug effect or combination of effects. For example, if a patient taking pertuzumab experiences drug-induced fatigue along with dysgeusia, nausea, and abdominal pain, he or she may reduce food intake, which increases weight loss.[13,14] The impairment of the ability to gather, prepare, and ingest food may occur following drug-induced cognitive, visual, movement, or gait disturbances.

During clinical trials, nutrition status is rarely an endpoint except for documentation of weight changes, glycemic control, or electrolyte abnormalities. When altered nutrient absorption, distribution, metabolism, excretion, or status is recognized as a drug-induced effect, it is usually identified in postmarketing cases, case series, or studies. Classic nutrient deficiency syndromes are rare, but lesser deficits may be more frequently manifest. This point highlights the value of routine nutrition-focused history taking and physical examination. The magnitude of change in biomarker or kinetic parameters (when available) will be relevant to the potential clinical significance of, and recommended intervention for, an interaction. For example, although the mechanism is unclear, symptomatic hypomagnesemia can result from treatment with the proton-pump inhibitor omeprazole.[15] Based on competition at several transporters as studied with an in vitro model, metformin may impair thiamin status.[16] Numerous medications can interfere with vitamin B_6 status, and others with vitamin D status.[17,18] The value of nutrient supplementation in the face of clinically significant drug-induced deficits requires more study for specific recommendations.[19,20]

Nutrition Status

Just as hepatic or renal function are determining factors in drug disposition and effect, so is a patient's nutrition status.[21,22] An evaluation of a drug's pharmacokinetic/pharmacodynamic profile is infrequently made with respect to nutrition status (ie, protein-energy malnutrition, obesity, micronutrient deficits). Protein-energy malnutrition and obesity can influence a drug's distribution and clearance as a result of altered body composition and function, which is rarely described for most drugs.[23]

Weight-based dosing of medication in particular can become challenging in patients toward extremes of body habitus.[22,24] Body surface area and "ideal" body weight are not considered appropriate metrics for drug dosing in these circumstances.[22] Drug dosing based on empiric body weight relative to height without taking body composition into account is not recommended, especially when a validated predictive equation for lean weight that accounts for body mass index (eg, the Duffull-Green equation) is available.[25,26] The resultant value may be more appropriate for weight-based dosing in obesity when taking into account the altered distribution of a drug.

Micronutrient deficits can also influence drug disposition and effect.[21,27] This type of interaction can include an influence on the function or stability of enzyme systems involved in drug metabolism.[21] For example, vitamin C deficiency can influence the action of barbiturates and other drugs through a pharmacokinetic mechanism,[28-30] and iron deficiency may reduce activity of the widely used CYP3A4.[31]

Specific Foods

Individual components of a food or those specific ingredients that may be consumed as dietary supplement products may influence drug disposition. For example, dietary protein and protein supplements can increase drug metabolism.[32] The effect may be specific to a protein source (eg, soy protein vs casein) at inducing transporters and enzymes.[33] Numerous beverages that contain a wide variety of polyphenols are known to influence drug bioavailability.[34] Grapefruit juice is one commonly recognized example.[35] Grapefruit juice components (eg, bergamottin, naringin) influence a number of drug-metabolizing enzymes and drug transporters (including CYP3A and OATP, respectively) to increase bioavailability of some drugs (eg, atorvastatin) and reduce bioavailability of others (eg, etoposide).[35-37]

Individual nutrients (eg, micronutrients) and associated substances (eg, polyphenols) can influence drug disposition, especially when they are found at pharmacologic doses in dietary supplements. Anthocyanins and the glycoside-free anthocyanidins, which are found in common berries, can interact with CYP enzymes and transporters.[38,39] Some of these flavonoids and other phytochemicals can be found at higher concentrations in dietary supplement products, and these supplements are therefore more cause for concern than food sources with regard to interactions.[40] About

12% to 45% of persons using dietary supplements concurrently with prescription medication are at risk for interaction, with up to 29% of those experiencing an interaction that is considered serious or clinically significant.[41-44] Dietary supplement ingredients may also influence nutrient disposition. For example, the transport of thiamin and folic acid can be reduced by polyphenols.[45] Based on in vitro data, thiamin, riboflavin, and pyridoxine can interfere with zinc intestinal transport.[46] As always, caution should be exercised in extrapolating any in vitro and in vivo data to clinical situations.

The gut microbiota may potentially influence drug bioavailability in the face of nutrition exposure. Studies of bacteria-drug interactions, including those supplied in probiotic products, continue to provide additional mechanistic data.[47] Specific nutrients and other constituents of food products differentially influence the many species of microorganisms found in the gut. While some food ingredients may be used for energy and growth, others may affect expression of the microbiome and numerous metabolites formed. For example, questions about the poor systemic bioavailability of polyphenols has led to the suggestion that their clinical benefits occur indirectly by interaction with the gut microbiota.[48] The mechanisms by which these substances involve the gut microbiota may include a prebiotic role in modulating microbial populations, a metabolic role of the microbiota to liberate bioavailable polyphenol metabolites, or an indirect effect via microbiota-derived gene-product metabolites. The prebiotic role would render an influence on inflammation in general.[49] A change in inflammatory mediators, whether based on microbial population or specific metabolites made available, may result in subsequent effects on drug transporters and metabolizing enzymes. The metabolites of the microbiota ("postbiotics") may in turn influence gene expression in the gut epithelium and beyond.[50,51]

Meals

The presence of a meal changes the physiologic conditions within the gut lumen into which drug is administered. Depending on the medication, the result may be a change in rate and/or extent of drug absorption, with the latter influence on bioavailability (represented by change in AUC) being potentially significant. Absorption across the intestinal mucosa is not the same as oral bioavailability (ie, amount of drug delivered to the systemic circulation or site of effect), as the latter is more difficult to predict given the first-pass effect.[52] However, food is reasonably well established to influence drug absorption and bioavailability.[53] This type of interaction can occur for a variety of physicochemical and physiologic reasons, including altered gastric emptying rate, proximal intestinal pH, bile flow, splanchnic blood flow, and enterocyte permeability, transport, and metabolism. Well-designed food-effect studies are useful in recognizing food-drug interactions and designing management strategies. The US Food and Drug Administration (FDA)–recommended test meal, which contains 800 to 1000 kcal with about 50% of energy from fat, is often—but not always—used for food-effect bioavailability studies. Therefore, to make an informed practice recommendation, it is important to note what test meal conditions have been used in a study. The antipsychotic ziprasidone offers a good example of how complex the meal effect might be. The drug's bioavailability is enhanced using the standard high-calorie/high-fat meal, but the effect is seen to a greater extent when a high-calorie/low-fat meal is used and a lower extent with a low-calorie/high-fat meal.[54,55] Beyond test-meal conditions, therapeutic diets prescribed in the clinical setting may influence drug disposition. For example, a modified Atkins diet has been reported to reduce serum concentrations of several antiepileptic drugs (by up to 46% in the case of lamotrigine), requiring close therapeutic monitoring.[56]

In the absence of clinical data, a drug's known physicochemical data can be used to predict drug disposition with a meal. Each drug's solubility and permeability characteristics (see Chapters 3 and 4) may help predict meal effects on bioavailability. Generally, drugs with low solubility but high permeability/metabolism (ie, BCS or BDDCS Class 2 agents) can have an increased bioavailability in the presence of food, whereas a negative effect is more likely for BCS or BDCCS Class 3 drugs.[57] No meal-effect is expected with BDDCS Class 1 drugs, and few data exist for Class 4 drugs (the least-represented group). A clinical study will provide data on the extent to which the change in bioavailability is clinically significant (eg, AUC change of 20% to 25%).

Each of the described types of drug interactions with nutrition is important, and any of them may certainly be at play in patients receiving medication through an EAD. However, the interaction with EN is typically the primary concern in enteral medication administration. With the confines of the EAD (see Chapter 1) for delivering both enteral feeds and medication, along with variability in drug preparation methods (see

Chapter 5), this focus is understandable. Given the wide variability in EN formulations and delivery methods, the potential for interaction goes beyond extrapolating from meal/food effect data and is deserving of further study and discussion.

Optimizing Drug Delivery and Enteral Nutrition

Introduction

In recent years, several excellent publications have provided valuable information on medication administration through enteral feeding tubes, including interactions with EN.[58-63] These are interactions that may occur in the enteral delivery device or within the GI lumen or at the gut mucosal epithelium. An appreciation of the complexity of medication administration in enterally fed patients has led to reference works with drug monographs.[64]

Historically, with an open enteral feeding system, there has always been an opportunity for admixing medication with the EN formula directly in the delivery container. A 2013 national survey revealed that 21% of nurse respondents still add drugs, including antimicrobials and electrolytes, directly to the EN formula.[65] Given the compatibility and stability concerns, this administration method is not recommended.[63] Adding medication directly to an EN formula requires knowledge of their compatibility together, the stability of each component, and the presumed therapeutic effectiveness of the drug when administered under conditions of typical use. The studies that have been performed over the years have been limited by the number of products evaluated, the heavy reliance on visual compatibility over chemical compatibility and stability, and the relevance of the in vitro findings for bioavailability.[66-71] Altered pH, osmolality, and viscosity of the admixtures were rarely described.[67,69] Although these older data with their limitations cannot be extrapolated to newer EN products or medications, the studies have provided some general insight into the product variables that may influence compatibility. These include liquid drug product pH (≤ 4 is generally more problematic) and alcohol content (can denature protein), as well as EN protein type (casein is more problematic) and fiber content (can form gel). Furthermore, in vitro incompatibility between drug and EN formula predicts tube clogging that cannot be flushed clear as well as drug concentrations that generally decline over time. Current recommendations support administration of appropriate medication through the same EAD as EN but do not support mixing the two in the delivery container.[63]

A general admonition to treat EN as a meal and temporally dose medication accordingly may make sense for the patients being fed intermittently with meal-like volumes/rates into the stomach. However, continuous feeds into the stomach or small bowel are less representative of a meal effect.[60] A number of articles have described the effects of administering both the drug and EN through the same EAD in this scenario, and these articles provide recommendations, albeit for only a handful of medications. (These potential drug-nutrition interactions with EN will be discussed later in this chapter.) The clinical decision points at the center of this discussion are (a) whether or not to hold the EN in order to administer the medication through the EAD, and (b) if EN *is* held, how long should it be interrupted before and after drug administration to avoid the interaction. An overriding clinical concern is that each interruption in feeding to accommodate drug administration risks inadequate delivery of nutrition. As a result, especially in acute care settings, the option of selecting an alternative medication or route of administration (despite cost and other implications) needs to remain viable.

In some cases, the presumed EN-drug interaction may actually be the result of an interaction between the medication and the access device that involves properties of the drug formulation, how it is prepared, and the physical dimensions and material of the feeding tube. For example, diazepam solution may adsorb to the feeding tube.[60] Lanthanum, sevelamer, and sucralfate are to be avoided altogether in patients receiving EN, given these drugs' limited water solubility and interaction with residual EN components, and the resulting high risk for a clogged feeding tube,[60] which would, of course, significantly interrupt and delay the patient's EN delivery.

A special case of potential tube clogging involves the proton pump inhibitors. These drugs reduce gastric acid secretion and are used in the management of patients with gastroesophageal reflux and peptic ulcer disease as well as stress-related mucosal damage. Potential tube obstruction using the enteric-coated products depends on the granule size of the product relative to the internal diameter of the EAD, which is generally problematic when the tube is less than 14 Fr.[72] Combining these products with water tends to increase the stickiness of the enteric-coated granules toward each other, which further increases occlusion risk. Fruit juices (eg, apple, orange) are to be avoided because they increase that stickiness even further, especially when their pH is less than that of the EN. Immediate-release proton pump inhibitors (commercially available or extemporaneously prepared in sodium bicarbonate solution using the USP method) are preferred for enteral feeding tube administration because their clinical effectiveness is maintained.[73] Suspensions made from lansoprazole solutabs or omeprazole immediate-release preparations are preferred when small-bore feeding tubes greater than 6 Fr are used.[72] Of course, the intravenous route is always an option for acutely ill patients.

Returning to reported interactions between EN and individual drugs, a thorough evaluation of the literature by an American Society for Parenteral and Enteral Nutrition (ASPEN) task force was presented at Clinical Nutrition Week in 2015, providing an update on the authenticity and significance of these interactions. Although not yet published, the task force's work has taken into account the limitations in the literature (case reports, small sample sizes, design) to offer a set of recommendations. Table 2-2 and the remainder of the chapter review the most frequently discussed drugs with a potential for interaction with EN.

Antiepileptic Drugs

Classic (eg, carbamazepine, phenytoin) and newer-generation (eg, lamotrigine, vigabatrin) antiepileptic agents, many of which have a narrow therapeutic index, are widely used for a number of neurologic disorders. Both carbamazepine and phenytoin are considered BDDCS Class 2 agents. Their solubility issues contribute to slow and variable GI absorption, but they are expected to be better absorbed in the presence of a meal. Liquid formulations (ie, suspensions) of these drugs are frequently used, especially for enterally fed patients.

In vitro studies using different solid dosage forms of *carbamazepine* revealed the lowest drug recovery in the presence of EN.[74] Single-dose carbamazepine suspension administered by nasogastric tube exhibited a 10% mean reduction in bioavailability compared with oral dosing in the fasted state, but with significant intersubject variability.[75] The studies did not account for the important roles played by the 10 Fr tube, administering undiluted suspension, or gut metabolism. An in vitro evaluation of multiple methods to prepare and administer carbamazepine suspension

Table 2-2. Selected Enteral Nutrition–Drug Interactions

Drug	Comments
Antiepileptic Drugs	
Carbamazepine	• No need to separate drug administration from timing of EN. • Dilute suspension, and flush EAD well before/after dose. • Closely monitor therapeutic drug effects.
Phenytoin	• No need to separate drug administration from timing of EN. • Dilute suspension, and flush EAD well before/after dose. • Closely monitor therapeutic drug effects.
Fluoroquinolones	
Ciprofloxacin	• Avoid drug administration soon after or before EN; separate from feeding by at least 2 hours.
Levofloxacin	• Avoid drug administration soon after or before EN; separate from feeding by at least 2 hours.
Moxifloxacin	• Avoid drug administration soon after or before EN; separate from feeding by at least 2 hours.
Ofloxacin	• Avoid drug administration soon after or before EN; separate from feeding by at least 2 hours.
Others	
Levodopa	• Separate drug administration from intermittent EN administration or protein administration by at least 2 hours. • Consider drug administration in daytime, with continuous EN at night.
Warfarin	• Separate drug administration from EN administration by at least 1 hour. • Dilute the drug in a small volume and administer quickly.

Abbreviations: EAD, enteral administration device; EN, enteral nutrition.

identified best drug recovery at the distal end of the feeding tube when the suspension was diluted (1:1 by volume) followed by flushing.[76] Drug loss was between 2% and 24% with no EN involved. Modified-release carbamazepine granules diluted in formula resulted in 50% to 100% tube occlusion rates in patients with 14- to 24-Fr EADs.[77] When suspended in water and administered rapidly, the granules still caused tube occlusion in a proportion of these patients.[77]

Sharp clinical observation revealed that patients receiving *phenytoin* suspension via nasogastric tube along with EN had subtherapeutic drug concentrations.[78] This finding led to a prospective study to determine whether EN truly interfered with drug absorption. Its conclusion that continuous EN by the nasogastric tube significantly interfered with absorption of phenytoin suspension regardless of whether the patient is stabilized on drug or EN first has been widely cited, as has the suggestion that withholding EN for 2 hours before and after drug administration will prevent the interaction.[78,79] The interaction was reported in subsequent cases.[80] A study performed in volunteers using phenytoin suspension seemed to suggest that the interaction varied with the EN formula.[81] However, neither the mechanism for the purported interaction nor best practices to prevent it have been made clear.[82] Withholding EN for 2 or more hours around the dose of phenytoin has not necessarily improved phenytoin absorption.[83] Clamping a gastrostomy tube for 1 hour after the dose of phenytoin and before restarting EN was shown to improve serum concentrations in a group of patients.[84] Of note, no description was provided of drug dilution, flushing protocol, or the EN regimen.

Many mechanisms, none of them definitive, have been suggested for the interaction between phenytoin and EN, and, because of limited data, there is no agreement on how to manage it.[85] Some have suggested that the interaction has nothing to do with EN and is related to the method of preparing and administering the drug through the EAD. An in vitro study of multiple methods of administration suggested not only that dilution of the suspension, with a flush before and after the dose, improves the delivery through a 16-Fr nasogastric tube but also the interaction may be with the feeding tube, and not the EN.[86] This lack of EN effect was reflected in patient case reports.[87] Another in vitro study evaluated a single dose of phenytoin suspension administered through a 20-Fr gastrostomy tube under various conditions.[88] Investigators described best drug recovery when the undiluted suspension was followed by a flush. The differences between the two in vitro studies include the type of EAD (ie, material, diameter, and surface area). Given the high pKa of phenytoin, a solubility effect of the relatively acidic EN and gastric pH has also been suggested.[89] There is additionally more binding to the tube at a lower pH. Missing from all these data are pharmacokinetic studies that examine bioavailability. This omission is important because of the nonlinear kinetics of phenytoin, with its erratic absorption in which a single dose may take over 24 hours to be absorbed.[90] Although conducted in healthy subjects, AUC analysis available from prospective randomized controlled trials suggest no difference in phenytoin bioavailability with EN.[91,92] Another pharmacokinetic analysis more closely representing clinical use, with continuous EN administered through a nasogastric tube, used two different phenytoin formulations in a single-dose crossover design.[90] The drug was diluted and the feeding tube was flushed before and after drug administration. The absolute bioavailability was about 90%, with greater variability with the suspension than the sodium salt, but similar to values seen in the fasted state.

The absorption profile of another anti-epileptic drug, *vigabatrin*, may be significantly reduced by a peptide-based infant formula when both are administered orally; however, no data are yet available for enteral administration.[93] This reduction in absorption may be related to an interaction at the epithelial transporter, based on an in vitro and in vivo study.[93]

The current data do not support withholding EN for any significant time to administer carbamazepine or phenytoin, but the drug suspension should first be diluted, and the tube should be flushed prior to and following drug administration. Additionally, patients receiving these anti-epileptic drugs will need to be more closely followed when receiving EN therapy. When considering the unproven practice of withholding EN, clinicians must be aware of the risks for the reduced delivery of nutrients or feeding intolerance with increased EN administration rates.

Fluoroquinolone Antimicrobials

The fluoroquinolone antimicrobials are valuable for treating a variety of infections caused by susceptible microorganisms. Critical to their clinical effectiveness is achieving adequate serum concentrations that remain above a defined AUC–to–minimum inhibitory concentration (MIC) for the organism. Interactions that reduce bioavailability run the risk for therapeutic failure. Multivalent cations (ie, aluminum, calcium, iron, magnesium, and zinc) chelate with the fluoroquinolones and significantly reduce bioavailability.[94,95] Temporal spacing of at least 2 to 4 hours may be adequate to alleviate the interaction with therapeutic doses of these minerals as found in antacids and supplements.[94-96] The interaction of ciprofloxacin, levofloxacin, moxifloxacin, or ofloxacin with an EN formulation that contains multivalent cations can result in significantly reduced bioavailability of the drug, and it takes place quickly.[97-101] The degree of interaction will depend on cation concentrations in the EN.[97] A molar ratio of cation to fluoroquinolone of 1–3:1 and elevated pH may play a role in maximally reducing drug bioavailability. Interpatient variability is significant, thereby limiting the predictability of the interaction in an individual patient.[98,100,102,103] It remains prudent to avoid administration of fluoroquinolones together with EN; no single best alternative (eg, separating by at least 2 to 4 hours, administering higher drug doses, or using the parenteral route) is known.[104]

Levodopa

Levodopa, widely used in the management of patients with Parkinson disease, competes with protein for intestinal absorption. This interaction can impair drug absorption, resulting in clinical exacerbations and a neuroleptic malignant-like syndrome, similar to the effect of a reduction in drug dose. This outcome has also been reported in acutely ill patients receiving EN through the gastric or postpyloric route.[105,106] Clinical exacerbations in enterally fed patients resolved with protein-dose reductions (to ≤1 g/kg) and/or separating drug administration from EN.[107,108] Although this interaction could be avoided by reducing protein intake or administration, the restriction of daily protein or shifting more protein to the evening (ie, "protein shifting") may result in nutritional deficits over time. Managing this interaction involves providing bolus feedings separated from levodopa administration by at least 2 hours, nighttime feedings with daytime medication, or an empiric increase in drug dose as needed.[106] In a pilot study of essential amino acid supplementation (16 g daily, distributed apart from meals and levodopa) to address protein restriction in patients with Parkinson disease managed with levodopa, no detrimental effects were seen after 6 months.[109]

The FDA recently approved a device for administration of the new suspension formulation of carbidopa/levodopa that delivers the drug continuously into the small bowel; the objective is to bypass the erratic gastric emptying in patients with Parkinson disease and minimize motor fluctuations and dyskinesia.[110] The expectation is that EN will be administered through the gastric access of the device. However, unless the EN is being administered as a bolus, which is unlikely given the high risk for aspiration in these patients, there will cease to be much separation of formula and drug. In the more clinically stable patient, the individualized dosing regimen of medication infuses over 16 hours in the day, with EN being administered over 8 hours at night despite some interaction at overlapping times. Given the disease-induced impairment of GI motility in parkinsonian patients, it is not clear whether this regimen plays any role in feeding tube disruption.[111]

Warfarin

Warfarin, an anticoagulant used to manage patients with venous thromboembolism or atrial fibrillation, works by inhibiting VKORC1 activity, thereby interfering with vitamin K activation and availability to carboxylate glutamate residues as required by several clotting factors for activation. As a result, there was an historic concern that vitamin K intake would interfere with the drug's anticoagulant effect, and the first reported treatment failures in patients receiving warfarin and EN were subsequently attributed to the vitamin K content of the formulations.[112,113] However, an interaction was still being reported after the manufacturers reformulated their EN products with much lower vitamin K content.[114-116] Current approaches do not support vitamin K restriction as a strategy to improve warfarin's effect.[117] In fact, consistent vitamin K intake helps maintain adequate anticoagulation.

An in vitro study published in 1989 revealed that a physicochemical (rather than a pharmacodynamic) interaction, likely due to the macromolecular fraction of EN, was the mechanism resulting in lower warfarin availability and clinical failure.[118] This finding seemed to be confirmed by patient case reports in which separating warfarin from EN administration by 1 to 3 hours mitigated the interaction.[119-121] Another in vitro study indicated that warfarin binds with the large, unfilterable component of EN, a problem that is seemingly worse in the presence of formulas with intact protein than with an amino acid–based formula.[120] A crossover case series further suggests the complexity of warfarin disposition in patients receiving EN.[122] This investigation indicated that withholding continuous EN for 1 hour before and after warfarin administration significantly improved the international normalized ratio response—with an overall difference of 0.87.[122,123] Another in vitro study identified a potential role of warfarin binding to a polyurethane feeding tube.[124] Therefore, in addition to holding the feed for an hour around the daily warfarin dose, the drug may be best delivered rapidly in a small volume with adequate flushing before and after.

Other Medications

A few other medications, including levothyroxine, penicillin V, and theophylline, will probably benefit from being administered separately from EN.[60] However, some types of medication are best administered in close proximity with EN, to take advantage of optimizing food-effect bioavailability. These drugs include atovaquone and posaconazole.[60]

Conclusion

All types of interactions between drugs and nutrition are important to consider in the patient receiving EN. In the absence of data on the effect of food or EN, it may be possible to predict the influence on the extent of drug absorption based on physicochemical properties.[125]

References

1. Greenblatt DJ, von Moltke LL. Drug-drug interactions: clinical perspective. In: Rodrigues AD, ed. *Drug-Drug Interactions.* 2nd ed. New York: Informa Healthcare; 2008:643–664.
2. Bohnert T, Patel A, Templeton I, et al. Evaluation of a new molecular entity as a victim of metabolic drug-drug interactions—an industry perspective. *Drug Metab Disp.* 2016;44:1399–1423.
3. Boullata JI. Drug and nutrition interactions: not just food for thought. *J Clin Pharm Ther.* 2013;38:269–271.
4. Boullata JI, Hudson LM. Drug-nutrient interactions: a broad view with implications for practice. *J Acad Nutr Diet.* 2012;112:506–517.

5. Chan LN. Drug-nutrient interactions. *JPEN J Parenter Enteral Nutr.* 2013; 37:450–459.

6. Jensen K, Ni Y, Panagiotou G, Kouskoumvekaki I. Developing a molecular roadmap of drug-food interactions. *PLoS Comput Biol.* 2015; 10:e1004048.

7. Talattof A, Price JC, Amidon GL. Gastrointestinal motility variation and implications for plasma level variation: oral drug products. *Mol Pharm.* 2016;13:557–567.

8. Dahlgren D, Roos C, Lundqvist A, et al. Regional intestinal permeability of three model drugs in human. *Mol Pharm.* 2016:13:3013–3021.

9. Drozdzik M, Groer C, Penski J, et al. Protein abundance of clinically relevant multidrug transporters along the entire length of the human intestine. *Mol Pharm.* 2014;11:3547–3555.

10. Sugihara M, Takeuchi S, Sugita M, et al. Analysis of intra- and intersubject variability in oral drug absorption in human bioequivalence studies of 113 generic products. *Mol Pharm.* 2015;12:4405–4413.

11. Kim SHJ, Jackson AJ, Hunt CA. In silico, experimental, mechanistic model for extended-release felodipine disposition exhibiting complex absorption and a highly variable food interaction. *PLoS One.* 2014; 9:e108392.

12. Piccolo KM, Boullata JI. The influence of polypharmacy on nutrition. In: Bendich A, Deckelbaum RJ, eds. *Preventive Nutrition.* 5th ed. New York: Humana Press; 2016:83–113.

13. Gordon MS, Matei D, Aghajanian C, et al. Clinical activity of pertuzumab (rhuMAb 2C4), a HER dimerization inhibitor, in advanced ovarian cancer: potential predictive relationship with tumor HER2 activation status. *J Clin Oncol.* 2006;24:4324–4332.

14. Agus DB, Sweeney CJ, Morris MJ, et al. Efficacy and safety of single-agent pertuzumab (rhuMAb 2C4), a human epidermal growth factor receptor dimerization inhibitor, in castration-resistant prostate cancer after progression from taxane-based therapy. *J Clin Oncol.* 2007;25:675–681.

15. Shabajee N, Lamb EJ, Sturgess I, Sumathipala RW. Omeprazole and refractory hypomagnesaemia. *BMJ.* 2008;337:173–175.

16. Liang X, Chien HC, Yee SW, et al. Metformin is a substrate and inhibitor of the human thiamine transporter, THTR-2 (SLC19A3). *Mol Pharm.* 2015;12:4301–4310.

17. Ueland PM, Ulvik A, Rios-Avila L, Midttun Ø, Gregory JF. Direct and functional biomarkers of vitamin B6 status. *Annu Rev Nutr.* 2015; 35:33–70.

18. Jones G. Extrarenal vitamin D activation and interactions between vitamin D_2, vitamin D_3, and vitamin D analogs. *Annu Rev Nutr.* 2013;33:23–44.

19. Morrow LE, Wear RE, Schuller D, Malesker M. Acute isoniazid toxicity and the need for adequate pyridoxine supplies. *Pharmacotherapy.* 2006;26:1529–1532.

20. Drain PK, Kupka R, Mugusi F, Fawzi WW. Micronutrients in HIV-positive persons receiving highly active antiretroviral therapy. *Am J Clin Nutr.* 2007;85:333–345.

21. Walter-Sack I, Klotz U. Influence of diet and nutritional status on drug metabolism. *Clin Pharmacokinet.* 1996;31:47–64.

22. Boullata JI. Drug disposition in obesity and protein-energy malnutrition. *Proceed Nutr Soc.* 2010;69:543–550.

23. Jacques KA, Erstad BL. Availability of information for dosing injectable medications in underweight or obese patients. *Am J Health-Syst Pharm.* 2010;67:1948–1950.

24. Pai MP. Drug dosing based on weight and body surface area: mathematical assumptions and limitations in obese adults. *Pharmacotherapy.* 2012;32:856–868.

25. Janmahasatian S, Duffull SB, Ash S, et al. Quantification of lean body-weight. *Clin Pharmacokinet.* 2005;44:1051–1065.

26. Beckman LM, Boullata JI, Fisher PL, Compher CW, Earthman CP. Evaluation of lean body weight equation by dual-energy X-ray absorptiometry measures. *JPEN J Parenter Enteral Nutr.* 2017;41:392–397.

27. Conney AH, Burns JJ. Factors influencing drug metabolism. *Adv Pharmacol.* 1962;1:31–58.

28. Richards RK, Kueter K, Klatt TJ. Effects of vitamin C deficiency on action of different types of barbiturates. *Proc Soc Exp Biol Med.* 1941; 48:403–409.

29. Conney AH, Bray GA, Evans C, Burns JJ. Metabolic interactions between L-ascorbic acid and drugs. *Ann N Y Acad Sci.* 1961;92:115–127.

30. Ginter E, Vejmolova J. Vitamin C-status and pharmacokinetic profile of antipyrine in man. *Br J Clin Pharmacol.* 1981;12:256–258.

31. Pai AB, Norenberg J, Boyd A, Raj D, Chan L-N. Effect of intravenous iron supplementation on hepatic cytochrome P450 3A4 activity in hemodialysis patients: a prospective open-label study. *Clin Ther.* 2007; 29:2699–2705.

32. Anderson KE. Effects of specific foods and dietary components on drug metabolism. In: Boullata JI, Armenti VT, eds. *Handbook of Drug-Nutrient Interactions.* 2nd ed. New York: Humana Press, 2010:243–265.

33. Ronis MJJ, Chen Y, Liu X, et al. Enhanced expression and glucocorticoid-inducibility of hepatic cytochrome P450 3A involve recruitment of the pregnane-X-receptor promoter elements in rats fed soy protein isolate. *J Nutr.* 2011;141:10–16.

34. Fleisher B, Unum J, Shao J, An G. Ingredients in fruit juices interact with dasatinib through inhibition of BCRP: a new mechanism of beverage-drug interaction. *J Pharm Sci.* 2015;104:266–275.

35. Bailey DG. Grapefruit and other fruit juices interactions with medicines. In: Boullata JI, Armenti VT, eds. *Handbook of Drug-Nutrient Interactions.* 2nd ed. New York: Humana Press, 2010:267–302.

36. Ando H, Tsuruoka S, Yanagihara H, et al. Effects of grapefruit juice on the pharmacokinetics of pitavastatin and atorvastatin. *Br J Clin Pharmacol.* 2005;60:494–497.

37. Dolton MJ, Roufogalis BD, McLachlan AJ. Fruit juices as perpetrators of drug interactions: the role of organic anion-transporting polypeptides. *Clin Pharmacol Ther.* 2012;92:622–630.

38. Sand PG, Dreiseitel A, Stang, M, et al. Cytochrome P450 2C19 inhibitory activity of common berry constituents. *Phytother Res.* 2010;24:304–307.

39. Dreiseitel A, Oosterhuis B, Vukman KV, et al. Berry anthocyanins and anthocyanidins exhibit distinct affinities for the efflux transporters BCRP and MDR1. *Br J Pharmacol.* 2009;158:1942–1950.

40. Egert S, Rimbach G. Which sources of flavonoids: complex diets or dietary supplements? *Adv Nutr.* 2011;2:8–14.

41. Peng CC, Glassman PA, Trilli LE, et al. Incidence and severity of potential drug-dietary supplement interactions in primary care patients: an exploratory study of 2 outpatient practices. *Arch Intern Med.* 2004; 164:630–636.

42. Lee AH, Ingraham SE, Kopp M, et al. The incidence of potential inter-actions between dietary supplements and prescription medications in cancer patients at a Veterans Administration hospital. *Am J Clin Oncol.* 2006;29:178–182.

43. Sood A, Sood R, Brinker FJ, et al. Potential for interactions between dietary supplements and prescription medications. *Am J Med.* 2008; 121:207–211.

44. Loya AM, González-Stuart A, Rivera JO. Prevalence of polypharmacy, polyherbacy, nutritional supplement use and potential product inter-actions among older adults living on the United States-Mexico border: a descriptive, questionnaire-based study. *Drugs Aging.* 2009;26:423–436.

45. Martel F, Monteiro R, Calhau C. Effect of polyphenols on the intestinal and placental transport of some bioactive compounds. *Nutr Res Rev.* 2010;23:47–64.

46. Tupe RS, Agte VV. Effect of water soluble vitamins on Zn transport of Caco-2 cells and their implications under oxidative stress conditions. *Eur J Nutr.* 2010;49:53–61.

47. Selwyn FP, Cheng SL, Klaassen CD, Cui JY. Regulation of hepatic drug-metabolizing enzymes in germ-free mice by conventionalization and probiotics. *Drug Metab Disp.* 2016;44:262–274.
48. Shen L, Ji H-F. Intestinal microbiota and metabolic diseases: pharmacological implications. *Trends Pharmacol Sci.* 2016;37:169–171.
49. Morais CA, de Rosso VV, Estadella D, Pisani LP. Anthocyanins as inflammatory modulators and the role of the gut microbiota. *J Nutr Biochem.* 2016;33:1–7.
50. Shukla SJ, Sakamura S, Huang R, et al. Identification of clinically used drugs that activate pregnane X receptors. *Drug Metab Disp.* 2011; 39:151–159.
51. Yan Q. Membrane transporter and drug development: relevance to pharmacogenomics, nutrigenomics, epigenetics, and systems biology. *Methods Mol Biol.* 2010;637:1–21.
52. Tian S, Li Y, Wang J, et al. ADME evaluation in drug discovery. 9: Prediction of oral bioavailability in humans based on molecular properties and structural fingerprints. *Mol Pharm.* 2011;8:841–851.
53. Fleisher D, Sweet BV, Parekh A, Boullata JI. Drug absorption with food. In: Boullata JI, Armenti VT, eds. *Handbook of Drug-Nutrient Interactions.* 2nd ed. New York: Humana Press; 2010:209–241.
54. Lincoln J, Stewart ME, Preskorn SH. How sequential studies inform drug development: evaluating the effect of food intake on optimal bioavailability of ziprasidone. *J Psychiatr Pract.* 2010;16:103–114.
55. Sutton SC, Nause R, Gandelman K. The impact of gastric pH, volume, and emptying on the food effect of ziprasidone oral absorption. *AAPS J.* 2017;19:1084–1090.
56. Kvernelend M, Taubøll E, Selmer KK, et al. Modified Atkins diet may reduce serum concentrations of antiepileptic drugs. *Acta Neurol Scand.* 2015;131:187–190.
57. Benet LZ. The role of BCS (Biopharmaceutics Classification System) and BDDCS (Biopharmaceutics Drug Disposition Classification System) in drug development. *J Pharm Sci.* 2013;102:34–42.
58. Magnuson BL, Clifford TM, Hoskins LA, Bernard AC. Enteral nutrition and drug administration, interactions, and complications. *Nutr Clin Pract.* 2005;20:618–624.
59. Williams NT. Medication administration through enteral feeding tubes. *Am J Health-Syst Pharm.* 2008;65:2347–2357.
60. Wohlt PD, Zheng L, Gunderson S, et al. Recommendations for the use of medications with continuous enteral nutrition. *Am J Health-Syst Pharm.* 2009;66:1458–1467.

61. Matysiak-Luśnia K, Łysenko L. Drug administration via enteral feeding tubes in intensive therapy—terra incognita? *Anaesthesiol Intens Ther.* 2014; 46:307–311.
62. Silva RF, Novaes CG, Rita M. Interactions between drugs and drug-nutrient in enteral nutrition: a review based on evidence. *Nutr Hosp.* 2014;30:514–518.
63. Boullata JI, Carrera AL, Harvey L, et al. ASPEN Safe practices for enteral nutrition therapy. *JPEN J Parenter Enteral Nutrition.* 2017;41:15–103.
64. White R, Bradnam V. *Handbook of Drug Administration via Enteral Feeding Tubes.* 3rd ed. London, UK: Pharm Press, 2015.
65. Guenter P, Boullata J. Nursing2013 survey results: Drug administration by enteral feeding tube. *Nursing.* 2013;43(12):26–33.
66. Cutie AJ, Altman E, Lenkel L. Compatibility of enteral products with commonly employed drug additives. *JPEN J Parenter Enteral Nutr.* 1983; 7:186–191.
67. Holtz L, Milton J, Sturek JK. Compatibility of medications with enteral feedings. *JPEN J Parenter Enteral Nutr.* 1987;11:183–186.
68. Strom JG, Miller SW. Stability of drugs with enteral nutrient formulas. *DICP Ann Pharmacother.* 1990;24:130–134.
69. Ortega de la Cruz C, Fernández Gallardo LC, Damas Fernández-Figares M, García Martínez E. Compatibilidad físico-química de medicamentos con nutrición enteral. *Nutr Hosp.* 1993;8:105–108.
70. Udeani GO, Bass J, Johnston TP. Compatibility of oral morphine sulfate solution with enteral feeding products. *Ann Pharmacother.* 1994; 28:451–455.
71. Crowther RS, Bellanger R, Szauter KEM. In vitro stability of ranitidine hydrochloride in enteral nutrient formulas. *Ann Pharmacother.* 1995; 29:859–862.
72. Wensel TM. Administration of proton pump inhibitors in patients requiring enteral nutrition. *P T.* 2009;34(3):143–160.
73. Conrad SA, Gabrielli A, Margolis B, et al. Randomized, double-blind comparison of immediate-release omeprazole oral suspension versus intravenous cimetidine for the prevention of upper gastrointestinal bleeding in critically ill patients. *Crit Care Med.* 2005;33:760–765.
74. Kassam RM, Friesen E, locock RA. In vitro recovery of carbamazepine from Ensure. *JPEN J Parenter Enteral Nutr.* 1989;13:272–276.
75. Bass J, Miles MV, Tennison MB, Holcombe BJ, Thorn MD. Effects of enteral tube feeding on the absorption and pharmacokinetic profile of carbamazepine suspension. *Epilepsia.* 1989;30:364–369.
76. Clark-Schmidt AL. Loss of carbamazepine suspension through nasogastric feeding tubes. *Am J Hosp Pharm.* 1990;47:2034–2037.

77. Riss JR, Kriel RL, Kammer NM, Judge MK, Montgomery MJ. Administration of Carbatrol to children with feeding tubes. *Pediatr Neurol.* 2002;27:193–195.
78. Bauer LA. Interference of oral phenytoin absorption by continuous nasogastric feedings. *Neurology.* 1982;32:570–572.
79. Bauer LA, Edwards WA, Dellinger EP, et al. Importance of unbound phenytoin serum levels in head trauma patients. *J Trauma.* 1983;23: 1058–1060.
80. Saklad JJ, Graves RH, Sharp WP. Interaction of oral phenytoin with enteral feedings. *JPEN J Parenter Enteral Nutr.* 1986;10:322–323.
81. Guidry JR, Eastwood TF, Curry SC. Phenytoin absorption in volunteers receiving selected enteral feedings. *West J Med.* 1989;150:659–661.
82. Au Yeung SCS, Ensom MHH. Phenytoin and enteral feedings: does evidence support an interaction? *Ann Pharmacother.* 2000;34:896–905.
83. Ozuna J, Friel P. Effects of enteral tube feeding on serum phenytoin levels. *J Neurosurg Nurs.* 1984;16:289–291.
84. Faraji B, Yu PP. Serum phenytoin levels of patients on gastrostomy tube feeding. *J Neurosci Nurs.* 1998;30:55–59.
85. Gilbert S, Hatton J, Magnuson B. How to minimize interaction between phenytoin and enteral feedings: two approaches. *Nutr Clin Pract.* 1996;11: 28–31.
86. Cacek AT, DeVito JM, Koonce JR. In vitro evaluation of nasogastric administration methods for phenytoin. *Am J Hosp Pharm.* 1986;43: 689–692.
87. Bader MK. Case study of two methods for enteral phenytoin administration. *J Neurosci Nurs.* 1993;25:233–242.
88. Splinter MY, Seifert CF, Bradberry JC, et al. Recovery of phenytoin suspension after in vitro administration through percutaneous endoscopic gastrostomy Pezzer catheters. *Am J Hosp Pharm.* 1990;47:373–377.
89. Splinter MY, Seifert CF, Bradberry JC, et al. Effect of pH on the equilibrium dialysis of phenytoin suspension with and without enteral feeding formula. *JPEN J Parenter Enteral Nutr.* 1990;14:275–278.
90. Doak KK, Haas CE, Dunnigan KJ, et al. Bioavailability of phenytoin acid and phenytoin sodium with enteral feedings. *Pharmacotherapy.* 1998; 18:637–645.
91. Krueger KA, Garnett WR, Cornstock TJ, et al. Effect of two administration schedules of an enteral nutrient formula on phenytoin bioavailability. *Epilepsia.* 1987;28:706–712.
92. Marvel ME, Bertino JS. Comparative effects of an elemental and a complex enteral feeding formulation on the absorption of phenytoin suspension. *JPEN J Parenter Enteral Nutr.* 1991;15:316–318.

93. Nøhr MK, Thale ZI, Brodin B, et al. Intestinal absorption of the anti-epileptic drug substance vigabatrin is altered by infant formula in vitro and in vivo. *Pharmacol Res Persp*. 2014;2:e00036.

94. Polk RE. Drug-drug interactions with ciprofloxacin and other fluoro-quinolones. *Am J Med*. 1989;87(Suppl 5A):76S–81S.

95. Lomaestro BM, Bailie GR. Quinolone-cation interaction: a review. *Ann Pharmacother*. 1991;25:1249–1258.

96. Lomaestro BM, Bailie GR. Effect of staggered dose of calcium on the bioavailability of ciprofloxacin. *Antimicrob Agents Chemother*. 1991;35: 1004–1007.

97. Mueller BA, Brierton DG, Abel SR, et al. Effect of enteral feeding with Ensure on oral bioavailabilities of ofloxacin and ciprofloxacin. *Antimicrob Agents Chemother*. 1994;38:2101–2105.

98. Cohn SM, Sawyer MD, Burns GA, et al. Enteric absorption of cipro-floxacin during tube feeding in the critically ill. *J Antimicrob Chemother*. 1996;38:871–876.

99. Burkhardt O, Stass H, Thuss U, et al. Effects of enteral feeding on the bioavailability of moxifloxacin in healthy volunteers. *Clin Pharmacokinet*. 2005;44:969–976.

100. Kees MG, Schaeftlein A, Haeberle HA, et al. Population pharmaco-kinetics and pharmacodynamics evaluation of intravenous and enteral moxifloxacin in surgical intensive care unit patients. *J Antimicrob Chemother*. 2013;1331-1337.

101. Wright DH, Pietz SL, Konstantinides FN, Rotschafer JC. Decreased in vitro fluoroquinolone concentrations after admixture with an enteral feeding formulation. *JPEN J Parenter Enteral Nutr*. 2000;24:42–48.

102. de Marie S, VandenBergh MFQ, Bujik SLCE, et al. Bioavailability of ciprofloxacin after multiple enteral and intravenous doses in ICU patients with severe Gram-negative intra-abdominal infections. *Intens Care Med*. 1998;24:343–346.

103. Mimoz O, Binter V, Jacolot A, et al. Pharmacokinetics and absolute bioavailability of ciprofloxacin administered through a nasogastric tube with continuous enteral feeding to critically ill patients. *Intens Care Med*. 1998;24:1047–1051.

104. Chui D, Cheng L, Tejani A. Clinical equivalency of ciprofloxacin 750 mg enterally and 400 mg intravenously for patients receiving enteral feeding: systematic review. *CJHP*. 2009;62:127–134.

105. Casier I, Jeanjean A, Hantson P. Postoperative hyperthermic syndrome following antiparkinsonian drugs withdrawal: the pitfalls of enteral refeeding. *Anaesth Intens Care*. 2013;41:814–815.

106. Whitman CB, Ablordeppey E, Taylor B. Levodopa withdrawal presents as fever in a critically ill patient receiving concomitant enteral nutrition. *J Pharm Pract.* 2016;29:574–578.
107. Cooper MK, Brock DG, McDaniel CM. Interaction between levodopa and enteral nutrition. *Ann Pharmacother.* 2008;42:439–442.
108. Bonnici A, Ruiner C-E, St-Laurent L, Hornstein D. An interaction between levodopa and enteral nutrition resulting in neuroleptic malignant-like syndrome and prolonged ICU stay. *Ann Pharmacother.* 2010;44:1504–1507.
109. Cucca A, Mazzucco S, Bursomanno A, et al. Amino acid supplementation in L-dopa treated Parkinson's disease patients. *Clin Nutr.* 2015;34: 1189–1194.
110. Seeberger LC, Hauser RA. Carbidopa levodopa enteral suspension. *Expert Opin Pharmacother.* 2015;16:2807–2817.
111. Krones E, Zollner G, Petritsch W. Knotting of percutaneous endoscopic jejunostomy feeding tubes in two patients with Parkinson's disease and continuous levodopa treatment. *Z Gastroenterol.* 2012;50:213–216.
112. O'Reilly RA, Rytand DA. Resistance to warfarin due to unrecognized vitamin K supplementation. *N Engl J Med.* 1980;3030:160–161.
113. Landau J, Moulds RFW. Warfarin resistance caused by vitamin K in intestinal feeds. *Med J Aust.* 1982;2:263–264.
114. Parr MD, Record KE, Griggith GL, et al. Effect of enteral nutrition on warfarin therapy. *Clin Pharm.* 1982;1:274.
115. Watson AJM, Pegg M, Green JRB. Enteral feeds may antagonize warfarin. *BMJ.* 1984;288:6416.
116. Martin JE, Lutomski DM. Warfarin resistance and enteral feedings. *JPEN J Parenter Enteral Nutr.* 1989;13:206–208.
117. Violi F, Lip GYH, Pignatelli P, Pastori D. Interaction between dietary vitamin K intake and anticoagulation by vitamin K antagonists: is it really true? *Medicine.* 2016;95:e2895.
118. Kuhn TA, Garnett WR, Wells BK, et al. Recovery of warfarin from an enteral nutrient formula. *Am J Hosp Pharm.* 1989;46:1395–1399.
119. Petretich DA. Reversal of Osmolite warfarin interaction by changing administration time. *Clin Pharm.* 1990;9:93.
120. Penrod LE, Allen JB, Cabacungan LR. Warfarin resistance and enteral feedings: 2 case reports and a supporting in vitro study. *Arch Phys Med Rehab.* 2001;82:1270–1273.
121. Krajewski KC, Butterfoss K. Achievement of therapeutic international normalized ratio following adjustment of tube feeds. *J Clin Pharmacol.* 2011;51:440–443.

122. Dickerson RN, Garmon WM, Kuhl DA, et al. Vitamin K-independent warfarin resistance after concurrent administration of warfarin and continuous enteral nutrition. *Pharmacotherapy.* 2008;28:308–313.
123. Dickerson RN. Warfarin resistance and enteral tube feeding: a vitamin K-independent interaction. *Nutrition.* 2008;24:1048–1052.
124. Klang M, Graham D, McLymont V. Warfarin bioavailability with feeding tubes and enteral formula. *JPEN J Parenter Enteral Nutr.* 2010; 34:300–304.
125. Gu C-H, Li H, Levons J, et al. Predicting effect of food on extent of drug absorption based on physicochemical properties. *Pharmaceut Res.* 2007;24:1118–1130.

Solubilization of Medication

Christel A.S. Bergström, PhD

Background

Drug solubility and drug permeability across the intestinal wall are the two major factors influencing drug absorption after oral administration. To obtain systemic exposure after oral intake, the dosage form must disintegrate, dissolve, and maintain a concentration in the intestinal fluid that is high enough to diffuse toward the gut epithelium and support drug absorption. The most important region of the gut for absorption of immediate-release (IR) dosage forms is the small intestine. This is due to the larger surface area of the small intestine as compared to the stomach and large intestine, the relatively long transit time as compared to the stomach, and the larger volume of resting water available for dissolution as compared to the large intestine.

Scientific advances over the last few decades have resulted in better ability to predict oral absorption and discern the individual contributions of drug dissolution, membrane permeability, net transport, and enzyme metabolism to oral bioavailability. A detailed description of gut absorption and its importance for bioavailability is provided in Chapter 4. The present chapter focuses on drug solubility and how excipients and the physiologic environment influence the solubility. Applications to drug administration via an enteral access device (EAD) will be noted, keeping in mind that it is not the route of administration foremost in the minds of the formulation scientists who designed the drug dosage form or the regulators who approved the marketed drug product.

The first sections of this chapter provide definitions and descriptions of physicochemical properties of importance for the resulting drug solubility. The second half of the chapter describes the physiologic conditions that have an impact on the solubility in each of the segments of the gastrointestinal (GI) tract (stomach, duodenum, jejunum, ileum, and colon). A brief description of the role of excipients and formulation to enable dissolution or increase solubility is included in the latter section.

Pertinent Definitions

Solution is defined as a mixture of two or more components that together constitute one liquid phase that is known to be homogeneous. The element that is the major component and which determines the state of the system is the *solvent*, whereas the component that is dissolved in the solvent is referred to as the *solute*. For our purposes, the unchanged drug solid is the solute, which is typically dissolved in a water-based system.

Dissolution is the process that describes the transfer of each of the many drug molecules from its solid form into solution. As an example, a single 200 mg tablet of ibuprofen contains approximately 600 quintillion (10^{18}) molecules. Dissolution is controlled by the affinity between the solute and the solvent and is dependent on conditions related to the environment (eg, temperature, pressure, ionic strength). The rate of dissolution is directly proportional to the surface area of the drug particle, solubility, salt formation, and solid-state properties.

The *solid state* of drug particles (eg, acicular, flake, and crystalline versus amorphous) refers to the unique shape of powdered drug, which influences dissolution. Drug molecules come together to form either an amorphous solid or a crystalline structure; the latter may be polymorphic. If a drug is polymorphic, only one form (the polymorph) will be thermodynamically stable.

Thermodynamic *solubility* is defined as the maximum amount of the solid compound that can be dissolved in the solvent at equilibrium. This amount is based on the energy required to break solid state bonds and the energy required to insert drug molecules among the water molecules. The thermodynamic solubility is equal to the saturated concentration of the substance in the solvent at a set temperature and pressure. For available drugs, it is often determined as the highest dose strength dissolved in 250 mL of water across a pH range (~1.0 to 7.5). The solubility value (mg/mL or mmol/L) should be provided together with factors affecting this value (conditions of the experiment such as pH, buffer composition and ionic strength, and temperature). The *intrinsic solubility* describes the solubility of the neutral (nonionized) compound in water at room temperature.

Nonsaturated solutions are those that are produced at concentrations below the thermodynamic solubility. This strategy is valuable to make a solution that diminishes the risk for crystallization and particle formation in the final product. Nonsaturated solutions are often used when preparing a drug for administration through an EAD.

Supersaturation is defined as a concentration that exceeds the saturated concentration (eg, the solubility value). Supersaturation is related to the kinetic solubility of the drug, where the higher-than-expected solubility concentration may be obtained as a result of a pH shift or formulation efforts.

A *solvate* describes a crystal form of a drug with molecules of solvent incorporated (embedded) into the complex. When water is the solvent, the complex is referred to as a hydrate.

The term *dose number* (D_O) refers to potential or practical solubility, calculated as the maximum oral dose commercially available divided by the product of the apparent equilibrium solubility and volume available for dissolution. A compound is highly soluble when the D_O is less than 1. For example, digoxin and griseofulvin have similar solubility but vary in maximum dose (0.5 mg vs 500 mg). As a result, their D_O values differ considerably: digoxin's D_O is ~0.08 (very soluble), whereas griseofulvin's D_O is ~133 (poorly soluble).

A *dispersion* is defined as solute particles scattered in a continuous phase. When the continuous phase is a liquid within which the particles are dispersed, the system may be referred to as a slurry or suspension. For example, dispersing a tablet or capsule contents in water allows mixing into a slurry but does not necessarily mean the drug goes into solution. Many liquid drug formulations and most enteral nutrition products are dispersions with properties distinct from those of solutions.

Dependence of Solubility on Physicochemical Properties

Solid State Form

The solubility of a drug is dependent on its inherent physicochemical properties as well as the physiologic environment in which the drug is placed. A critical physicochemical property of each active pharmaceutical ingredient (API) is its aqueous solubility because a drug must dissolve in an aqueous environment. Aqueous solubility is necessary to create a

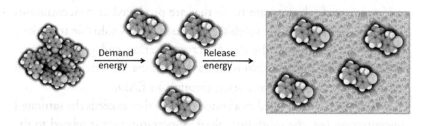

Figure 3-1. The dissolution process. The drug molecule needs to dissociate from its solid (step 1: demands energy), and, at the same time, the water needs to loosen up its tight structure and form a cavity large enough to incorporate the drug (demands energy). Thereafter, the drug is inserted into the water and interacts with the surrounding water molecules (step 2: releases energy).

concentration gradient within the gut, which provides a chance for the drug to be absorbed. The thermodynamics behind solubility are shown in Figure 3-1.

A prerequisite for the drug molecule to dissolve in an aqueous solvent is that the molecule dissociates from its crystal lattice. This process is dependent on the intermolecular bonds formed between the drug molecules in the crystal lattice. Compounds with strong intermolecular bonds and/or a complex binding pattern with a large number of interaction points between the many drug molecules in the crystal lattice often show a limited capability of dissociating from their solid form and, as a result, have high melting points (ie, T_m >200°C). These compounds (eg, hydrochlorothiazide with a T_m of ~275°C) are referred to as "brick dust" molecules, mainly to visualize the strong and dense packing of the molecules in the solid that limits their dissolution in the surrounding medium.[1]

At the same time that a drug compound needs to dissociate from its crystal lattice, the surrounding solvent needs to prepare for incorporating a new molecule. The larger the cavity that needs to be formed, the larger the energy penalty for the formation is. To decrease the energy penalty associated with the cavity formation, additives that loosen the tight water structure (eg, hydrotropic salts, cosolvents) can be included in the aqueous solvent; this technique is one way to improve the aqueous solubility of drug molecules. Finally, to be soluble, the dissociated, free drug molecule needs to be inserted in the solvent cavity through interaction with the surrounding water molecules.

Hydrophobic compounds have limited capacity to interact with the water phase, in accordance with *similia similibus solvuntur* (ie, "like dissolves like"), and such compounds are therefore solubility-limited by poor hydration. These compounds are typically lipophilic drugs with a high partition coefficient (logP) between octanol and water (ie, logP >3). Poorly soluble compounds restricted in solubility by poor hydration are referred to as "grease ball" molecules (eg, spironolactone [T_m ~135°C, logP ~3]) because of their high hydrophobicity and lack of interaction with the water.[1] Between "brick dust" and "grease ball" compounds are intermediates that are limited by both the solid state and the lipophilicity (ie, T_m >200°C and logP >3). For example, the practically insoluble drug danazol has a T_m of 226°C and logP of 4.5. The relationship between T_m, logP, and solubility (logS) is nicely described by the following general solubility equation established by Yalkowsky and coworkers:[2]

$$logS = 0.5 - 0.01(T_m - 25) - logP \qquad \text{(Eq. 3-1)}$$

Nearly a quarter of all drugs have a logS at a value of –4 or less (eg, the approximate logS of danazol is –6). Generally, as lipophilicity (represented by logP) increases, aqueous solubility (represented by logS) decreases. The lipophilicity of a drug molecule represents its affinity for a water-immiscible organic phase (eg, n-octanol) in comparison to the aqueous environment.[3] The logP and the pH-dependent lipophilicity (logD) are typically determined using n-octanol and water, where each phase is saturated with the other. The concentration of the analyte is determined in both phases and used to calculate the lipophilicity. The logP reflects the partitioning of the compound at a pH where it is neutral, whereas the logD varies with pH (which is typically recorded alongside the logD value).[4] The latter is a result of the distribution of ionizable species, which depends on the pH and the drug's pKa. The pH-related lipophilicity (logD) is more applicable to clinical drug administration given low gastric pH and a more alkaline pH in the jejunum. New drug compounds are evaluated to determine their pKa (eg, by acid-base titrations) and lipophilicity (eg, by shake-flask method, high-performance liquid chromatography–ultraviolet [HPLC-UV] technology).[5] In the end, a balance between water solubility and lipophilicity at the gut absorption site is important.

Apart from crystalline forms, amorphous solids have a higher free energy, which translates into higher sorption of moisture, higher solubility, and greater dissolution rate. Although an amorphous form dissolves faster, it may convert to a more stable crystalline form under different conditions. If preparing an amorphous drug, conditions that allow crystal formation, including solvates, will need to be avoided.

Dissolution

The thermodynamics of the dissolution process presented in a simple form in Figure 3-1 can be described as a more detailed thermodynamic sequence (Figure 3-2),[6] which takes into account the Gibbs net free energy (ΔG). Free energy is a measure of the energy available to perform work in a system, decreasing during a spontaneous process until an equilibrium is reached ($\Delta G = 0$). For the dissolution process to take place, the change in free energy (ΔG) needs to be a negative value. For a drug to go through various thermodynamic steps from solid state all the way to solution, the series of free energy values should be negative. The relationship between the intrinsic solubility and the change in Gibbs free energy is as follows:

$$\Delta G_{sol} = \Delta G_{sub} + \Delta G_{hydr} = -RT\ln S_0 V_m \qquad \text{(Eq. 3-2)}$$

where ΔG_{sol} is the Gibbs free energy for solution; ΔG_{sub} is the Gibbs free energy for sublimation; ΔG_{hydr} is the Gibbs free energy for hydration; R is the molar gas constant; T is the temperature (in Kelvin); S_0 is the intrinsic solubility (in molar); and V_m is the molar volume. An organic solvent can be used as an intermediate between the gaseous and hydrated state in the experimental assessment of the hydration process, and in such cases Eq. 3-2 will be transformed to the following:

$$\Delta G_{sol} = \Delta G_{sub} + \Delta G_{solv} + \Delta G_{tr} = -RT\ln S_0 V_m \qquad \text{(Eq. 3-3)}$$

where ΔG_{solv} is the Gibbs free energy for solvation in organic solvent and ΔG_{tr} is the Gibbs free energy for the transfer of the molecule from the organic solvent to water. If the organic solvent used is octanol and if the logP value of the compound is determined, the ΔG_{tr} can be replaced by the following:

$$\Delta G_{tr} = 2.303RT\log P \qquad \text{(Eq. 3-4)}$$

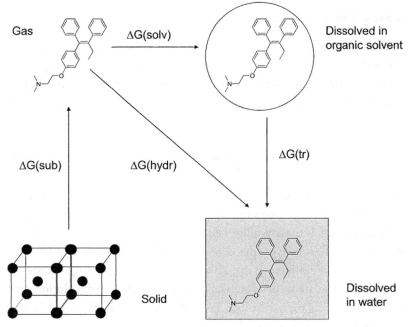

Figure 3-2. Thermodynamic cycle of solvation. It is difficult to calculate the solvation step from solid to solution. To enable calculation of the amount dissolved, step-wise addition of the different processes involved (dissociation, hydration/solvation) can be used. Abbreviations: ΔG_{hyd}, Gibbs free energy of hydration; ΔG_{solv}, Gibbs free energy of solvation; ΔG_{sub}, Gibbs free energy of sublimation; ΔG_{tr}, Gibbs free energy of transfer. Reprinted with permission of Elsevier from reference 6: Bergström CAS, Larsson P. Computational prediction of drug solubility in water-based systems: Qualitative and quantitative approaches used in the current drug discovery and development setting. *Int J Pharm.* 2018;540(1–2):185–193.

The above equations enable calculation of the Gibbs free energy of all three steps of the thermodynamic process. In turn, the result gives an indication of how easily a drug will go into solution.

Dependence of Solubility on Physiologic Conditions

Ultimately, absorption may be limited by dissolution, as well as low cell-membrane permeability. Absorption may even be limited by solubility itself, if the dose is too large to dissolve in the intestinal fluid available.

Dissolution and Solubility

The quicker the dissolution of drug molecules, the better the condition for absorption. The close relationship between the process of drug dissolution and the drug's solubility is described by the Noyes-Whitney equation, including modifications by Nernst and Brunner (adjusted for sink condition),[7]

$$\frac{dm}{dt} = DA\frac{S}{Vh} \qquad \text{(Eq. 3-5)}$$

indicative of the influences on dissolution rate (dm/dt), where D is the diffusion coefficient in the solvent; A is the surface area of the undissolved drug material; S is the solubility value; V is the volume; and h is the thickness of the diffusion layer adjacent to the undissolved solid particle.

Factors that influence the solubility of a drug (drug-related or environment-related) therefore also directly influence its dissolution rate. In addition, drug particle size and particle surface area affect the dissolution rate. These factors are all considered when designing an oral dosage form of each drug under development. Disintegration, dispersion, and micronization are factors that increase the surface area and hence are important to consider when designing IR formulations. For example, the porosity (ie, the unfilled space) of a tablet may influence the disintegration and thereby the dispersion of the tablet material and dissolution of the drug. This is one approach to allow some products to disperse relatively easily in water.

Transit Time and Volume

The GI tract physiology is of importance when it comes to drug dissolution in vivo. A limiting factor is the amount of time a drug spends in different GI regions. Transit times through the different compartments of the GI tract are highly variable and may differ significantly among individuals, but, in general, the overall transit time for ingested solids in the main GI compartments is as follows: stomach, 0 to 2 hours; small intestine (duodenum, jejunum, and ileum), 3 to 4 hours; and large intestine, 8 to 18 hours.[8] Thus, compounds that slowly dissolve will not have time enough to completely dissolve in the stomach or small intestine. Also, drugs that are administered through a postpyloric EAD (ie, into the duodenum or jejunum, bypassing the stomach) are given less time to dissolve in the gut environment. Another factor affecting the amount of drug dissolved is the volume of fluid present. Often, a volume of 250 mL of water is used to calculate whether solubility will be limiting absorption, assuming that the patient will drink a large glass of water when ingesting the medication.[9] However, water is rapidly absorbed, and the resting volume of water in the stomach, small intestine, and large intestine is significantly lower (<50 mL, 105 mL, and 13 mL, respectively).[8,10] Now, imagine the patient being enterally fed. Because the volumes of enteral nutrition (EN) in the GI tract vary depending on the administration method, the volume (let alone colloidal structures) into which a drug is administered will also vary—or may be unknown.

Gut pH

The solubility of protolytes (salt forms of a drug) depends on the pH of the solution and the drug pKa and is described by the Henderson-Hasselbalch equation.[11] The relationship is presented for a weak base in equation 3-6:

$$pKa = pH + \log\frac{S - S_0}{S_0} \qquad \text{(Eq. 3-6)}$$

where S is the solubility at the pH inserted in the equation. Solubility for a weak base (often found as a hydrochloride salt) will increase logarithmically below the pKa of the compound, whereas the solubility for a weak acid (often found as a sodium or potassium salt) increases above the pKa. For zwitterions (which contain both a positively charged and negatively charged group), the solubility will be the lowest at the isoelectric point, in between the two pKa values. Examples of pH-dependent solubility profiles are provided in Figure 3-3.

   There is a strong pH gradient in the GI tract, and pH levels also show high interindividual variability. The fasted pH of gastric fluid is 1 to 3.5, whereas the small intestine has a pH interval of 6 (duodenum) to 8 (ileum), the ascending colon has a pH interval of 5.5 to 7.5, and the descending colon has a somewhat narrower pH interval of 7 to 8.[8] Recent studies have also identified considerable interindividual variability in the pH of the stomach (1.8 to 6.4),[12] and duodenum (3.4 to 8.3),[13] whereas the observed interindividual variability of the pH in the colon is narrower.[14] For ionizable

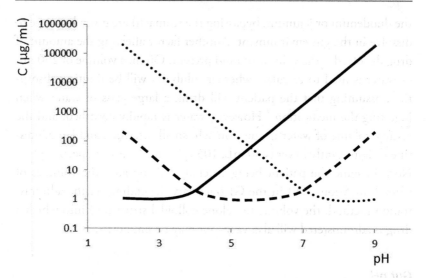

Figure 3-3. The pH-dependent solubility of ionizable drugs. Examples of pH-dependent solubility (concentration in µg/mL) profiles of a weak acid with pKa of 4 (solid line), a weak base with pKa of 7 (dotted line), and a zwitterion with pKa of 4 and 7 (dashed line). In the gastrointestinal tract, compounds are exposed to a pH interval of approximately 1 to 8.

compounds, the physiologic solubility can therefore be assumed to vary significantly between patients, even before any disease or medication that may further alter pH is considered. The variability in pH may be of greatest importance for those compounds whose pKa is in the pH range of 4 to 5, where such pH differences would have the most significant impact. In addition, ionizable compounds that have a D_O close to 1 (where the whole dose is expected to dissolve in the 250 mL of water administered)[9] are also at risk for precipitation by these pH changes. In particular, when intestinal fluids have a higher-than-average pH, that would be detrimental for poorly soluble, weak bases with pKa values of 5 to 6. Conversely, patients whose intestinal fluids have a lower-than-average pH would have lower solubility of weak acids with pKa values of 5 to 6.

The Biopharmaceutical Classification System (BCS) attempts to classify drugs into one of four groups by solubility and permeability: Class 1, high solubility/high permeability; Class 2, low solubility/high permeability; Class 3, high solubility/low permeability; and Class 4, low solubility/low permeability.[9] GI tract fluids are much more complex in composition than water alone, even in the fasted state. The complexity increases in the fed state. A BCS Class 2, weak-acid drug may act more like a Class 1 molecule if it is introduced into the more alkaline environment of the small intestine.

Bile

Bile excreted into the duodenum will form mixed micelles or vesicles composed of bile salts, cholesterol, and phospholipids. Bile also shows large variability in both the concentration of the different components and the release pattern between individuals. The components form lipoidal nanoaggregates of a variety of forms and sizes.[15] Common to all these structures is that they arrange their polar atoms to face the surrounding water and hence include a hydrophobic core structure in micelles (or lipid bilayers of vesicles). This environment can help to solubilize poorly water-soluble, highly lipophilic, compounds and thereby increase the dissolved amount to a great extent.[16,17] The concentration of the components determines the level of solubilization; therefore, solubility in the fed state, where the concentration of bile is higher, is typically greater than solubility in the fasted state. Of course, bile secretion may vary depending on the presence of disease or altered feeding patterns. For particular medicines, dosing the IR medication with food is recommended, to benefit from the natural solubilization that comes with the higher levels of lipids and bile when the patient is in the prandial state. However, it should be noted that food or EN also affects other factors of importance for drug absorption and distribution, and administering drugs with food/EN is not always an appropriate approach to increase absorption. In some cases, lipophilic, poorly water-soluble compounds are formulated as lipid-based dosage forms to achieve the solubility advantage associated with lipids in food while reducing the risk for other food-related effects on the drug absorption pattern (eg, effects related to gastric emptying, motility, viscosity of intestinal content).[18]

Manipulating Drug Formulations to Optimize Gut Solubility

A large fraction of drug compounds show poor water solubility, and approximately 40% to 50% of all marketed oral compounds are defined as being poorly soluble.[19,20] Poor water solubility is in this case related to the dose; by standard definition, the maximum dose strength is not dissolved in the 250 mL of water across the pH interval 1.0 to 6.8.[9,21]

Different methods to increase the solubility in intestinal fluid are therefore used when designing drug formulations with the purpose to increase the concentration that is driving absorption. These techniques mainly involve (a) salt formation to make use of the higher solubility of the ionized species; (b) lipid-based formulations, where solubilization is increased; (c) solid-state transformations, where a more soluble solid form (typically the amorphous form) is administered; and/or (d) carriers such as cyclodextrins or mesoporous materials that may make use of either solubilization or amorphization. These "solubility enhancement" designs incorporated into a commercial drug product need to be considered when preparing a drug for administration through an EAD.

If salt formation is an option, it is typically the primary choice to increase solubility because it involves a relatively straightforward production process in which the salt is formulated with typical IR excipients needed for rapid disintegration and dispersion.

Lipid-based formulations use an approach that is similar to the naturally occurring process in the intestine where lipids act as a hydrophobic reservoir that can solubilize lipophilic drugs. Most lipid-based formulations are digested by lipases in the small intestine, which drive a restructuring of the nanoaggregates or lipid droplets. Therefore, the solubilization capacity is constantly changing, which results in a certain extent of supersaturation in combination with the solubilization effect. Based on these two different processes, the drug concentration in the intestine should become higher and can significantly support absorption of the formulated drug. For very "lipid-loving" compounds, the administration of the drug as a lipid-based formulation may even trigger direct absorption to the lymphatic system. This pathway may be used to escape first-pass hepatic metabolism, and it is even more attractive if the target for the therapy is within the lymphatic system.[18,22]

Synthesis of cocrystals and amorphization are methods to disturb strong intermolecular interactions in the crystal lattice, hence increasing the dissolution rate and hopefully achieving supersaturation.[23,24] The interest in using the amorphous material has increased, probably because the amorphous formulations may result in significant supersaturation and the molecules are then presented in their free form and are readily available for absorption (in contrast, for example, to lipid-based formulations where a fraction of the molecules are "bound" by the hydrophobic interior). However, the amorphous form is a metastable phase, which strives to recrystallize to its stable polymorph; therefore, the amorphized compound will need to be physically stabilized. Typically, this is achieved by adding pharmaceutical polymers such as cellulose derivatives or polyvinyl alcohols or polyethylene glycol. By carefully selecting which polymer(s) to use, the amorphous form can be stabilized in its dry form (ie, to maintain the amorphous form during storage) and then obtain a "spring" (quick dissolution) and "parachute" (extended time frame for supersaturation) dissolution profile when immersed in water.[25] Stability of drugs at supersaturation is generally better in intestinal fluids than in gastric fluids.[26]

Different carrier systems can be used to deliver the compound either in a more soluble solid form or by acting as a solubilizer. Examples of the former are mesoporous carriers in which the amorphous form can be loaded in and stabilized by the nano-sized pores. The system then acts in a manner similar to that of other polymer-based amorphous formulations where the rapid release is obtained. To maintain this high concentration, stabilization is typically required and obtained by the addition of polymers. In another type of carrier system, cyclodextrins act as solubilizer. These cyclic oligosaccharides have a polar outer surface that makes them readily soluble in water, but their cores are hydrophobic. The hydrophobic core can then be utilized by lipophilic compounds, which can bind the hydrophobic part of the molecule in the cyclodextrin core, thereby minimizing the unfavorable interactions with water.

Finally, some drugs are formulated as prodrugs to overcome poor properties, in essence creating a BCS Class 1 compound. The molecule attached to the active drug to improve absorption is then detached after absorption to release the active pharmaceutical ingredient.

Given the complexity of all these formulation designs, attempts to crush and dilute oral products in minimal fluid prior to EAD administration may significantly alter the intended effect.

Summary

The concentration of a medication in the intestine after intake of an oral IR dosage form depends on a large number of factors and is the result of the interplay between the drug molecule, the excipients, and the patient's physiology. The most important molecular properties for drug solubility are T_m, logP, and pKa. From the physiology perspective, the amount that is finally dissolved and readily available for absorption depends on transit times through the different GI compartments, the pH of those compartments, the resting volume of water, and the degree of bile secretion. Based on the recent literature, the interindividual variability is expected to be high for all these physiologic responses; the dissolution and solubility is therefore also expected to differ significantly between patients.

Interpatient variability in the physiologic factors affecting drug absorption is likely increased when medication is administered by EAD in patients receiving EN, and the use of drug therapies in such patients requires close monitoring. It should also be noted that preparing slurries (eg, crushed tablets in liquid) and administering such dispersed medicines through an EAD may significantly affect the performance of the formulation as well. For example, the supersaturation effect may be lost before administering the dose. To some extent, the physiologic effects can be controlled by formulation strategies. In many cases, the formulation of the drug is designed to enable absorption and provide significant bioavailability after oral administration of poorly soluble drugs. These formulation strategies are designed to make use of the physiologic environment and processes naturally occurring in the intestine or enable delivery through the usage of more soluble solid dosage forms.

References

1. Bergström CA, Charman WN, Porter CJ. Computational prediction of formulation strategies for beyond-rule-of-5 compounds. *Adv Drug Deliv Rev*. 2016;101:6–21. doi:10.1016/j.addr.2016.02.005.
2. Jain N, Yalkowsky SH. Estimation of the aqueous solubility I: application to organic nonelectrolytes. *J Pharm Sci*. 2001;90:234–252.
3. van de Waterbeemd H, Abagyan R, Ferenczy GG, et al. Glossary of terms used in computational drug design. *Int Union Pure Appl Chem*. 1997;69: 1137–1152.
4. Comer J, Tam K. Lipophilicity profiles: theory and measurement. In: Testa B, van de Waterbeemd H, Folkers G, Guy R, eds. *Pharmacokinetic Optimization in Drug Research*. Weinhein, Germany: Wiley-VCH; 2001: 275–304.
5. Bergström CA, Holm R, Jørgensen SA, et al. Early pharmaceutical profiling to predict oral drug absorption: current status and unmet needs. *Eur J Pharm Sci* . 2014;57:173–199.
6. Bergström CAS, Larsson P. Computational prediction of drug solubility in water-based systems: Qualitative and quantitative approaches used in

the current drug discovery and development setting. *Int J Pharm.* 2018; 540(1–2):185–193.

7. Noyes AA, Whitney WR. The rate of solution of solid substances in their own solutions. *J Am Chem Soc.* 1897;19:930–934.

8. Sjogren E, Abrahamsson B, Augustijns P, et al. In vivo methods for drug absorption—comparative physiologies, model selection, correlations with in vitro methods (IVIVC), and applications for formulation/API/ excipient characterization including food effects. *Eur J Pharm Sci.* 2014; 57:99–151.

9. Amidon GL, Lennernäs H, Shah VP, Crison JR. A theoretical basis for a biopharmaceutic drug classification: the correlation of in vitro drug product dissolution and in vivo bioavailability. *Pharm Res.* 1995;12:413–420.

10. Schiller C, Fröhlich CP, Giessmann T, et al. Intestinal fluid volumes and transit of dosage forms as assessed by magnetic resonance imaging. *Aliment Pharmacol Ther.* 2005;22:971–979.

11. Hasselbalch KA. Die Berechnung der Wasserstoffzahl des Blutes aus der freien und gebunden Kohlensäure desselben, und die Sauerstoffbindung des Blutes als Funktion der Wasserstoffzahl. *Die Biochemische Zeitung.* 1916;78:112–144.

12. Schneider F, Grimm M, Koziolek M, et al. Resolving the physiological conditions in bioavailability and bioequivalence studies: comparison of fasted and fed state. *Eur J Pharm Biopharm.* 2016;108:214–219.

13. Riethorst D, Mols R, Duchateau G, et al. Characterization of human duodenal fluids in fasted and fed state conditions. *J Pharm Sci.* 2016;105: 673–681.

14. Diakidou A, Vertzoni M, Goumas K, et al. Characterization of the contents of ascending colon to which drugs are exposed after oral administration to healthy adults. *Pharm Res.* 2009;6:2141–2151.

15. Riethorst D, Baatsen P, Remijn C, et al. An in-depth view into human intestinal fluid colloids: intersubject variability in relation to composition. *Mol Pharm.* 2016;13:3484–3493.

16. Persson EM, Gustafsson AS, Carlsson AS, et al. The effects of food on the dissolution of poorly soluble drugs in human and in model small intestinal fluids. *Pharm Res.* 2005;22:2141–2151. doi:10.1007/ s11095-005-8192-x.

17. Fagerberg JH, Bergström CA. Intestinal solubility and absorption of poorly water soluble compounds: predictions, challenges and solutions. *Ther Deliv.* 2015;6:935–959.

18. Feeney OM, Crum MF, McEvoy CL, et al. 50 years of oral lipid-based formulations: provenance, progress and future perspectives. *Adv Drug Deliv Rev.* 2016;101:167–194. doi:10.1016/j.addr.2016.04.007.

19. Benet LZ, Wu C-Y, Custodio JM. Predicting drug absorption and the effects of food on oral bioavailability. *Bull Tech Gattefossé.* 2006;99:9–16.

20. Bergström CA, Andersson SB, Fagerberg JH, Ragnarsson G, Lindahl A. Is the full potential of the biopharmaceutics classification system reached? *Eur J Pharm Sci.* 2014;57:224–231.

21. European Medicines Agency. Guideline on the Investigation of Bioequivalence. http://www.ema.europa.eu/docs/en_GB/document_library/Scientific _guideline/2010/01/WC500070039.pdf. Accessed November 21, 2017.

22. Trevaskis NL, Kaminskas LM, Porter CJ. From sewer to saviour—targeting the lymphatic system to promote drug exposure and activity. *Nat Rev Drug Discov.* 2015;14:781–803.

23. Kuminek G, Cao F, Bahia de Oliveira da Rocha A, Goncalves Cardoso S, Rodriguez-Hornedo N. Cocrystals to facilitate delivery of poorly soluble compounds beyond-rule-of-5. *Adv Drug Deliv Rev.* 2016;101:143–166. doi:10.1016/j.addr.2016.04.022.

24. Taylor LS, Zhang G. Physical chemistry of supersaturated solutions and implications for oral absorption. *Adv Drug Deliv Rev.* 2016;101:122–142. doi:10.1016/j.addr.2016.03.006.

25. Augustijns P, Brewster ME. Supersaturating drug delivery systems: fast is not necessarily good enough. *J Pharm Sci.* 2012;101:7–9.

26. Bevernage J, Hens B, Brouwers J, et al. Supersaturation in human gastric fluids. *Eur J Pharm Biopharm.* 2012;81:184–189.

4

Oral Bioavailability

Hans Lennernäs, PhD

Introduction and Definitions

Oral administration of medication and subsequent gastrointestinal (GI) drug absorption dominates contemporary drug therapy. This drug delivery route is safe, physiologically efficient, and easily accessible, with less discomfort for the patient than other routes of administration (eg, intramuscular, subcutaneous). In the United States, the top 50 prescription drugs that are oral products account for 58% of all units sold and 44% of total revenues.[1,2]

Recent approaches to drug discovery and subsequent formulation development have yielded additional, highly potent and selective drugs that have challenging biopharmaceutical properties, such as low aqueous solubility, sometimes in combination with limited and highly variable intestinal absorption and bioavailability. These challenging drugs with low solubility require advanced formulation strategies to enable successful and predictable GI drug absorption, bioavailability, and clinical use.

The care of many patients with a functional GI tract in hospital and some in home care requires medication administration through an enteral access device (EAD). The same EADs are used to administer medications, enteral nutrition (EN), and individual nutrients to patients with different diseases and conditions. The EADs clinically are classified by site of insertion (eg, nasal, oral, percutaneous) and GI location of the distal end (eg, stomach, duodenum, jejunum) (see Chapter 1). The choice of an enteral access route depends on several factors, including the patient's concurrent diseases and/or injuries, the presence or risk of impaired gastric motility and/or aspiration, and the anticipated duration of EN therapy.

This chapter presents the topic of oral bioavailability based on administration of an intact oral dosage form, with added points of relevance

Table 4-1. Selected Definitions

Term	Definition
Absorption	The movement of an intact drug molecule across the enterocyte's apical membrane. Absorption requires a balance of a drug's physicochemical properties and the gastrointestinal tract physiology or pathophysiology as well as enterocyte transport proteins. Transporters engage in bimolecular interaction and therefore exhibit saturable kinetics.
Bioavailability	The extent to which an orally administered active pharmaceutical ingredient (API) from a pharmaceutical dosage form reaches the systemic circulation from which clinical effects subsequently arise. Bioavailability is often defined as the fraction (F) of the drug dose eventually exposed to the bloodstream. This exposure is calculated by the area under the concentration-time curve (AUC) obtained from experimental study.
First-pass effect	Description of the extraction (E_G, E_H) of a drug following oral or enteral administration by the gut and hepatic metabolizing enzymes and efflux transporters prior to reaching the systemic circulation.
Permeability	The capacity of a drug to cross a cell membrane including at the gut epithelium. Permeability can be described by the rate of absorption (in cm/s) following direct measurement of the effective intestinal permeability (P_{eff}). Together with a drug's solubility, dissolution rate, and gut transit (see Chapter 3), permeability determines the extent of drug absorption.
Biopharmaceutical Classification System (BCS)	BCS divides drugs into four different classes based on solubility and intestinal permeability: Class 1, high solubility/high permeability; Class 2, low solubility/high permeability; Class 3, high solubility/low permeability; and Class 4, low solubility/low permeability.

to enteral drug administration included. Several key terms used in this chapter are defined in Table 4-1.

The science that describes oral bioavailability needs to be carefully interpreted for bioavailability with EAD drug administration, as the bioavailability may be altered in a manner that influences the therapeutic outcome. The distinctive drug absorption processes that occur to various degrees along the GI tract must be thoroughly understood to accurately predict absorption, bioavailability, and treatment effect.

In the clinical setting, the extemporaneous formulation approaches used for delivering a drug through GI access devices must be tailored to the challenging biopharmaceutical properties of the drug's active pharmaceutical ingredient (API) and product formulation features. Even if liquid formulations are optimal to use for enteral delivery, their use is not always feasible, as many approved oral pharmaceutical products are only available in solid formulations (ie, tablets, capsules). As a consequence, a solid formulation with the selected API and excipients is often crushed (or capsules opened) and mixed with water prior to administration. These dispersions are then administered through the EAD with several limitations on how they affect GI absorption, bioavailability, clinical effect, and/or safety. When liquid formulations are available, whether a commercial product or an extemporaneously compounded preparation is preferred will depend on the medication and the formulation's influences on bioavailability. In some cases, *ex tempore* (ie, extemporaneously prepared) formulations and enteral drug administration of existing oral products may lead to treatment failure or toxicity.

The practical pathway to bioavailability of an oral drug formulation (API plus excipients) involves a number of barriers: acidic gastric juices, the complex enzyme and secretion-filled environment of the small bowel, the presence of a diverse microbiota, and the gut mucosal epithelium. Crossing the apical membrane of these enterocytes (ie, absorption) is aided by permeability and uptake transporters, but it can be opposed by drug metabolizing enzymes and efflux transporters. The portal vein then allows the drug that escapes drug extraction to travel to the liver, where it encounters additional drug metabolizing enzymes and efflux transporters (see Figure 4-1). The fraction of the drug not extracted (ie, metabolized, transported out) will contribute to systemic bioavailability. For an oral drug to be 100% bioavailable, it must be 100% absorbed. However, 100% absorption does not necessarily translate to 100% bioavailability because of the intervening barriers. In fact, the oral bioavailability of most drugs is less than 100%.

The dynamic GI luminal composition, volumes of GI fluids, and hydrodynamic conditions generated by GI motility, secretion, and absorption are controlled by endocrine and neural factors.[3-10] These factors strongly

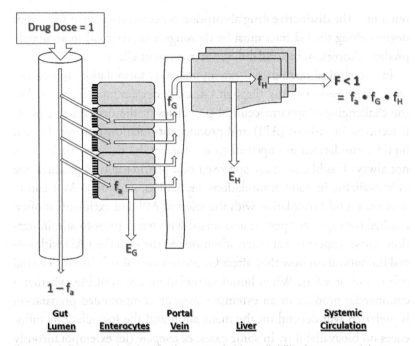

Figure 4-1. The steps involved in the systemic bioavailability from an oral drug dose. E_G, gut extraction; E_H, hepatic extraction; F, bioavailable fraction; f_a, the fraction absorbed; f_G, the fraction escaping gut extraction; f_H, the fraction escaping hepatic extraction.

influence release and dissolution of the API from any dosage form. However, the effect of dissolution on GI absorption is also modulated by a plethora of other factors involved in the drug absorption process (see Chapter 3).[3-5] For instance, the overall impact of dissolution, precipitation, and/or redissolution on GI drug absorption is strongly influenced by the effective intestinal permeability, most likely mediated by improved sink conditions. In a similar fashion, capacity-limited processes such as enzymatic intestinal biotransformation, carrier-mediated transport, and/or efflux processes through the intestinal wall, metabolism in the intestinal mucosa, and lymphatic transport must all be considered to determine the impact of drug form and formulation on absorption and bioavailability.[3-10]

Depending on the composition of the reformulated pharmaceutical product, different biopharmaceutical, physiologic, and pathophysiologic factors will determine the overall rate and extent of GI absorption and bioavailability of the administered drug(s). When comparing gastric and proximal small intestinal (duodenum, jejunum) delivery, the major differences are (a) the impact of gastric emptying and luminal condition (eg, luminal pH, bile salt concentration) and (b) the fact that the stomach is not a major absorption region compared with the proximal small intestine.[3,5] It is also important to consider whether the reformulated drug(s) are given without nutrient supply (recommended) or with it. The factors involved in the fasted and fed states, and their interplay, will be discussed.

The Influence of Permeability on Absorption and Bioavailability

When a drug formulation is delivered in any way to the GI tract, the rate and extent of the drug's absorption are determined by its transit through the absorption regions of the small and large intestine, drug release and dissolution kinetics, stability and binding processes in the GI lumen, and effective regional intestinal permeability (P_{eff}).[1,2,11–13] The Biopharmaceutical Classification System (BCS) provides a scientific basis for identifying the fundamental rate-limiting biopharmaceutical factors of intestinal drug absorption (ie, solubility and P_{eff}).[14–16] Together with the in vitro dissolution kinetics of crystals of the drug compound in the pharmaceutical product, the BCS accounts for three absorption factors from which the rate and extent of intestinal drug absorption can be predicted for immediate-release (IR) dosage forms. Drug regulatory aspects related to in vivo performance of pharmaceutical dosage forms have been the driving force in the development of the BCS, but it can be useful in decision-making about drug administration via EADs. Accordingly, the IR pharmaceutical products for BCS Class 1 drugs are the preferred solid dosage form to be used in *ex tempore* formulation for enteral drug administration. Drugs from the three remaining BCS classes need some consideration and adjustment to their physicochemical and biopharmaceutical properties before an enteral drug delivery treatment strategy is developed.

General Theoretical Considerations About Gastrointestinal Drug Absorption and Bioavailability

The GI barriers to oral drug absorption, and hence bioavailability, can be considered biological and physiologic. They include the gut lumen pH, enzymes, bile salts, transit time, mucus layer, unstirred water layer, local surface pH and enzymes, villi, epithelial cells, and epithelial cell membrane. Bioavailability is a key clinical pharmacokinetic variable for characterizing the fraction (F) of a given dose that reaches the systemic circulation in an unchanged and pharmacologically active form. These theoretical considerations are fully applicable to enteral drug delivery through any EAD.

Bioavailability following oral or enteral dosing mainly depends on three general but rather complex serial processes (refer to Figure 4-1): the fraction of the dose absorbed (f_a), the first-pass extraction of the drug in the gut wall (E_G), and the first-pass extraction of the drug in the liver (E_H):[14,17]

$$F = f_a(1 - E_G)(1 - E_H)$$ (Eq. 4-1)

Different factors determine the f_a and E_G of drugs and are themselves divided into three broad categories: (a) pharmaceutical factors, such as choice of excipients and method of manufacturing; (b) biopharmaceutical and physicochemical factors of the drug molecule itself, such as solubility and solid-state forms (see Chapter 3); and (c) physiologic, biochemical, and pathophysiologic factors in the GI tract.

f_a

According to scientific and regulatory definitions, f_a is the fraction of the dose transported across the apical cell membrane (absorbed) into the cellular space of the enterocyte/colonocyte.[14,17] The enterocyte is the dominating cell for absorption in the GI tract. The rate (mass of drug absorbed over time), M(t), and the cumulative mass of drug absorbed (relative to drug dose administered), D, following administration directly into the GI tract is described by the following equation:

$$f_a = \frac{M(t)}{D}$$ (Eq. 4-2)

These parameters are influenced by the following key biopharmaceutical factors: dose/dissolution ratio, adsorption to the tube material, occlusion in the tube, precipitation, chemical and/or enzymatic degradation in the lumen, luminal complex binding, interaction with infused nutrients and pharmaceutical excipients, intestinal transit, and effective intestinal permeability. In addition, drug metabolism by the gut micro-biota in the lumen may sometimes reduce the f_a, especially for drugs sensitive to hydrolytic and other reductive enzymatic reactions.[18] An additional important consideration that affects GI absorption is whether the approved oral formulation is designed to provide a clinical and safety release rate that may be destroyed if the solid formulation is crushed and dissolved as a part of the formulation. The f_a can be further theoretically defined at any time (t) as follows:

$$f_a = \frac{M(t)}{D} = \int_0^t \int_A \int \cdot C_{lumen} \cdot P_{eff} \cdot dAdt \qquad \text{(Eq. 4-3)}$$

where C_{lumen} is the free reference concentration of the drug in the intesti-nal lumen, A is the available intestinal surface area, and P_{eff} is the average value of the effective intestinal permeability along the intestinal region where absorption occurs.[14] It therefore becomes obvious that, aside from concentration and permeability, the transit time in the major absorption regions is one of the key variables along with available absorption time and radius of the intestine.[19] From equation 4-3, it is clear that the P_{eff}, dissolved and free drug concentrations, and the intestinal transit are the key variables controlling the overall rate and extent of absorption, and the equation is applicable regardless of the intestinal epithelial transport mechanism(s).[13–16] The factors controlling absorption following delivery of an enteral dose are displayed in Figure 4-2. It is expected that different degrees of dilution of oral products with high viscosity might affect the dissolution rate for BCS Class 2 and Class 4 drugs, as the sink conditions might be reduced because of slower bulk diffusion.[20,21]

E_G and E_H

Once the drug has reached the intracellular site in the enterocyte, it may be metabolized by phase I enzymes, predominantly CYP3A4, and may be vulnerable to other enzymatic processes such as phase II conjugation by glucuronides, sulfates, and/or glutathione. The enzymatic capacity of the small intestine to metabolize drugs, often working in tandem with efflux transporters, can be expressed in pharmacokinetic terms as the extraction ratio (proportion of presented drug extracted) of the intes-tine (E_G).[14,17] However, the CYP3A4 activity has sharp regional differ-ences, with the highest expression in the proximal small intestine, a

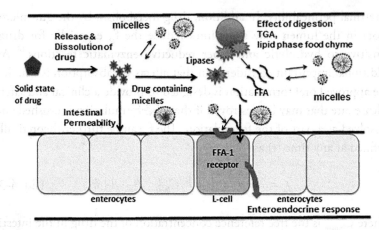

Figure 4-2. A summary of the main biopharmaceutical processes (solubility, dissolution, and intestinal permeability) affecting gastrointestinal (GI) drug absorption following a direct delivery of a solid and immediate-release dosage form. The drug delivery through these access ports needs to consider the composition of nutrients in the fluid and their digestive components. These substances may influence drug absorption through a strong enteroendocrine response that influences GI motility and GI transit, or more directly interfere with absorption. FFA = free fatty acids; TGA = triglycerides.

reduced expression in distal small intestine, and almost no expression in the colon.[22-26] The regional differences in CYP3A4-mediated gut wall metabolism are crucial to consider, especially for the assessment of interactions with other drugs and some nutrients. Efflux transporters (eg, P-glycoprotein, multidrug resistance–associated protein [MRP], breast cancer resistance protein [BCRP]) all vary in terms of specific protein content expression, with regional differences of their own. Accordingly, with any drug administered through a postpyloric EAD placed into a patient (eg, following bariatric surgery), the bioavailability may increase because the E_G may have been reduced.[27] The fraction of absorbed drug that escapes efflux and/or metabolism in the small intestine $(1 - E_G)$ may undergo additional metabolism and/or biliary secretion (ie, efflux) in the liver (E_H) before reaching the systemic circulation. It is important to consider that both a drug and a metabolite (most often a conjugate) do not necessarily have to be eliminated if they are secreted back into the intestinal lumen because they can undergo enterohepatic circulation. The E_H is dependent on blood flow (Q_H), protein binding (f_u), the blood/plasma ratio (C_b/C_p), and the intrinsic clearance of enzymes and/or transporters (Cl_{int}), and it is often based on the well-stirred assumption, as shown by equation 4-4:[17]

$$E_H = \frac{f_u \cdot Cl_{int}}{Q_H + f_u \cdot Cl_{int}} \qquad \text{(Eq. 4-4)}$$

where the intrinsic clearance (Cl_{int}) assumes no extrahepatic metabolism or renal clearance. It is also recognized that transport mediated by membrane proteins in hepatocytes must be included in models that predict and explain liver extraction.[28,29] These membrane transporters may influence uptake into hepatocytes and/or canalicular efflux transport into bile. These processes are expected to play a crucial in vivo role in the local concentration-time profile in the vicinity of the intracellular enzymes in the liver.[28–30]

Physiologic and Pathophysiologic Factors in Gastrointestinal Drug Absorption and Bioavailability

Stomach

Gastric drug absorption is generally limited, especially when compared to absorption in the small intestine.[3] For some drugs, absorption from the large intestine is extensive and important for the success of modified-release (eg, extended- or sustained-release) oral dosage forms.[1,2,31] Accordingly, gastric emptying determines the onset of absorption because it controls the transfer of the drug in any form to the major site of intestinal absorption.[16,19] The emptying rate from the stomach is mainly affected by the digestive state, the properties of the dosage form, fluid volume, disease state, posture, and any concomitantly administered drugs.[32–37] Variable gastric emptying has been recognized to have a major impact on the absorption rate for drugs with high intestinal permeability and a short terminal half-life, to such an extent that it might influence the therapeutic outcome of the drug.[38–40] The influence of gastric emptying is therefore important to consider, mainly as a factor for the onset of effect for drugs delivered through EADs placed in the stomach. It is also important to consider that patients with a gastric access device may have slow and delayed emptying because of the high lipid or fiber content in the EN formula they receive as well as their posture. With poor gastric emptying, patients may need occasional gastric suction to address nausea and elevated volume, which may lead to loss of a drug (ie, partial withdrawal of the given dose) and, consequently, reduced absorption and bioavailability of the administered drug(s).

Gastrointestinal Motility

GI motility is a highly variable physiological process in both the fasted and fed states. It also has a strong impact on GI drug absorption in patients who are administered drugs through an EAD. Based on an extensive motility-dependent compartmental absorption and transit mechanistic analysis, it was concluded that the interplay between fluid volume and GI motility needs further in vivo studies to better understand and predict how these processes determine the plasma concentration-time exposure.[19] This information will help predict differences in drug absorption and bioavailability in patients fed continuously compared with those fed intermittently. The digestive condition is determined by the luminal absence or presence of infused nutrients (and their digestion and absorption).[34,35,37]

The GI tract is not only an organ for digestion/absorption and immunology, it is also the body's largest endocrine organ.[34,35,37] In addition to regulating satiety and food intake, the enteroendocrine system plays a fundamental role in orchestrating postprandial physiology, and it is central to the regulation of glucose, lipid, and protein homeostasis. The digested food or EN components at their low molecular weights can influence chemosensors (receptors) on the L-cells and other specialized endocrine cells in the small intestine (Figure 4-2).[41-43] These nutrients bind and act through the G-protein-coupled receptors at the luminal side of enteroendocrine cells,[37] and certain gut hormones are released rapidly. Different hormones are released depending on where in the GI tract the digested food components are acting via the chemoreceptors.[41-43] For example, the ileal brake decreases appetite and slows down the transit of chyme through the GI system by way of the enteroendocrine system.[44,45] This normal physiologic response in the postprandial state will impact absorption in patients with a gastric EAD.

The interdigestive peristalsis is initiated in the antrum and propagates distally, passing through the pylorus and then further down the small intestine before finally ending up in the ileum.[46-49] This motility pattern is called the *interdigestive migrating myoelectric complex* (IMMC). The IMMC cycle typically takes 90 to 120 minutes, but its duration is highly variable, ranging from 50 minutes to 3 hours.[48-50] The IMMC cycle is interrupted by food and becomes reinitiated when the stomach is empty again.[48,50]

In earlier clinical pharmacokinetic studies, it was proposed that the fasted state is not as uniform or standardized as is often anticipated. For drugs such as acetaminophen, tetracycline, phenacetin and levodopa, considerable variation in absorption rate following administration of conventional dosage forms has been demonstrated.[22,51-55] Fluctuations in the plasma concentration-time curve related to variations in the absorption rate are most pronounced for drugs such as levodopa, which has a high absorption rate (due to a high P_{eff}) and a short terminal half-life. In this case, it has been suggested that the variable gastric emptying contributes significantly to the clinical problems with fluctuation in the antiparkinsonian effect. The fluctuations are, however, markedly reduced when levodopa is administered by continuous intraduodenal infusion.[23-25] The gastric emptying half-life in the fasted state has been shown to be highly dependent on the volume in the stomach and the phase of the IMMC cycle, and it ranges from a few minutes to more than 1 hour.[19,26]

As already mentioned, the volume of the water administered concomitantly with the drug is an important factor for the gastric emptying rate in the fasted state.[19,26] In a study where fasted healthy volunteers were enterally intubated, the gastric emptying rate of a large volume (200 mL) was faster than that of a small volume (50 mL). Note that larger volumes may be needed when diluting viscous or hypertonic liquid drug products for EAD administration. Furthermore, it was found that the most pronounced difference between the emptying rates of the two volumes was achieved when the volumes were administered in the first quiescent IMMC phase.[19,26] This observation shows that there is a considerable variability in the gastric emptying rate in the fasted state. Gastric emptying in the fasted mode is also influenced by properties of the fluid administered simultaneously with the drug formulation, such as pH, osmolality, and energy content.[3,18]

Small Intestine

The small intestine's function is to digest the chyme emptied from the stomach by secretion of various digestive enzymes and luminal mixing, followed by absorption across the intestinal mucosa. Because of its large surface area, the small intestine has the highest capacity for the uptake of nutrients and drugs. Transit in the small intestine is affected by a complex interaction between anatomy, motility, secretion, gut sensing and endocrine response, and absorption. The motility of the small intestine is separated into two distinct phases, which are dependent on the digestive state.[19,46,47]

The fed state is characterized by segmental and propulsive contractions, the segmental contractions being the most frequent. Their purpose is to mix and facilitate absorption by spreading out the luminal content throughout the small intestine. However, it has been proposed that gastric emptying rate is the main factor that influences the spread of particles/fragments in the small intestine. This hypothesis is supported by the observation that there is minor further spreading once the solids have left the stomach.[56] In the fed state, nutrients bind and act through the G-protein-coupled receptors at the luminal side of enteroendocrine cells,[37] and certain gut hormones are released rapidly and have feedback control of GI secretion and motility.

The motility of the small intestine in the fasted mode is similar to the fasted motility pattern of the stomach. The first period is quiescent; the second phase has an erratic contractility; and the third phase is characterized by intense activity, which is associated with a rapid transit of chyme in the distal direction. The IMMC is then continuously propagated distally until it reaches the ileum, where the movement is stagnated and only seldom gets to the distal part of the ileum.[46-48] The spreading of intestinal content in the small intestine seems to be regrouped when the material is approaching the ileocecal sphincter. This sphincter seems to control emptying into the colon and prevent the back-flux of colonic material into the distal ileum. The phenomenon of stagnation in the ileocolonic region and the factors controlling the transit in this region of the alimentary tract demand further study.[19,56-58] The small intestinal transit time has been demonstrated to be around 3 hours and tends to be very consistent, although a time range from less than 1 hour up to 8 hours has been reported.[3,19,56,59] No effect of the dosage form or digestive state of the alimentary tract has been found. It has also been shown that the intraindividual variability in the small bowel transit of a tablet is of the same magnitude as the interindividual variability.[56,59,60] Various age-related changes in a number of physiologic functions may have an impact on the performance of the formulation (eg, GI transit, luminal dissolution rate).[61] Such differences deserve further research to establish drug delivery strategies through EADs for specific age groups and, especially, to adjust for any effect(s) of disease(s).

Colon

The main functions of the colon are to absorb water and electrolytes; to store and transport slugs, which become more solid when they approach the distal part of colon; and to ferment the microflora in the lumen. The length of the colon is approximately 125 cm and can be divided into several segments. The region of the large bowel assumed to be the optimal site for drug absorption encompasses the cecum, the ascending colon, and first half of the transverse colon. In distal parts, except for the rectum, the feces are too solid for adequate drug dissolution.[62]

Unlike the small intestine, the transit time through the colon is highly variable.[3,19,59,60,63-66] This variability can have a major influence on the bioavailability of drugs with an incomplete and slow colonic absorption as well as those used in controlled-release products. Oral solids take about 20 to 30 hours to pass through the colon, but the transit time can range from 1 hour to more than 60 hours. The intraindividual variability in the transit time of a tablet through the colon has been found to be of the same magnitude as the interindividual variability.[59,60,63-66]

Microbiota

Even as it maintains the absorption of drugs and nutrients, the GI tract also acts as an efficient barrier against potentially hazardous bacteria and toxins. Gut-associated lymphoid tissue (GALT), the largest immunologic tissue in the body, is located in the intestine.[67] The single epithelial layer in the intestine, composed mainly of enterocytes and colonocytes, performs the crucial task of regulating the balance between efficient absorption and optimal protection, and affects the permeability of drugs.

The gut microbiota is essential for correct intestinal function and therefore plays an important role in health and disease. It has been estimated that the human body plays host to 10^{14} bacteria (10 times more than the "resident" eukaryotic cells)—and the vast majority are located within the gut.[68] These bacteria form a complex ecosystem that influences the host and is a prerequisite for health and normal physiology. The microbiota differ in composition and concentration along the GI tract.[68] The stomach contains fewer bacteria due to its low pH, and bacteria levels in the jejunum are modest because of the inhibitory action by bile/pancreatic secretion. The bacterial composition in the ileum approaches that of the colonic microbiota. The concentration of bacteria in the colon is high due to the organ's higher pH, abundance of nutrients, and less aggressive peristalsis. The human colon may be regarded as a continuously running fermenter, generating 10^{12} organisms per gram of feces. The fermentation by intestinal microorganisms of nondegradable carbohydrates, such as nonstarch polysaccharides and oligosaccharides, produces short-chain fatty acids (predominantly butyrate, propionate, and acetate). These fatty acids are absorbed by the epithelium and metabolized in the colonic epithelium, liver, and peripheral tissue. The epithelium in the colon receives approximately 70% of its energy supply from fatty acids in the colonic lumen.[69]

The diverse physiologic processes of the GI tract are finely tuned and in balance to optimize the well-being of the host and play a highly significant role in the permeability of drugs across the small and large intestine.

Intestinal Permeability

Physiologic Relevance

The P_{eff} of a drug compound describes the transport rate across the rate-limiting region of a barrier such as the intestinal mucosa. The P_{eff} can be applied regardless of membrane transport mechanism. In the intestine, the rate-limiting step for passive lipoidal diffusion is often the apical membrane, due to its composition and properties.[70,71]

The P_{eff}, together with solubility, dissolution rate, and GI transit, is one of the key biopharmaceutical variables that determine the in vivo rate and extent of intestinal drug absorption in humans and animals.[11-14] The physicochemical properties of the drug compound and the complex physiologic and biochemical conditions of the GI tract will also strongly affect intestinal P_{eff} in vivo. Depending on the transport mechanism(s) involved, variations in GI physiology may affect the P_{eff} differently.[3,10-12,19,60,61] It is important to consider that intestinal P_{eff} may depend on multiple, parallel transport processes such as passive transcellular diffusion, carrier-mediated absorption, and carrier-mediated efflux.

Paracellular diffusion is considered a minor transport route for drugs with molecular weight (MW) larger than 250 to 300.[71,72] Smaller compounds, such as urea and creatinine (MW of 60 and 131, respectively), have been shown to be absorbed via this route in vivo in humans.[71,72] The available surface area for paracellular intestinal absorption has been estimated to be about 0.01% of the total surface area of the small intestine. The quantitative importance of the paracellular route for the macroscopic intestinal absorption of hydrophilic compounds in vivo is not yet fully clear. Several in vitro investigations have demonstrated that the paracellular route is important for the intestinal absorption of various hydrophilic compounds. However, in vivo studies have suggested that this route makes only a minor contribution to the overall intestinal absorption of drugs. The fact that the relationships among various absorption mechanisms differ along the intestinal tract complicates the construction of models designed to predict the rate and extent of intestinal absorption.

The use of any preclinical model designed to predict human intestinal drug absorption has to start with a validation against corresponding human in vivo data. We have developed methods for performing regional, single-pass perfusions of the proximal jejunum and distal rectum in vivo in humans. These methods have been extensively used to determine the effective permeability of various compounds.[11–13] The jejunum is the major absorbing region for most drugs in most mammals. It also has the largest surface area and is the site of the most active carrier-mediated transport in the gut.[3,11–13] Human in vivo jejunal permeability values for 42 compounds (29 drugs) have been determined over a period of 18 years and are presented in Table 4-2.[11–13]

In Vivo Determination

In humans, P_{eff} is best determined by performing a single-pass perfusion of a specified region of the intestine—often in the jejunum—using a perfusion tube system (eg, Loc-I-Gut; Pharmacia, Inc.).[11–13] Drug transport (ie, absorption) across the membrane of the perfused jejunal region is the difference between the mass entering and the mass leaving that intestinal segment:

$$dM/dt = Q_{in}C_{in} - Q_{out}C_{out} = Q(C_{in} - C_{out}) \quad \text{(Eq. 4-5)}$$

Table 4-2. The Biopharmaceutics Classification System Grouping of 31 Drugs Based on Human Effective Permeability

Drug	Human In Vivo Permeability[a]	BCS Class	Laboratory
α-Methyldopa	0.10	3	UU
Amiloride	1.6	1	UU
Amoxicillin	0.30	3	UU
Antipyrine	5.60	1	UU
Atenolol	0.20	3	UU
Carbamazepine	4.30	2	UU
Cephalexin	1.56	2	UM
Cimetidine	0.26	3	UU
Cyclosporine	1.61	2	UM
Desipramine	4.50	1	UU
Enalaprilat	0.20	3	UU
Enalapril maleate	1.57	(1)[b]	UM
Fexofenadine	0.07	3	UU
Fluvastatin	2.40	1	UU
Furosemide	0.05	4	UU
Hydrochlorothiazide	0.04	3	UU
Inogatran	0.03	3	UU
Isotretinoin	0.99	2	UU
Ketoprofen	8.70	1	UU
Levodopa	3.40	(1)[b]	UU
Lisinopril	0.33	3	UU
Losartan	1.15	3	UU
Metoprolol	1.34	1	UU
Naproxen	8.50	1	UU
Piroxicam	6.65	2	UM
Propranolol	2.91	1	UU
Ranitidine	0.27	3	UM
Terbutaline	0.30	3	UU
Valacyclovir	1.66	(1)[b]	UM
R-Verapamil	6.80	1	UU
S-Verapamil	6.80	1	UU

Abbreviations: BCS, Biopharmaceutics Classification System; P_{eff}, effective intestinal permeability; UM, University of Michigan; UU, Uppsala University.

[a]Each P_{eff} value was determined in vivo in the proximal jejunum in humans with a single-pass approach at pH 6.5 and under isotonic conditions. Twenty-four of the drugs were evaluated at Uppsala University, Sweden, and five were evaluated at the University of Michigan. Human P_{eff} was determined at a concentration that was based on the most common clinical dose dissolved in 250 mL. For low-solubility concentrations, the highest possible drug concentrations were applied.

[b]High permeability due to carrier-mediated absorption; currently not included in BCS Class 1.

Source: Data are from references 11–13.

where C_{in} and C_{out} are the inlet and outlet drug concentrations, respectively, and Q is the flow through the tube at physiologic rates. The mass balance relationship has previously been proposed to describe the transport rate of the drug (absorbed mass) across the whole mucosal barrier according to Fick's first law:[70,71]

$$dM/dt = A \cdot P_{eff} \cdot (C_{ref-lumen} - C_{ref-blood}) \qquad \text{(Eq. 4-6)}$$

where A is the surface area of the mucosal membrane; P_{eff} is the effective permeability; and the reference concentrations $C_{ref-lumen}$ and $C_{ref-blood}$ are on the two opposite sides of the intestinal mucosa. Based on the discussion in the previous section, in which the apical cell membrane was considered to be rate-limiting, $C_{ref-cytosol}$ can replace $C_{ref-blood}$ to improve the relationship.[13,14,73]

P_{eff} and other variables are calculated from the steady-state level in the perfusate leaving the intestinal segment. The compounds of interest in the perfusate (drug solute and nonabsorbable marker) within the intestinal segment achieve equilibrium after approximately 50 to 60 minutes. Based on a residence time distribution analysis, the hydrodynamics within the perfused jejunal segment were best described by a well-mixed model.[11,73,74] P_{eff} is then calculated using the outlet concentration as a reference concentration, according to equation 4-7:

$$P_{eff} = \frac{Q_{in} \cdot (C_{in} - C_{out})}{C_{out} \cdot 2\pi r l} \qquad \text{(Eq. 4-7)}$$

where Q_{in} is the inlet perfusate rate (the perfusion flow rate entering the jejunal segment); C_{in} and C_{out} are the inlet and outlet perfusate concentrations of the drug, respectively; r is the radius (r = 1.75 cm); and l is the length of the jejunal segment (10 cm). In all experiments, the stability and adsorption of the drugs are carefully assessed (at 37°C for 180 minutes), and no degradation or adsorption have been detected for any of the drugs investigated.

Incidentally, in rats, steady-state P_{eff} is usually calculated using the parallel-tube model, since they are perfused from an entrance at one end of the intestinal segment to exit at the other end (ie, open system) with drug concentrations expected to decrease exponentially along the segment (ie, not well mixed):[11,75]

$$P_{eff} = \frac{Q_{in} \cdot \ln(C_{out}/C_{in})}{A} \qquad \text{(Eq. 4-8)}$$

where C_{in} and C_{out} are the concentrations of each tested compound, corrected for inlet and outlet fluid-transport, respectively; Q_{in} is the perfusion flow rate; and A is the mass transfer surface area within the intestinal segment $(2\pi rl)$, which is assumed to be a cylinder with a height of 10 cm.[11–14,73–75] In the dog and pig models, the permeability is calculated using the well-stirred model (equation 4–7) because it is assumed that the hydrodynamics are similar to the corresponding model in the human intestine.

In Vitro Determination

The apparent permeability (P_{app}) represents the appearance rate of the drug calculated from the mass transport rate across the membrane. Calculations of the apparent permeability using excised intestinal segments or cell mono layer (eg, Caco-2 cell model) are made according to equation 4–9:

$$P_{app} = \frac{dQ}{dt} \cdot \frac{1}{A \cdot C_0}$$ (Eq. 4–9)

where dQ/dt is the steady-state appearance rate of the compound in the receiver compartment; A is the exposed tissue area; and C_0 is the donor concentration of the drug.[3,4]

Clinical Relevance

During the past decades, significant efforts have been made to investigate the effect of transport carrier-mediated efflux on the pharmacokinetics of drugs and their metabolites.[3,11,13,76–84] Most of our understanding of the mechanisms behind intestinal efflux is derived from cell culture studies and gene knockout animal models.[78–84] Unfortunately, direct kinetic comparisons of transport variables under the complicated circumstances of in vivo settings in humans are rare.[3,11,13,81] The in vivo pharmacokinetic evaluation of the quantitative importance of drug transporters suffers from the lack of good in vivo probe molecules and specific transport inhibitors. However, experimental clinical studies have proposed that P-glycoprotein (P-gp)–mediated efflux at the intestinal barrier has a limited effect on the plasma exposure.[11–13] A number of reports have investigated in detail the clinical importance and concluded that P-gp inhibition in isolation will not result in clinically important alterations in plasma drug exposure. Conversely, P-gp transport may be of significance in barrier tissues (tumors, lymphocytes, brain), resulting in attenuated efficacy.[85-88]

It is well known that the intestinal absorption potential of drugs that are mainly transported by passive diffusion may be predicted from molecular properties, such as polar surface area, hydrogen bonding, logP, logD, and MW.[89-93] Hence, we require better *in silico* models that can predict permeability for chemical structures outside the established chemical space and which can then be used to define the relationship between physicochemical descriptors and permeability.[3] The values for in vivo jejunal human permeability (P_{eff}) from perfusion studies for 22 chemically and structurally diverse compounds were correlated in a multivariate data analysis that included both experimentally determined lipophilicity values obtained using the pH-metric technique and calculated molecular descriptors.[6,71] One of the models obtained from this multivariate analysis was used to predict the log P_{eff} values for an external validation set composed of 34 compounds. The data correlated well with human absorption data for the same compounds, further validating the in vivo human permeability data set, as does the observation that passive diffusion is the dominant mechanism for the in vivo intestinal absorption of many drugs.[89-93] In this analysis, the cutoff polar surface area value for low and high permeability was less than 100 Å^2 (high $P_{eff} > \approx 1.0 \times 10^{-4}$ cm/s and $f_a > 90\%$).

Correlation of Human Jejunal Permeabilities with Preclinical Permeability Models

In medication development, there is a strong demand for the accurate and rapid characterization of biopharmaceutical processes such as solubility, dissolution, luminal stability, intestinal permeability, and first-pass metabolism in the gut and liver.[3,4,14,16,72,75,80,81] Several preclinical models have been used to address drug characteristics including permeability.

Rat-Human Comparison

The single-pass intestinal perfusion in rats is a common and validated in situ absorption model. Jejunal, ileal, and colonic P_{eff} has been measured using a single-pass intestinal perfusion method in anesthetized rats in situ at a perfusion rate of 0.2 mL/min.[3,4,14,16,72,75] A number of drugs from different BCS classes (summarized in Table 4-1) have been investigated in human jejunum.[10–13] An intestinal perfusion experiment is usually done with the drug at a concentration where it is in solution.[11–13] All the investigated drugs were stable and demonstrated no sign of degradation or adsorption to the catheters. When treating patient with EADs, chemical degradation and adsorption to the tube material are important factors to investigate prior to any clinical use.[1,2,11–13]

The viability of this intestinal transport model was assessed by testing a range of physiologic function. For example, ^{14}C-PEG 4000, an established nonabsorbable and fluid flux marker compound, was used to monitor whether the intestinal barrier was intact. In addition, the carrier-mediated cotransport of Na$^+$/D-glucose was examined.[11–13] Antipyrine was included as a marker for passive transcellular transport and used as an indicator of extensive changes of mesenteric blood flow.[13]

For passively transported compounds, the rank order in perfused proximal jejunal segments of both humans and rats was similar.[6,13,72,73,75,94] The human P_{eff} for drugs transported by passive diffusion were higher in humans in vivo than in the rats in situ, irrespective of the permeability classification of the drug.[6,72,73,75] Plausible reasons for the lower rat intestinal P_{eff} value include differences in the effective absorptive area within the perfused segment and/or species differences affecting partitioning into the membrane, membrane diffusion coefficient, and/or diffusion distance.[6,72,73,75] The anesthesia may somewhat slow passive diffusion across the jejunal barrier and explains some of the quantitative differences between these two species. Compounds that are transported via a carrier, such as levodopa and D-glucose, deviated from this linear relationship between the two single-pass perfusion models, which clearly demonstrates that drugs transported through membrane transport protein(s) should be characterized by transport mechanism(s) and kinetics, and then subsequently evaluated to establish a scaling factor for the transport kinetics. However, both human and rat P_{eff} values accurately predict the quantitative amount of drug absorbed in vivo in humans.[6,72,73,75,94] Also, in the rat jejunum, there are no age-related changes in passive or carrier-mediated absorption of drugs and nutrients.[94]

Single-pass perfusion in the rat provides permeability data that may be applied to classify drugs according to the BCS and the potential clinical use for enteral drug delivery. In vivo human studies for drugs administered through various types of EADs have also shown that the human and rat intestines absorb drugs in a very similar fashion.[1–4,11–13,94–96]

Although the small intestinal permeability data from the two species are highly correlated and have similar transporter expression patterns, the expression levels and patterns for metabolizing enzymes in the intestine are quite distinct.[3,4,6,13,72,73,75,80,81,94] A rat model, therefore, may be used to accurately predict oral drug absorption in the small intestine of humans, especially for a drug transported by lipoidal passive diffusion. However, predictions of drug metabolism and ultimate bioavailability are significantly less accurate.

The Ussing Chamber

In the Ussing chamber model, an intestinal specimen can be mounted, and then the in vitro transport and metabolism of drugs and metabolites can be monitored from apical and basolateral sides.[94,96–100] The P_{eff} for compounds transported by both passive lipoidal diffusion and carrier-mediated mechanisms across rat jejunal segments mounted in an Ussing chamber have been compared with corresponding human data.[98,99] P_{eff} and rank order were the same in excised rat jejunal segments (in vitro) and in human jejunum (in vivo) for passively transported compounds. Data from the two models were highly correlated ($r^2 = 0.95$) when both low- and high-P_{eff} drugs (transported by passive diffusion) were compared.[98,99]

Jejunal permeability data have been examined for nine *passively* absorbed drugs, which were classified according to the BCS as low- or high-permeability drugs. Permeability data from single-pass perfusions correlated highly with data from the Ussing chamber model in the rat.[101] However, there were deviations between the two absorption models, which were related to the physicochemical and permeability characteristics of the compounds. The P_{eff}/P_{app} ratio increased from about 1.0 for the low-permeability compounds (eg, terbutaline, atenolol, creatinine) to approximately 4.7 for those with the highest permeability (eg, antipyrine, naproxen). This finding was in accordance with correlations of human in situ and rat in vitro permeability, correcting for the intrinsic P_{eff} difference of 3.6 between humans and rats.[94,96–101]

Intestinal P_{eff} values for *carrier-mediated* transport compounds such as D-glucose, levodopa, and L-leucine were approximately 5- to 15-fold higher in the in vivo human model.[94,98,99] This higher value might partially be explained by the total absence of blood flow and/or a less-pronounced concentration gradient across the jejunal barrier in vitro. In addition, the in vitro P_{eff} values for the compounds transported via carriers might also be affected by the supply of cofactors, which are crucial for optimal function of the transport protein.[6,72,75,98,99]

Although there seems to be a high correlation between in vivo and in vitro permeability for drugs absorbed by passive transcellular diffusion along the intestine for the human, rat, and dog, it seems like there is a significant deviation for drugs transported by intestinal membrane transport proteins.[1–4,6,72,75,94–96,98,99] When directly comparing human in vivo jejunal permeability data with permeability data obtained from a Caco-2 cell model (a human colonic cell line), the best correlations were obtained for drugs absorbed by passive diffusion.[94,102,103] Results obtained solely from cell culture studies (eg, Caco-2 cells) may have led to an overinterpretation of the importance of efflux carriers on the intestinal absorption process.[78–88,94,102,103] Many drugs that were initially believed to undergo significant efflux in vitro were later shown to be completely absorbed in vivo.[11–13,73,82,87] However, one important function of the efflux transporter P-gp is to secrete hydrophilic conjugates formed intracellularly.[85,86,87] Furthermore, data based solely on cell culture studies (using Caco-2 cells) suggested that the in vitro permeability of fexofenadine, a substrate for P-gp and an uptake transporter (organic anion transporting polypeptide [OATP]), was increased in the absorptive direction by approximately 2- to 3-fold (from $\sim 0.3 \times 10^{-6}$ to 1.5×10^{-6} cm/s) in the presence of various P-gp-inhibitors (eg, verapamil, ketoconazole, and GF-120918) and that low passive diffusion was the main reason for the incomplete and highly variable rate and extent of intestinal absorption.[13,104–106] Interestingly, in vivo jejunal permeability in humans ($P_{eff} \sim 0.07 \times 10^{-4}$ cm/s) was affected neither by ketoconazole nor verapamil at clinical doses.[13,104–106] This finding suggests that the Caco-2 model did not accurately predict the in vivo absorption kinetics and mechanisms in human jejunum. However, the in vitro data predicted a drug-drug interaction that also occurs in vivo, probably in the liver.[80,81] The results from this study also emphasize that improved knowledge of in vitro and in vivo correlations are crucial when data from in vitro methods alone are used in physiologically based pharmacokinetic modeling and prediction of in vivo absorption and bioavailability of drugs in early drug development. Furthermore, clinically relevant drug-drug interactions for transport proteins are of increasing interest in clinical development and usage.[85–87] The in vivo role of P-gp-mediated efflux has not been fully evaluated because of the lack of good substrates and because passive diffusion often contributes significantly to the overall barrier transport. Overinterpretation of the role played by cellular efflux rather than first-pass gut wall/liver metabolism may also help explain why investigations of this topic are insufficient.[85–88]

Conclusion

This chapter summarizes some of the most pertinent factors affecting drug bioavailability from the GI tract, including intestinal permeability and GI motility and transit. These factors will, to a large extent, affect the intra- and interpatient variability in both the rate and extent of absorption of the drug formulation delivered through the EAD. To optimize the various treatments through enteral drug delivery, mainly liquid and oral IR dosage forms should be the basis for the necessary *ex tempore* formulation. Accordingly, the BCS provides an excellent knowledge-based tool to apply when planning which oral drug formulation should be used for optimized enteral drug delivery through various devices.

References

1. Dahlgren D, Roos C, Lundqvist A, et al. Regional intestinal permeability of three model drugs in human. *Mol Pharm.* 2016;13:3013–3021.
2. Dahlgren D, Roos C, Johansson P, et al. Regional intestinal permeability in dogs: biopharmaceutical aspects for development of oral modified-release dosage forms. *Mol Pharm.* 2016;13:3022–3033.
3. Sjögren E, Abrahamsson B, Augustijns P, et al. In vivo methods for drug absorption—comparative physiologies, model selection, correlations with in vitro methods (IVIVC), and applications for formulation/API/excipient characterization including food effects. *Eur J Pharm Sci.* 2014; 16:57:99–151
4. Kostewicz ES, Abrahamsson B, Brewster M, et al. In vitro models for the prediction of in vivo performance of oral dosage forms. *Eur J Pharm Sci.* 2014;16;57:342–366.
5. Koziolek M, Grimm M, Schneider F, et al. Navigating the human gastrointestinal tract for oral drug delivery: uncharted waters and new frontiers. *Adv Drug Deliv Rev.* 2016;101:75–88
6. Cao X, Gibbs ST, Fang L, et al. Why is it challenging to predict intestinal drug absorption and oral bioavailability in human using rat model? *Pharm Res.* 2006;23:1675–1686.

7. Bonlokke L, Hovgaard L, Kristensen HG, Knutson L, Lennernäs H. Direct estimation of the in vivo dissolution of spironolactone, in two particle size ranges, using the single-pass perfusion technique (Loc-I-Gut) in humans. *Eur J Pharm Sci.* 2001;12:239–250.

8. Bonlokke L, Hovgaard L, Kristensen HG, et al. A comparison between direct determination of in vivo dissolution and the deconvolution technique in humans. *Eur J Pharm Sci.* 1999;8:19–27.

9. Carlert S, Akesson P, Jerndal G, et al. In vivo dog intestinal precipitation of mebendazole: a basic BCS class II drug. *Mol Pharm.* 2012;9:2903–2911.

10. Dahan A, Beig A, Lindley D, Miller JM. The solubility-permeability interplay and oral drug formulation design: two heads are better than one. *Adv Drug Deliv Rev.* 2016;101:99–107

11. Dahlgren D, Roos C, Sjögren E, Lennernäs H. Direct in vivo human intestinal permeability (P_{eff}) determined with different clinical perfusion and intubation methods. *J Pharm Sci.* 2015;104:2702–2726.

12. Lennernäs H. Human in vivo regional intestinal permeability: importance for pharmaceutical drug development. *Mol Pharm.* 2014;11:12–23.

13. Lennernäs H. Intestinal permeability and its relevance for absorption and elimination. *Xenobiotica.* 2007;37:1015–1051.

14. Amidon GL, Lennernäs H, Shah VP, Crison JR. A theoretical basis for a biopharmaceutic drug classification: the correlation of in vitro drug product dissolution and in vivo bioavailability. *Pharm Res.* 1995;12:413–420.

15. Kasim NA, Whitehouse M, Ramachandran C, et al. Molecular properties of WHO essential drugs and provisional biopharmaceutical classification. *Mol Pharm.* 2004;12:85–96.

16. Lennernäs H, Abrahamsson B. The use of biopharmaceutic classification of drugs in drug discovery and development: current status and future extension. *J Pharm Pharmacol.* 2005;57:273–285.

17. Wu CY, Benet LZ, Hebert MF, et al. Differentiation of absorption and first-pass gut and hepatic metabolism in humans: studies with cyclosporine. *Clin Pharmacol Ther.* 1995;58(5):492–497.

18. Koziolek M, Garbacz G, Neumann M, Weitschies W. Simulating the postprandial stomach: physiological considerations for dissolution and release testing. *Mol Pharm.* 2013;10:1610–1622.

19. Talattof A, Price JC, Amidon GL. Gastrointestinal motility variation and implications for plasma level variation: oral drug products. *Mol Pharm.* 2016;13:557–567.

20. Cao F, Amidon GL, Rodriguez-Hornedo N, Amidon GE. Mechanistic analysis of cocrystal dissolution as a function of pH and micellar solubilization. *Mol Pharm.* 2016;13:1030–1046.

21. Krieg BJ, Taghavi SM, Amidon GL, Amidon GE. In vivo predictive dissolution: comparing the effect of bicarbonate and phosphate buffer on the dissolution of weak acids and weak bases. *J Pharm Sci.* 2015;104: 2894–2904.

22. Wade DN, Mearrick PT, Birkett DJ, Morris J. Variability of L-dopa absorption in man *Aust N Z J Med.* 1974;4:138–143.

23. Kurlan R, Nutt JG, Woodward WR, et al. Erratic gastric emptying of levodopa may cause "random" fluctuations of Parkinsonian mobility. *Neurology.* 1988;38:419–421.

24. Nutt JG, Woodward WR, Hammerstad JP, Carter JH, Anderson JL. The "on-off" phenomenon in Parkinson's disease: relation to levodopa absorption and transport. *N Engl J Med.* 1984;310:483–484.

25. Bredberg E, Tedroff J, Aquilonius SM, Paalzow L. Pharmacokinetics and effects of levodopa in advanced Parkinson's disease. *Eur J Clin Pharmacol.* 1990;39:385–389.

26. Oberle RL, Chen T-S, Lloyd C, et al. The influence of the interdigestive migrating myoelectric complex on the gastric emptying of liquids. *Gastroenterology* 1990;99:1275–1282.

27. Azran C, Wolk O, Zur M, et al. Oral drug therapy following bariatric surgery: an overview of fundamentals, literature and clinical recommendations. *Obes Rev.* 2016;17:1050–1066.

28. Takada T, Weiss HM, Kretz O, Gross G, Sugiyama Y. Hepatic transport of PKI166, an epidermal growth factor receptor kinase inhibitor of the pyrrolo-pyrimidine class, and its main metabolite, ACU154. *Drug Metab Dispos.* 2004;32:1272–1278.

29. Enokizono J, Kusuhara H, Sugiyama Y. Involvement of breast cancer resistance protein (BCRP/ABCG2) in the biliary excretion and intestinal efflux of troglitazone sulfate, the major metabolite of troglitazone with a cholestatic effect. *Drug Metab Dispos.* 2007;35:209–214.

30. Ghibellini G, Vasist LS, Leslie EM, et al. In vitro-in vivo correlation of hepatobiliary drug clearance in humans. *Clin Pharmacol Ther.* 2007;81: 406–413.

31. Davis SS, Wilding IR. Oral drug absorption studies: the best model for man is man! *Drug Discov Today.* 2001;6:127–130.

32. Faas H, Steingoetter A, Feinle C, et al. Effects of meal consistency and ingested fluid volume on the intragastric distribution of a drug model in humans—a magnetic resonance imaging study. *Aliment Pharmacol Ther.* 2002;16:217–224.

33. Keller J, Binnewies U, Rösch M, et al. Gastric emptying and disease activity in inflammatory bowel disease. *Eur J Clin Invest.* 2015;45:1234–1242.

34. Little TJ, Feinle-Bisset C. Effects of dietary fat on appetite and energy intake in health and obesity—oral and gastrointestinal sensory contributions. *Physiol Behav.* 2011;104:613–620.

35. Nauck M. Incretin therapies: highlighting common features and differences in the modes of action of glucagon-like peptide-1 receptor agonists and dipeptidyl peptidase-4 inhibitors. *Diabetes Obes Metab.* 2016;18:203–216.

36. Olausson, E. A. Alpsten M, Larsson A, Mattsson H, Andersson H, Attvall S. Small particle size of a solid meal increases gastric emptying and late postprandial glycaemic response in diabetic subjects with gastroparesis. *Diabetes Res Clin Pract.* 2008;80:231–237.

37. Sam AH, Troke RC, Tan TM, Bewick GA. The role of the gut/brain axis in modulating food intake. *Neuropharmacology.* 2012;63:46–56.

38. Nyholm D, Askmark H, Gomes-Trolin C, et al. Optimizing levodopa pharmacokinetics: intestinal infusion versus oral sustained-release tablets. *Clin Neuropharmacol.* 2003;26:156–163.

39. Nyholm D, Lennernäs H. Irregular gastrointestinal drug absorption in Parkinson's disease. *Expert Opin Drug Metab Toxicol.* 2008;4:193–203.

40. Nyholm D, Lennernäs H, Johansson A, Estrada M, Aquilonius SM. Circadian rhythmicity in levodopa pharmacokinetics in patients with Parkinson disease. *Clin Neuropharmacol.* 2010;33:181–185.

41. Engelstoft MS, Egerod KL, Holst B, Schwartz TW. A gut feeling for obesity: 7TM sensors on enteroendocrine cells. *Cell Metab.* 2008;8:447–449.

42. Engelstoft MS, Egerod KL, Lund ML, Schwartz TW. Enteroendocrine cell types revisited. *Curr Opin Pharmacol.* 2013;13:912–921.

43. Rebello CJ, O'Neil CE, Greenway FL. Gut fat signaling and appetite control with special emphasis on the effect of thylakoids from spinach on eating behavior. *Int J Obes (Lond).* 2015;39:1679–1688.

44. Maljaars PW, Peters HP, Mela DJ, Masclee AA. Ileal brake: a sensible food target for appetite control. A review. *Physiol Behav.* 2008;95:271–281.

45. Maljaars PWJ, van der Wal RJP, Wiersma T, et al. The effect of lipid droplet size on satiety and peptide secretion is intestinal site-specific. *Clin Nutr.* 2012;31:535–542.

46. Kerlin P, Phillips S. Variability of motility of the ileum and jejunum in healthy humans. *Gastroenterology.* 1982;82:694–700.

47. Kerlin P, Zinsmeister A, Phillips S. Relationship of motility to flow of contents in the human small intestine. *Gastroenterology.* 1982;82:701–706.

48. Kellow JE, Borody TJ, Phillips SF, Tucker RL, Haddad AC. Human interdigestive motility: variations in patterns from esophagus to colon. *Gastroenterology.* 1986;91:386–395.

49. Rees WD, Malagelada JR, Miller JL, Go VLW. Human interdigestive and postprandial gastrointestinal motor and gastrointestinal hormone patterns. *Dig Dis Sci.* 1982;27:321–329.

50. Code CF, Marlett JA. The interdigestive myo-electric complex of the stomach and small bowel of dogs. *J. Physiol.(Lond)* 1975;246:289–309.

51. Clements JA, Heading RC, Nimmo WS, Prescott LF. Kinetics of acetaminophen absorption and gastric emptying in man. *Clin Pharmacol Ther.* 1978;24:420–431.

52. Evans MA, Broe GA, Triggs EJ, et al. Gastric emptying rate and the systemic availability of levodopa in the elderly parkinsonian patient. *Neurology.* 1981;31:1288–1294.

53. Heading RC, Nimmo WS, Prescott LF, Tothill P. The dependence of paracetamol absorption on the rate of gastric emptying. *Br J Pharmacol.* 1973;7:415–421.

54. Prescott LF. Gastrointestinal absorption of drugs. *Med Clin N Am.* 1974; 58:907–916.

55. Robertson DRC, Renwick AG, Wood ND, et al. The influence of levodopa on gastric emptying in man. *Br J Clin Pharmacol.* 1990;29:47–53.

56. Coupe AJ, Davis SS, Evans DF, Wilding IR. Correlation of the gastric emptying of nondisintegrating tablets with gastrointestinal motility. *Pharm Res.* 1991;8:1281–1285.

57. Khosla R, Davis SS. Gastrointestinal transit of non-disintegrating tablets in fed subjects. *Int J Pharm.* 1989;53:107–117.

58. Mojaverian P, Reynolds JC, Ouyang A, et al. Mechanism of gastric emptying of a nondisintegrating radiotelemetry capsule in man. *Pharm Res.* 1991;8:97–100.

59. Birkebaek NH, Memmert K, Mortensen J, Dirksen H, Christensen MF. Fractional gastrointestinal transit time: intra- and interindividual variation. *Nucl Med Comm.* 1990;11:247–252.

60. McConnell EL, Fadda HM, Basit AW. Gut instincts: explorations in intestinal physiology and drug delivery. *Int J Pharm.* 2008;364:213–226.

61. Merchant HA, Liu F, Orlu Gul M, Basit AW. Age-mediated changes in the gastrointestinal tract. *Int J Pharm.* 2016;16:303–308.

62. Wilson CG, Washington N, Hardy JG, Bond SW. The influence of food on the absorption of acyclovir: a pharmacokinetic and scintigraphic assessment. *Int J Pharm.* 1987;38:221–225.

63. Price JMC, Davis SS, Wilding IR. The effect of fibre on gastrointestinal transit times in vegetarians and omnivores. *Int J Pharm.* 1991;76:123–131.

64. Metcalf AM, Phillips SF, Zinsmeister AR, et al. Simplified assessment of segmental colonic transit. *Gastroenterology.* 1987;92:40–47.

65. Hardy JG, Wilson CG, Wood E. Drug delivery to the proximal colon. *J Pharm Pharmacol.* 1985;37:874–877.

66. Hardy JG, Healey JNC, Lee SW, Reynolds JR. Gastrointestinal transit of an enteric-coated delayed-release 5-aminosalicylic acid tablet. *Aliment Pharmacol Therap.* 1987;1:209–216.

67. Brayden DJ, Jepson MA, Baird AW. Keynote review: intestinal Peyer's patch M cells and oral vaccine targeting *Drug Discov Today.* 2005;10:1145–1157.

68. Luckey TD. Introduction to intestinal microecology. *Am J Clin Nutr.* 1972;25:1292–1294.

69. Wong, JM, de Souza R, Kendall CW, Emam A, Jenkins DJ. Colonic health: fermentation and short chain fatty acids. *J Clin Gastroenterol.* 2006;40:235–243.

70. Lande MB, Donovan JM, Zeidel ML. The relationship between membrane fluidity and permeabilities to water, solutes, ammonia, and protons. *J Gen Physiol.* 1995;106:67–84.

71. Lennernäs H. Does fluid flow across the intestinal mucosa affect quantitative oral drug absorption? Is it time for a reevaluation? *Pharm Res.* 1995;12:1573–1582.

72. Fagerholm U, Nilsson D, Knutson L, Lennernäs H. Jejunal permeability in humans in vivo and rats in situ: investigation of molecular size selectivity and solvent drag. *Acta Physiol Scand.* 1999;165:315–324.

73. Lennernäs H. Human intestinal permeability. *J Pharm Sci.* 1998;87: 403–410.

74. Lennernäs H, Lee ID, Fagerholm U, Amidon GL. A residence-time distribution analysis of the hydrodynamics within the intestine in man during a regional single-pass perfusion with Loc-I-Gut: in-vivo permeability estimation. *J Pharm Pharmacol.* 1997;49:682–686.

75. Fagerholm U, Johansson M, Lennernäs H. Comparison between permeability coefficients in rat and human jejunum. *Pharm Res.* 1996;13: 1336–1342.

76. Berggren S, Gall C, Wollnitz N, et al. Gene and protein expression of P-glycoprotein, MRP1, MRP2, and CYP3A4 in the small and large human intestine. *Mol Pharm.* 2007;4:252–257.

77. Englund G, Rorsman F, Ronnblom A, et al. Regional levels of drug transporters along the human intestinal tract: co-expression of ABC and SLC transporters and comparison with Caco-2 cells. *Eur J Pharm Sci.* 2006;29:269–277.

78. Englund G, Jacobsson A, Rorsman F, et al. Efflux transporters in ulcerative colitis: Decreased expression of BCRP (ABCG2) and Pgp (ABCB1). *Inflamm Bowel Dis.* 2007;13(3):291–297.

79. Collett A, Higgs NB, Sims E, Rowland M, Warhust G. Modulation of the permeability of H2 receptor antagonists cimetidine and ranitidine by P-glycoprotein in rat intestine and the human colonic cell line Caco-2. *J Pharmacol Exp Ther.* 1999;288:171–178.

80. Collett A, Tanians-Hughes J, Carlson GL, Harwood MD, Warhust G. Comparison of P-glycoprotein-mediated drug-digoxin interactions in Caco-2 with human and rodent intestine: relevance to in vivo prediction. *Eur J Pharm Sci.* 2005;26:386–393.

81. Chiou WL, Chung SM, Wu TC, Ma C. A comprehensive account on the role of efflux transporters in the gastrointestinal absorption of 13 commonly used substrate drugs in humans. *Int J Clin Pharmacol Ther.* 2001;39:93–101.

82. Bourdet DL, Thakker DR. Saturable absorptive transport of the hydrophilic organic cation ranitidine in Caco-2 cells: role of pH-dependent organic cation uptake system and P-glycoprotein. *Pharm Res.* 2006;23:1165–1177.

83. Bourdet DL, Pritchard JB, Thakker DR. Differential substrate and inhibitory activities of ranitidine and famotidine toward human organic cation transporter 1 (hOCT1; SLC22A1), hOCT2 (SLC22A2), and hOCT3 (SLC22A3). *J Pharmacol Exp Ther.* 2005;315:1288–1297.

84. Bourdet DL, Pollack GM, Thakker DR. Intestinal absorptive transport of the hydrophilic cation ranitidine: a kinetic modeling. *Pharm Res.* 2006;23(6):1178–1187.

85. Fenner KS, Troutman MD, Kempshall S, et al. Drug-drug interactions mediated through P-glycoprotein: clinical relevance and in vitro-in vivo correlation using digoxin as a probe drug. *Clin Pharmacol Ther.* 2009; 85(2):173–181.

86. Cook JA, Feng B, Fenner KS, et al. Refining the in vitro and in vivo critical parameters for P-glycoprotein, [I]/IC50 and [I2]/IC50, that allow for the exclusion of drug candidates from clinical digoxin interaction studies. *Mol Pharm.* 2010;5;7(2):398–411.

87. Lee CA, Cook JA, Reyner EL, Smith DA. P-glycoprotein related drug interactions: clinical importance and a consideration of disease states. *Expert Opin Drug Metab Toxicol.* 2010;6(5):603–619.

88. Greiner B, Eichelbaum M, Fritz P, et al. The role of intestinal P-glycoprotein in the interaction of digoxin and rifampin. *J Clin Invest.* 1999; 104:147–153.

89. Winiwarter S, Bonham NM, Ax F, Hallberg A, Lennernäs H, Karlen A. Correlation of human jejunal permeability (in vivo) of drugs with experimentally and theoretically derived parameters. A multivariate data analysis approach. *J Med Chem.* 1998;41:4939–49.

90. Winiwarter S, Ax F, Lennernäs H, et al. Hydrogen bonding descriptors in the prediction of human in vivo intestinal permeability. *J Mol Graph Model.* 2003;21:273–287.

91. Lipinski CA, Lombardo F, Dominy BW, Feeney PJ. Experimental and computational approaches to estimate solubility and permeability in drug discovery and development settings. *Adv Drug Deliv Rev.* 2001;46:3–26.

92. Smith D, Artursson P, Avdeef A, et al. Passive lipoidal diffusion and carrier-mediated cell uptake are both important mechanisms of membrane permeation in drug disposition. *Mol Pharm.* 2014;2;11(6):1727–1738.

93. Sugano K, Kansy M, Artursson P, et al. Coexistence of passive and carrier-mediated processes in drug transport. *Nat Rev Drug Discov.* 2010; 9(8):597–614.

94. Lennernäs H. Animal data: the contributions of the Ussing chamber and perfusion systems to predicting human oral drug delivery in vivo. *Adv Drug Deliv Rev.* 2007;59(11):1103–1120.

95. Tannergren C, Bergendal A, Lennernäs H, Abrahamsson B. Toward an increased understanding of the barriers to colonic drug absorption in humans: implications for early controlled release candidate assessment. *Mol Pharm.* 2009;6(1):60–73.

96. Sjöberg Å, Lutz M, Tannergren C, et al. Comprehensive study on regional human intestinal permeability and prediction of fraction absorbed of drugs using the Ussing chamber technique. *Eur J Pharm Sci.* 2013;48(1):166–180.

97. Nejdfors P, Ekelund M, Jeppsson B, Weström BR. Mucosal in vitro permeability in the intestinal tract of the pig, the rat, and man: species-and region-related differences. *Scand J Gastroenterol.* 2000;35(5):501–507.

98. Ungell AL, Nylander S, Bergstrand S, Sjöberg A, Lennernäs H. Membrane transport of drugs in different regions of the intestinal tract of the rat. *J Pharm Sci.* 1998;87(3):360–366.

99. Lennernäs H, Nylander S, Ungell AL. Jejunal permeability: a comparison between the Ussing chamber technique and the single-pass perfusion in humans. *Pharm Res.* 1997;14(5):667–671.

100. Ussing HH, Zerahn K. Active transport of sodium as the source of electric current in the short-circuited isolated frog skin. *Acta Physiologica Scand.* 1951;23(2–3):110–127.

101. Berggren S, Hoogstraate J, Fagerholm U, Lennernäs H. Characterization of jejunal absorption and apical efflux of ropivacaine, lidocaine and bupivacaine in the rat using in situ and in vitro absorption models. *Eur J Pharm Sci.* 2004;21(4):553–560.

102. Sun D, Lennernäs H, Welage LS, et al. Comparison of human duodenum and Caco-2 gene expression profiles for 12,000 gene sequences tags and

correlation with permeability of 26 drugs. *Pharm Res.* 2002;19(10): 1400–1416.

103. Lennernäs H, Palm K, Fagerholm U, Artursson P. Comparison between active and passive drug transport in human intestinal epithelial (Caco-2) cells and human jejunum in vivo. *Int J Pharm.* 1996;127:103–107.

104. Petri N, Borga O, Nyberg L, Hedeland M, Bondesson U, Lennernäs H. Effect of erythromycin on the absorption of fexofenadine in the jejunum, ileum and colon determined using local intubation in healthy volunteers. *Int J Clin Pharmacol Ther.* 2006;44(2):71–79.

105. Petri N, Tannergren C, Rungstad D, Lennernäs H. Transport characteristics of fexofenadine in the Caco-2 cell model. *Pharm Res.* 2004;21(8): 1398–1404.

106. Tannergren C, Petri N, Knutson L, et al. Multiple transport mechanisms involved in the intestinal absorption and first-pass extraction of fexofenadine. *Clin Pharmacol Ther.* 2003;74(5):423–436.

5

Drug Preparation and Administration with a User Guide to the Monographs

Joseph Boullata, PharmD

Introduction

Before administering medication through a patient's enteral access device (EAD), clinicians must consider multiple safety issues. Any necessary drug must be prepared and administered appropriately for the patient to meet therapeutic goals without raising the risk for complications. Errors, such as using an unsuitable drug formulation, incorrect preparation technique, or inappropriate administration site, have significant consequences. Obstruction of the patient's feeding tube, therapeutic failure, and drug toxicity including fatality have all been documented. Numerous errors can occur in a single patient requiring enteral medication.[1-4] Additionally, depending on the degree of exposure, some drugs may pose a hazard to the caregiver preparing the medication. The safety risk can also include oral medications intended for enteral administration that are inadvertently administered intravenously—25% to 40% of such errors result in sentinel events.[5-8] This chapter provides direction in drug order review, drug preparation, and drug administration for the enterally fed patient to reduce risk. This discussion is followed by a user guide to the monographs available in the second part of this book.

Medication Errors

Case reports and observational studies of enteral medication error, as well as multiple surveys have documented inappropriate drug preparation and administration practices. The blame for the errors has often been focused solely on the caregiver at the end of the process—usually the nurse. However, it is critical to appreciate that the drug administration

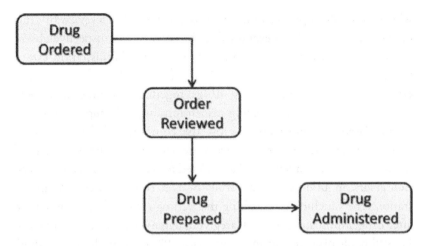

Figure 5-1. Interdisciplinary cascade leading to drug administration.

process begins with the prescriber and involves the pharmacist before the nurse or other caregiver handles the medication (Figure 5–1). Enteral medication errors can occur at each step (drug order, review, preparation, administration).[9]

Our nursing colleagues have expressed many concerns with drug manipulation at the point of care.[10] Crushing, splitting, or chewing of oral products can result in a variety of unintended outcomes for the patient. The nurse/provider may also be harmed if he or she is exposed to the drug product while manipulating it. This risk is especially notable when the drug preparation areas at their disposal are inadequate. The nurse may also have limited access to drug information sources, improper instructions on how to prepare a medication for administration, and, often, a lack of appropriate or clean devices for doing so.

Like nurses, prescribers and pharmacists recognize the limitations of available enteral drug products and challenges to their administration.[11,12] Although well over 90% of survey respondents (almost exclusively nurses) are confident in the appropriateness and effectiveness of their technique for drug preparation and administration, as many as one to three inappropriate techniques are identified per respondent.[13–20]

Apart from survey results and the occasional case reports after an enteral medication–related error, prospective observational studies provide the best insight into medication handling (ie, preparation and administration) practices. Again, the focus has been on clinicians, including nurses, whereas the role of pharmacists involved in drug regimen review or drug preparation has not been examined as thoroughly. In prospective observational studies, enteral medication preparation/administration errors made by nurses approach an astonishing 60% of doses.[21] Preparation errors include crushing/mixing drugs together, crushing modified-release dosage forms, not shaking suspensions, not diluting medications appropriately, and not wearing protective equipment.[21–23] Enteral drug preparation and administration errors occurred in over three-quarters of intensive care unit patients, and accounted for nearly 50% of all medication errors, in an observational study of over 10,000 doses.[23] Administration errors include not flushing the feeding tube before, between, or after drug administration.[21,22] Caregiving parents who received counseling still made observed dosing errors with 40% of their children's liquid medication.[24,25]

Prevention of all these errors remains the key to patient safety.[26] A systems approach can help reduce the risk for medication error.[27] This approach includes working with all stakeholders involved in any of the steps involved in caring for patients who may require enteral medication. This group develops and maintains policies and procedures around enteral medication preparation and administration. The documents must be clear about the responsibilities and tasks of prescribers, pharmacists, and nurses. An organization's policies and procedures should incorporate guidance documents and be consistent with published best practices across departments. Beyond federal law, state law, and USP mandates are the relevant clinical practice guidance documents. For example, the American Society for Parenteral and Enteral Nutrition guidance document "Safe Practices for EN Therapy" includes an entire section on medication.[28] Policies and procedures should also describe how all clinicians within the organization receive education and competency assessments.

Any identified enteral drug errors in an organization are best reviewed in a timely manner by an oversight committee, which can then recommend systems improvements to create a safer environment. It is critical to include policies and procedures that address enteral drug order review, preparation, labeling, dispensing, and administration. Safe practices have been recommended to address the error concerns in the steps of the enteral drug process and are incorporated into the following sections.[28]

Drug Order Review

Pharmacists play a critical role in the order review process by identifying each new drug order and assessing it within the full medication profile in the context of the patient's clinical status. This step is performed to ensure the appropriateness of each medication, communicate any potential discrepancies with the prescriber, and offer suitable alternatives. Pharmacists are familiar with reviewing a patient's ordered medications and intervening to resolve any orders that are inappropriate for the patient. They routinely consider whether drugs are ordered for *oral* or *enteral* administration. Because these are two distinct routes of administration, the pharmacist should always know the patient's current oral status (ie, *nil per os* [NPO] or NPO except medication) and feeding tube status.

Interventions that clarify or change medication orders after a thorough pharmacist review will need to be documented in the patient's health record. The pharmacist will consider and address both *patient*-related factors and *drug*-related factors when reviewing orders and making interventions (Table 5-1).

Table 5-1. Drug Order Review Query

Patient-related factors
- Is patient able to take medication by mouth?
- Are there any anatomical or functional abnormalities in the gastrointestinal tract that may interfere with drug absorption?
- What is the patient's enteral access device? (Assess entry point, distal site, and French size.)
- What is the current status of that enteral access device (position and patency)?

Drug-related factors
- Dosage form:
  o Is it immediate-release or modified-release (eg, enteric-coated, sustained-release, extended-release)?
  o Will modification of the dosage form alter drug-release characteristics?
- Drug:
  o What is the primary site of dissolution and absorption (if known)?
- Liquid formulation:
  o Is it intended for oral administration?
  o What is the osmolality and viscosity of the product or extemporaneously compounded preparation (if known)?

Patient-Related Factors

When reviewing an order, the pharmacist will identify whether the patient can take medication by mouth or requires enteral drug administration, as well as any anatomical or functional abnormalities present in the patient's gastrointestinal (GI) tract that may preclude drug absorption. The pharmacist will need to retrieve health record documentation of the patient's current EAD if that information is not part of the medication profile. The documentation should describe the EAD by its entry point and distal end, rather than just by the brand name. The pharmacist then considers the location of the distal end of the feeding tube, as well as the tube's diameter and length, identifies documentation verifying the initial placement and current positioning of the distal end of the feeding tube, and confirms tube patency. Dual-lumen EADs (see Chapter 1) are now frequently used in clinical practice; therefore, the pharmacist will need to identify which lumen (and distal site) will be used for drug administration. Ideally, to make the pharmacist review as efficient as possible, both the enteral feeding formulation and the flushing regimen administered through the EAD are part of the medication profile.

Drug-Related Factors

With rare exceptions, oral drug dosage forms are *not* designed for the physiologic constraints imposed by the patient requiring enteral nutrition (EN). When the enteral delivery system—including the access device—is used for drug administration, many questions arise, and evidence-based answers are relied upon as available.

The pharmacist's review process should identify any medication order that will require a preparation step (eg, appropriate crushing, diluting, mixing) prior to administration (see next section). The drug *dosage form* must be appropriate for enteral feeding tube administration (ie, immediate-release). Any solid dosage forms must be avoided if opening it (ie, capsule) and/or crushing it (ie, tablet) would result in a significant change in the absorption profile of the active pharmaceutical ingredient (API). Each ordered medication should be evaluated for its expected inherent solubility and release characteristics. If modifying the medication's dosage form would alter the release of API(s), an alternative dosage form, drug, or route of administration must be seriously considered.

The drug and its *formulation* both need to be appropriate based on the location of the distal end of the feeding. Among other things, the noted location should not bypass the primary site of drug dissolution and absorption. This factor is important regardless of whether a commercial product or an extemporaneous preparation is ordered. Hyperosmolar liquid drug preparations need to be carefully considered in context of the distal end of the tube. Oral preparations with an osmolality that exceed ~600 mOsm/kg contribute to adverse effects (eg, slowed gastric emptying, cramps, abdominal distension, pain, and diarrhea), especially in vulnerable patients.[29,30] This value approximates the upper end of physiologic osmolality found in healthy jejunum in the fed state. Many liquid medications have an osmolality that exceeds 1000 mOsm/kg due to various additives (eg, polyol sweeteners, propylene glycol).[31-33] Some of these liquid products are also highly viscous. Viscosity is an important consideration, especially for a narrow and lengthy tube through which the dose must traverse to reach the patient's gut. In addition to the resistance to flow encountered when administering a dose of viscous medication, such products can increase the cumulative risk for tube obstruction because they are more difficult to flush. Higher-viscosity products may also decrease gastric emptying.

Drug Preparation

Preparation refers to any step that will be required of the pharmacy, the nurse, or the caregiver at home to alter the dosage form from how it is made available prior to administration. This alteration could be as simple as diluting a medication in water or as complex as compounding an extemporaneous formulation.

Solids

For drugs accessible in solid forms, use only conventional, immediate-release, commercially available drug dosage forms for enteral administration. A fine powder can be obtained from these products by emptying capsule contents or crushing tablets. Film-coated tablets may prove more difficult to crush sufficiently. Modified-release dosage forms should be avoided.

For tablets that disperse easily, an alternative to crushing is to place the dose in the barrel of an enteral syringe (eg, 30 mL) and then replace the plunger, drawing up adequate purified water (eg, 10 to 30 mL) to allow a slurry to form in a few minutes—this method sometimes requires agitation. This technique avoids the risks of using a separate mixing container (ie, potential loss of drug or exposure to hazardous particulates from crushing). About half of all drugs in tablet form are considered dispersible within a 5-minute timeframe.[34]

Multiple sources can be reviewed to determine whether a solid dosage form can be crushed.[35] Many are listed as "Do Not Crush" because they have modified-release characteristics (eg, enteric-coated, sustained-release); others are listed because of hazards including teratogenicity and allergenicity. Open crushing creates significant amounts of aerosolized particulate matter ($>10^6$ particles/m^3).[36] Closed systems may be preferable for crushing tablets, especially for hazardous drugs.

Liquids

When using oral liquids for enteral administration, first consider the available commercial liquid product(s). Otherwise, seek an official USP formula or a published extemporaneous formula with adequate stability and sterility data. The ultimate safety and efficacy of the extemporaneous preparation depends on appropriate formulation and pharmaceutical judgment. To compound responsibly, appropriate methods are based on available data from the primary literature or compilations of those data.[37–41] The significance of stability and sterility data may be different for drug preparations intended for immediate use than for those stored 24 hours or longer. If the latter is considered (eg, to make a batch for one or more patients), information on stability and microbial growth under specific environmental conditions (light, temperature, humidity, and packaging material) and appropriate beyond-use date (BUD) will be required. Ideally, the compounded preparation should be stable (using a stability-indicating assay) beyond visual compatibility. Any preparation that requires compounding should ensure both physical and chemical stability and, ideally, provide data on final pH, osmolality, and viscosity. In a 2006 literature review and investigation of 83 liquid dosage forms, 7.2% of extemporaneously compounded preparations from existing dosage forms investigated exhibited stability concerns.[42] When present, these issues are often related to interactions between the API and excipients in the commercial product. In a more recent evaluation (2013), instability concerns for extemporaneously compounded preparations were managed with further manipulation.[43]

Notably, because many of the commercially available oral liquid products and "recipes" for extemporaneous preparations are designed with the intent of oral administration, they usually incorporate commercial flavoring agents, diluents, and thickening vehicles intended for the sensibilities of the oral route, which then contribute significantly to final osmolality and viscosity. Unfortunately, the final osmolality and viscosity values of the finished preparations are rarely reported. Whereas palatability is considered more important than osmolality or viscosity for oral delivery, the opposite is true for enterally administered medication.

USP Chapter <795> provides enforceable guidance for compounding nonsterile preparations, from simple to more complex.[44] Included are sections on responsibilities, the compounding process, facilities, equipment, storage, packaging, and documentation. These requirements are incorporated for medications that are prepared well in advance (ie, not for immediate use). For potentially hazardous medication, only trained personnel should prepare them in compliance with Occupational Safety and Health Administration, National Institute for Occupational Safety and Health, and USP Chapter <800> guidance.[45] Whether or not medications are potentially hazardous, personnel should avoid environmental cross-contamination, such as using the same mortar and pestle without cleaning between medications. Finally, if unable to use the available solid dosage form to make a liquid preparation, consider a therapeutic alternative.

Dilution

For preparation of dosage forms, USP requires *purified water*[44] (ie, water that is free of chemical or biological contaminants following source water selection, distillation, and filtration[46]). Drinking water (ie, bottled, tap, or well water) may be contaminated and is therefore not recommended for drug preparation.[28,47] Dilute each medication with purified water (eg, Sterile Water for Irrigation, USP) before administration to improve delivery of fine powders and reduce liquid osmolality and viscosity, especially for longer small-bore feeding tubes (see Tables 5–2 and 5–3). Generally, 15 to 30 mL of water is adequate to disperse an appropriate tablet or for a powdered drug. Dissolution should be adequate for a fine powder

Table 5-2. Preparing a Solid Dosage Form for Enteral Administration[a]

Capsule
- Open capsule(s) and completely empty the dry powder contents comprising the prescribed dose into a container (eg, medicine cup).
- Add volume of diluent (ie, purified water) and mix well.
- Draw up the mixture into an enteral syringe, using appropriate attachments as needed.
- Rinse additional water in container as needed to collect all visible powder particles and draw up into the enteral syringe.
- Cap the end of the syringe.
- Gently agitate to disperse the particles.

Tablet (crush)
- Crush tablets comprising the prescribed dose to a fine powder (preferably in a closed system).
- Add volume of diluent (ie, purified water) and mix well.
- Draw up the mixture into an enteral syringe, using appropriate attachments as needed.
- Rinse additional water in container as needed to collect all visible tablet particles and draw up into the enteral syringe.
- Cap the end of the syringe.
- Gently agitate to disperse the particles.

Tablet (disperse)
- Remove the enteral syringe plunger and place prescribed dose of dispersible tablet(s) into the barrel.
- Replace the plunger and draw up a volume of diluent (ie, purified water).
- Cap the end of the syringe.
- Gently agitate to disperse the tablet.

All preparations
- Label the enteral syringe for dispensing . . . *unless prepared outside the pharmacy for immediate use.*
- Collect all prepared medications due at the time for the single patient and carry them to the bedside for administration.

[a]Assumes the correct drug, dosage form, and formulation for the patient.

of small enough drug-particle size, but solubility depends on other factors as well (see Chapter 3). Dilution of the medication (dry or liquid) and irrigation (flushing) of the feeding tube with water is critical to ensure drug delivery through to the distal end of the EAD and to the patient. Suspensions will be easier to deliver once they are well diluted. For example, nearly 90% of the drug dose is not delivered to the end of a

Table 5-3. Preparing an Oral Liquid Dosage Form for Enteral Administration[a]

- Draw the prescribed dose up into an enteral syringe, using appropriate attachments as needed.
- Draw in some air prior to drawing up the volume of diluent (ie, purified water).
- Cap the end of the syringe.
- Gently agitate for adequate mixing.
- Label the enteral syringe for dispensing . . . *unless prepared outside the pharmacy for immediate use.*
- Collect all prepared medications due at the time for the single patient and carry them to the bedside for administration.

---

[a]Assumes the correct drug, dosage form, and formulation for the patient.

nasogastric tube if phenytoin suspension is not diluted or flushed.[48] The optimal degree of dilution likely depends on the viscosity and osmolality of the liquid medication. The viscosity of suspensions can be reduced significantly by 1:1 (v:v) dilution followed by a flush of the same total volume. This approach allowed for the successful delivery of carbamazepine suspension through nasogastric tubes.[49] When undiluted, even with some postdose flush, posaconazole suspension exhibited reduced absorption via nasogastric tube.[50,51] The higher viscosity of a drug preparation typically decreases the dissolution rate of drug particles. While this may be appropriate to maintain stability during transport and storage, it may be counterproductive if the preparation is introduced directly into the small bowel lumen. Therefore, dilution serves to enhance dissolution as well as delivery of the drug to the distal end of the EAD. Compared with suspensions, a solution may allow drug adsorption to the plastic container (eg, clonazepam).[42] At least a 1:1 volume dilution is expected to be adequate for viscous liquid drugs; however, depending on the osmolality of a liquid drug product, a dilution volume as high as 10:1 may be necessary to reduce the final osmolality. Whether these drug dilutions can be prepared in advance will depend on the duration of stability. Some drugs (eg, captopril) may undergo first-order oxidation in aqueous solution.[42]

Additional Considerations

Aside from selecting the appropriate drug and the acceptable commercial product (or extemporaneous preparation) at a suitable dilution, additional considerations may yet influence drug bioavailability in the enterally fed patient.

The ultimate systemic bioavailability of an oral drug depends on three processes: the fraction absorbed from the gut lumen into the enterocytes; the extraction (enzymatic metabolism or efflux transport) at the gut; and the extraction at the liver. These processes are in turn determined by three factors that are important to our discussion of drug preparation for enteral administration: physicochemical properties (eg, solubility), pharmaceutical elements (eg, excipients in the formulation), and physiologic influences (eg, variability in gut function). Even the seemingly simple act of crushing a commercial tablet and diluting it with purified water may pose a risk if the drug's bioavailability is ultimately influenced by factors such as the eventual particle size, interaction related to inherent excipients or water contaminants, or time of exposure (if drug degradation accelerates). Particle granularity using typical methods of crushing will differ by drug.[36] Many drug products contain APIs with poor water solubility that are formulated with specific excipients (eg, solubilizers, co-precipitates, surfactants) intended for intact oral administration. Breaking down this well-designed product and diluting the ingredients prior to administration runs the risk of altering the final disposition of the drug. In some cases (eg, amiloride, hydrocortisone), the pure powder form of the API can be more stable in an extemporaneous oral liquid than if the commercial tablets are used.[42]

Complexation and unavailability for absorption of an API can occur in the preparation of the dosage form as well as in GI fluid. This issue is more likely to affect excipient-containing liquid dosage forms. Given the complexity of a single API and its excipients, the interaction potential of combining *multiple* medications and their respective excipients is inevitably greater. Unless data suggest otherwise, the significant physicochemical risk for incompatibility and instability is expected to alter solubility and bioavailability. Given the numerous compounds (APIs and excipients), it is impossible to assign an equation for the multiple and complex reactions (rates, reaction orders, etc) involved. The many likely parallel or consecutive reactions would be unpredictable and impossible to evaluate. Therefore, the combination or mixing together of enteral medications is best avoided altogether. In the ideal world, all drugs could be made in a liquid preparation at neutral pH, with the drug fully dissolved, a low viscosity and osmolality, well-characterized absorption and bioavailability, and long-term stability that allows for preparation of batches in advance. However, in reality, each medication is unique, and the single, ideal liquid preparation is not available. Furthermore, the EN formula itself is not an ideal solvent, and medication is therefore not added to it. When evaluated, adding medication to EN has been shown to alter not only physicochemical properties but also bioavailability.[52-54]

Each institution should make good use of their available nonsterile pharmacy compounding services so that the frontline care provider is not burdened with drug preparation. The exception would be those medications with such poor (or undefined) stability that they need to be administered within minutes (less than 30) of preparation. The nurse should prepare those nonhazardous medications with limited stability in a dedicated clean area of the medication room. Otherwise, drug preparation should be left to trained pharmacy personnel responsible for preparing medications that require significant manipulation.

Labeling and Dispensing

What the pharmacy will prepare and/or dispense will need to be consistent with organizational staffing. Certainly, if the pharmacy prepares medication in advance for the clinician (or a caregiver at home), the dispensed drug container will be properly labeled (patient identifiers, drug name, dose, schedule, manufacturer name, lot, and BUD). If the dispensed preparation has been compounded, the organization's compounding record number is also included on the label.

Depending on compatibility and stability concerns, the pharmacy may dispense a drug that requires further preparation prior to administration. At the minimum, appropriate directions for preparation and administration should be provided—for example, as a label affixed to the container being dispensed. This instruction may be for a commercial unit-dose product that the nurse must prepare further (eg, dilution). Alternatively, instructions may be for unit doses prepared in the pharmacy in a suitable container. For example, dry powder medication (pure drug or product with excipients) could be labeled with directions to dilute it with water or, alternatively, to create a stable slurry of the dry powder in an appropriate diluent; a commercially available liquid or extemporaneously compounded liquid could be labeled with directions to administer as is or to dilute further just prior to administration.

Drug Administration

Administration refers to using an appropriate enteral device (eg, ENFit syringe) to deliver the medication through an EAD into the patient's GI tract (see Chapter 1). It also involves the timing of drug delivery with respect to the enteral feeding regimen, other medication, and flushing protocols.[55,56]

This distal step in the process requires an order specifying the route (ie, enteral) and site (eg, jejunostomy tube) of drug administration. Postpyloric administration can be a particular concern for antimicrobials or drugs with a narrow therapeutic index if bioavailability is altered. Enteral feeding is briefly held during drug administration times. The nurse (or nonclinician caregiver in some settings) then identifies the medication administration port of the enteral access (traced from the patient). The EAD is flushed with purified water (at least 15 mL for adult patients; a smaller flush for volume-restricted or pediatric patients) before the first medication at a scheduled administration time. The medication is then administered separately through the appropriate access site, using a clean enteral syringe (which may be the same enteral syringe used to prepare the dose). After administering the dose, an additional volume of water (eg, 15 mL) is drawn up in the enteral syringe as a rinse to be administered as a flush and to help ensure that the entire drug dose is delivered from the syringe through the EAD. After administering the last medication and flushing the EAD with water, continuous feeding is restarted in a timely manner (see Chapter 2). This process is repeated for each scheduled medication administration time throughout the day, within the patient's tolerable volume status—which will be lower in fluid-restricted patients and in pediatrics. Clinicians (or caregivers) with questions about drug preparation and administration should consult with a pharmacist with specific expertise.

* * * * *

Using the Monographs

Part II of this reference book contains drug monographs, the contents of which have been given considerable attention. This section of the chapter describes the parts of the monograph; provides the rationale for the included data; and offers suggestions about how best to use that information.

Parts of the Monograph

The first part of each monograph contains some basic information on the API (Figure 5–2a), whereas the second part provides practical information on enteral administration and nutrition considerations (Figure 5–2b). Most of the information in the first part of a monograph represents commonly available pharmaceutical data as found in a wide variety of sources, although not routinely together in one place.[57–59] Information in the second part of a monograph often relates to specific stability, compatibility, bioavailability, and nutrition-interaction data. When acknowledged in the primary source, the specific nutrition formulation studied as well as the complete reference for each study will be provided.

The name of each *API* is provided, including the salt form(s) when present. Combination products have therefore not been included in these monographs. Dosage forms of each medication contain the API and excipients. Selected *oral products* commercially available in the United States are listed, with preference given to innovator products for which data are most likely to be available. Generic product formulations likely differ in their included excipients, which may influence stability and compatibility but are not expected to significantly influence bioavailability or nutrition interactions.

The *physicochemical* data relevant to evaluating appropriateness of a *drug* for a site of administration or interaction potential with EN are provided. Included are molecular weight of pure drug, pKa, and water solubility. A critical property of an API is its water solubility (g/L = mg/mL) because water solubility predicts how well the API will dissolve in an aqueous environment (see Table 5-4). Water solubility, in turn, is necessary for drug absorption, but rates of dissolution (ie, drug particles going into solution [alternatively referred to as *solubilization* for dispersions such as suspensions]) vary even among APIs with good aqueous solubility. Amorphous structures usually dissolve faster, whereas drugs that exist in crystalline form(s), although more stable, often have slower dissolution rates. Slower dissolution rates risk giving time for API complexation/precipitation that may reduce bioavailability. The Noyes-Whitney and the Nernst-Brunner equations that describe dissolution assume a well-stirred bulk fluid volume beyond the unstirred boundary layer where molecules are first breaking off the drug particles. This assumption may not be met when the drug is mixed in small volumes of

Acyclovir

Product Availability

Solid	• Tablet: 400 mg, 800 mg (Zovirax® [Mylan]; others)
	• Capsule: 200 mg (Zovirax® [Mylan]; others)
Liquid	• Oral suspension: 200 mg/5 mL (Zovirax® [Mylan]; others)

Physicochemical (drug)

Molecular weight:	Permeability:	Water solubility:
• 225.21	• LogP –1.56	• Base 2.5 mg/mL (37°C)
	• LogD –1.76 (pH 7.4)	• Na-salt 100 mg/mL
pKa:	Classification:	
• 2.27, 9.25	• BCS Class 3 or 4; BDDCS Class 4	

Pharmaceutical (product)

Solid	• Tablets disperse in water (20 mL) within 2 minutes
Liquid	• Suspension:
	o pH 6.2
	o Osmolality: 874 mOsm/kg (measured 1:4 dilution with
	sterile water); 4205 mOsm/kg (calculated based on
	measurement of 1:5 dilution with sterile water)[1]
	o Viscosity 282 mPa·s
	o May contain glycerin and sorbitol
	o Maintain at controlled room temperature (do not refrigerate).
Note	• Capsules and oral suspension are considered bioequivalent.

Pharmacokinetic (patient)

Absorption	• Specific site not known; t_{max} within 2 hours after oral dose
	• Bioavailability ~10%–30% (variable, incomplete).
Transport	• Substrate for MATE1 efflux; OAT1 and OCT1 uptake
	• Plasma protein binding ~9%–33%
	• V_d ~0.69 L/kg
Metabolism	• Minimal hepatic metabolism to 9-CMMG and
	8-hydroxy-acyclovir
	• Most is eliminated unchanged in urine.
	• Cl ~327 mL/min/1.73 m²

Figure 5-2a. Example of active pharmaceutical ingredient information in a drug monograph (Acyclovir).

diluent and introduced directly into the small bowel (ie, no sink conditions; crystallization may occur instead). The higher the water solubility is, the better the concentration gradient to drive absorption is. Of course, the drug in an aqueous solution ideally maintains a balance of being soluble yet also permeable across cell membranes. Another physicochemical property is the lipid solubility of an API as an indicator of potential cell

Enteral Administration and Nutrition Considerations

Compatibility, Stability, and Bioavailability Considerations
- Tablet contents are absorbed when administered into duodenum.[2]
- Specific excipients (sodium lauryl sulfate and/or sodium caprate) can act as permeability enhancers for acyclovir, when included.[3]
- Acyclovir is unstable (HPLC analysis) in sucrose/maltitol or fructose/glucose solutions.[4]
- Commercial suspension combined (1:1) with Osmolite 1.2, under simulated clinical conditions, would result in clogging an 8 Fr, but not a 20 Fr, feeding tube.[1]
- Solid dispersions of acyclovir with multiple hydrophilic carriers resulted in enhanced dissolution and permeability.[5]
- Several amino acid ester prodrugs of acyclovir (eg, valine → valacyclovir) improve bioavailability by enhancing transport.[6]

Drug-Nutrition Interactions
- Drug may influence nutrition status directly or indirectly:
  - CNS: headache, encephalopathy, confusion, ataxia, paresthesia
  - GI: nausea, vomiting, diarrhea, elevated LFTs
  - Metabolic: hemolysis, anemia, transient elevation of BUN
  - Other: peripheral edema, myalgia
- Influence of malnutrition or obesity on drug disposition:
  - The body weight–normalized volume of distribution (L/kg) is much smaller in obesity and suggests that the drug is best dosed based on a lean body weight.[7]
- No known influence of food on oral absorption or bioavailability.

Recommendations

Gastric	• Disperse tablet in water (20 mL) prior to administration. • Avoid using the suspension for enteral access device administration. • No need to hold EN beyond the time required to flush-administer-flush.
Postpyloric	• As above. • Monitor for any unexpected change in effect.
Other	• As with all antimicrobials, consider parenteral alternative for acutely ill patients to ensure therapeutic concentrations.

Figure 5-2b. Example of compatibility, stability, bioavailability, and nutrition-interaction data in a drug monograph (Acyclovir).

membrane permeability. The *LogP* values represent a drug's partition coefficient, where positive values indicate lipid solubility, as well as its susceptibility to extraction. A LogP with a negative value indicates poor lipid solubility where absorption will depend more on small molecular weight and transporters. The *LogD* values represent a drug's distribution

Table 5-4. Defining Drug Solubility

Definition	Solubility, mg/mL
Very soluble	≥1000
Freely soluble	100–1000
Soluble	33–100
Sparingly soluble	10–33
Slightly soluble	1–10
Very slightly soluble	0.1–1
Practically insoluble	<0.1

coefficient, taking into account pKa and physiologic pH as well as the degree of lipid solubility at that pH. This coefficient may better reflect in vivo drug behavior, with higher values predicting membrane permeability and enzymatic extraction. When values for LogP and LogD have been estimated, rather than measured, the term *calc* is included.

When available, the *Biopharmaceutics Classification System (BCS)* or *Biopharmaceutics-Drug Disposition Classification System (BDDCS)* drug class is also listed in this section. Where debate over methods exists, more than one class may be listed. This information is relevant for predicting meal effects and interaction potential when clinical data are unavailable. For example, BDDCS Class 2 agents (low solubility, extensive metabolism/high permeability [eg, carbamazepine, glyburide]) are predicted to have an increased bioavailability in the presence of a meal, whereas bioavailability is reduced for BDDCS Class 3 drugs (high solubility, poor metabolism/low permeability [eg, captopril, doxycycline]). This classification is followed by *pharmaceutical* data relevant to evaluating the appropriateness of a *product* for EAD administration. As available, this information includes cautions in preparation for solids, and osmolality and viscosity for liquids. Keep in mind that data may be manufacturer-dependent.

The next section includes select *pharmacokinetic* data on the API that allows for interpretation or limitations of patient information. If no data on the specific site of absorption are available, the approximate time to maximum drug concentration (t_{max}) values provided can suggest early vs later sites of absorption in the GI tract. Of course, absorption site is just one of the factors that determine this parameter (t_{max}). The site (or window) of drug absorption is often not available in Food and Drug Administration–approved drug labeling, but it can be implied in the available literature. Although species differences make it difficult to extrapolate from animal data, there are additional in vitro and in vivo regional permeability methods available.[60,61] An excellent review on postpyloric drug administration was able to provide recommendations for 70 of 124 medications evaluated.[62] This review included recommendations for drugs to avoid administering by EAD altogether (eg, cyclosporine, isotretinoin), and those appropriate for the gastric enteral route only (eg, aspirin, ferrous sulfate). Cautions for postpyloric administration involve risks for increased absorption (eg, azathioprine, ciprofloxacin, fluconazole, pravastatin, zinc) or decreased absorption (eg, allopurinol, baclofen, calcium, gabapentin, lopinavir-ritonavir, sirolimus). All this information can be used to make best judgments about optimizing drug bioavailability for the patient with an EAD. This section of the monograph also includes known values for drug bioavailability (as the percentage of dose administered); volume of distribution (V_d), in L or L/kg; and clearance (Cl), most often in mL/min or mL/kg/h; usually, these data are derived in healthy adults.

The section on *enteral administration and nutrition considerations* provides more practical information. The data may be limited for some drugs, requiring reliance on the characteristics found in the first part of the respective monograph. When available, the information on the compatibility and stability of extemporaneous preparations allows for interpretation of expected bioavailability with enteral administration. Information on compatibility and stability will serve as a guide as to whether and how a drug can be prepared for enteral administration. A drug in solution needs to be chemically stable as well as soluble. *Compatibility* refers to the absence of physical or chemical reactions when a drug is combined with other material, whereas *stability* refers to the absence of drug degradation or loss over time. Typically, a drug loss of 10% or more from baseline is indicative of instability of a preparation. As available, the monograph's compatibility and stability data of preparations will include use of the pure API as well as commercial forms. Ideally, the physical changes in interfacial tension between drug particles after preparation would be studied. It is, however, more practical to evaluate any changes in physicochemical properties of the preparation just prior to administration as well as any changes to drug stability. Of course, pharmacokinetic studies would be required to evaluate the resultant bioavailability with enteral administration or from formulations under development. A drug dissolved in solution is required for but does not guarantee absorption (see Box 5-1). Dissolution is predictive of bioavailability because, generally, bioavailability is best for aqueous solutions relative to aqueous suspensions and, especially, solid dosage forms.

Box 5-1. Dissolution → Bioavailability

A drug with good solubility may still take a long time to hydrate and dissolve. In other words, a drug's solubility (mg/mL) is not necessarily indicative of the dissolution rate (mmol/s). Therefore, unless an active pharmaceutical ingredient (API) has a very high solubility, most drug absorption still depends on the dissolution rate. An aqueous medium accelerates the dissolution step, unless dilution of cosolvents actually reduces solubility. The drug may undergo complexation, precipitate out, or be degraded. Despite improving stability, complexation worsens bioavailability. Complexation or precipitate may occur ex vivo or in the gut lumen. Solubility is influenced by whether the drug is a salt or free form, whether its solid state is crystalline or amorphous. For the crystalline solid form of the API and excipient to go into solution, the attraction between solute and solvent must become greater than the attraction between solute particles. Solubility is generally predicted to improve with a number of factors, including higher temperature (but not for sodium sulfate) and the sodium (or potassium) salt of weak acids. The latter increases the diffusion layer pH, which then accelerates (in the stomach) dissolution and contributes to improving absorption. The acidic salts (eg, hydrochloride) of weak-base drugs dissolve more rapidly in gastric and intestinal fluid than the free base by greatly reducing pH in the diffusion layer. Several physiologic factors also influence the dissolution rate. These factors include the presence of food, fluid, and secretions. Drug-related factors affecting the dissolution rate include particle size, wettability, and solubility. A smaller particle size can increase solubility, but only up to a point of about 1 μm—in particles smaller than 1 μm, solubility is reduced because of the electrical charge on the particles. The pH of the solvent selected can improve solubility. For weak acids, solubility is improved at 2 pH units above the pKa where the respective drug species is ionized, whereas solubility for weak bases is improved at 2 pH units below the pKa. Unfortunately, absorption depends more on the unionized state.

The *drug-nutrition interaction* section provides information on the known influence of food or food components on drug absorption. Available data consider the influence of nutrition on gut physiology, drug dissolution, and bioavailability. In the absence of specific data related to EN, the influence of food on drug bioavailability offers a view on the potential influence of concurrent tube feeding. This section also describes additional drug-nutrition interactions (see Chapter 2). For example, medications may influence nutrition status, including the status of specific nutrients. A patient's nutrition status in turn may influence the disposition and effect of a drug.

The *recommendations* provided at the end of each monograph are a best appraisal based on the evidence available; however, each clinician will need to review and interpret the available data. The recommendations cannot always be based on sufficient or specific evidence, but they reflect a totality of the evidence available. The user may therefore come to a somewhat different recommendation based on an interpretation of the limited data at hand.

The editor welcomes additional information for the monographs to make future revisions and editions more valuable to users and their patients. Feel free to direct published data or other nonproprietary and disclosable information to the editor or publisher.

References

1. Emami S, Hamishehkar H, Mashayekhi, S, et al. Errors of oral medication administration in a patient with enteral feeding tube. *J Res Pharm Pract.* 2012;1(1):37–40.
2. Schier JG, Howland MA, Hoffman RS, Nelson LS. Fatality from administration of labetalol and crushed extended-release nifedipine. *Ann Pharmacother.* 2003;37:1420–1423.
3. Dickerson RN, Tidwell AC, Brown RO. Adverse effects from inappropriate medication administration via a jejunostomy feeding tube. *Nutr Clin Pract.* 2003;18:402–405.
4. Madigan SM, Courtney DE, Macauley D. The solution was the problem. *Clin Nutr.* 2002;21:531–532.
5. Institute for Safe Medication Practices. Willingness of staff to give oral meds IV is disconcerting. *ISMP Acute Care Med Safety Alert Newsletter.*

May 20, 1998. https://www.ismp.org/newsletters/acutecare/articles /19980520.asp. Accessed November 20, 2017.

6. Guenter P, Hicks RW, Simmons D, et al. Enteral feeding misconnections: a consortium position statement. *Jt Comm J Qual Patient Saf.* 2008;34: 285–292.

7. Institute for Safe Medication Practices. Avoiding inadvertent IV injection of oral liquids. *ISMP Acute Care Med Safety Alert Newsletter.* August 23, 2012. https://www.ismp.org/newsletters/acutecare/showarticle.aspx?id=29. Accessed November 20, 2017.

8. Institute for Safe Medication Practices. A successful ENFit launch still won't stop all incidents of oral medications given intravenously. *ISMP Acute Care Med Safety Alert Newsletter.* August 13, 2015. https://www .ismp.org/newsletters/acutecare/showarticle.aspx?id=115. Accessed November 20, 2017.

9. Cornish P. "Avoid the crush": hazards of medication administration in patients with dysphagia or a feeding tube. *CMAJ.* 2005;172:871–872.

10. Paparella S. Identified safety risks with splitting and crushing oral medications. *J Emerg Nurs.* 2010;36:156–158.

11. Arimanickam G. Tube feeding and drugs in intensive care unit. *Anaesth Intensive Care.* 2011;39:776.

12. Stegemann S. Drug administration via enteral tubing: an unresolved but increasing challenge. *Expert Opin Drug Deliv.* 2015;12:159–161.

13. Leff RD, Roberts RJ. Enteral drug administration practices: report of a preliminary survey. *Pediatrics.* 1988;81:549–551.

14. Mateo MA. Nursing management of enteral tube feedings. *Heart Lung.* 1996;25:318–323.

15. Schmieding NJ, Waldman RC. Nasogastric tube feeding and medication administration: a survey of nursing practices. *Gastroenterol Nurs.* 1997; 20:118–124.

16. Belknap DC, Seifert CF, Peterman M. Administration of medications through enteral feeding catheters. *Am J Crit Care.* 1997;6:382–392.

17. Seifert CF, Johnston BA. Drug administration through enteral feeding catheters [letter]. *Am J Health-Syst Pharm.* 2002;59:378–379.

18. Seifert CF, Johnston BA. A nationwide survey of long-term care facilities to determine the characteristics of medication administration through enteral feeding catheters. *Nutr Clin Pract.* 2005;20:354–362.

19. Hanssens Y, Woods D, Alsulaiti A, et al. Improving oral medicine administration in patients with swallowing problems and feeding tubes. *Ann Pharmacother.* 2006;40:2142–2147.

20. Guenter P, Boullata J. Nursing2013 survey results: drug administration by enteral feeding tube. *Nursing.* 2013;43(12):26–35.

21. Bertsche T, Nieman D, Mayer Y, et al. Prioritizing the prevention of medication handling errors. *Pharm World Sci.* 2008;30:907–915.

22. Joos E, Mehuys E, Van Bocxlaer J, et al. Drug administration via enteral feeding tubes in residential care facilities for individuals with intellectual disability: an observational study. *J Intellect Disab Res.* 2015; 59:215–225.

23. Sohrevardi SM, Jarahzadeh MH, Mirzaei E, et al. Medication errors in patients with enteral feeding tubes in the intensive care unit. *J Res Pharm Pract.* 2017;6:100–105.

24. Yin HS, Mendelsohn AL, Wolf MS, et al. Parents' medication administration errors. *Arch Pediatr Adolesc Med.* 2010;164:181–186.

25. Yin HS, Dreyer BP, Moreira HA, et al. Liquid medication dosing errors in children: role of provider counseling strategies. *Acad Pediatr.* 2014;14: 262–270.

26. Institute for Safe Medication Practices. Preventing errors when administering drugs via an enteral feeding tube. *ISMP Acute Care Med Safety Alert Newsletter.* May 6, 2010. https://www.ismp.org/newsletters/acutecare/articles/20100506.asp. Accessed November 20, 2017.

27. Boullata JI. Safe practices for enteral and parenteral nutrition. In: Seres DS, Van Way CW, eds. *Nutrition Support for the Critically Ill.* New York: Humana Press; 2016:229–241.

28. Boullata JI, Carrera AL, Banchik LH, et al. ASPEN safe practices for enteral nutrition therapy. *JPEN J Parenter Enteral Nutr.* 2017;41:15–103.

29. Niemiec PW, Vanderveen TW, Morrison JI, Hohenwarter MW. Gastrointestinal disorders caused by medication and electrolyte solution osmolality during enteral nutrition. *JPEN J Parenter Enteral Nutr.* 1983;7: 387–389.

30. Atakent Y, Ferrara A, Bhoqal M, Klupsteen M. The adverse effects of high oral osmolal mixtures in neonates: a review and study of the osmolality of calcium preparations. *Clin Pediatr.* 1984;23:487–491.

31. Obladen M, Mutz A. Oral medication in preterm infants? Physical properties of liquid drugs [German]. *Montasschr Kinderheilkd.* 1985;133: 669–674.

32. Dickerson RN, Melnik G. Osmolality of oral drug solutions and suspensions. *Am J Hosp Pharm.* 1988;45:832–834.

33. Fernández Polo A, Cabañas Poy MJ, Clemente Bautista S, et al. Osmolality of oral liquid dosage forms to be administered to newborns in a hospital. *Farm Hosp.* 2007;31:311–314.

34. Martin TP, Hayes P, Collins DM. Tablet dispersion as an alternative to formulation of oral liquid dosage forms. *Aust J Hosp Pharm.* 1993;23: 378–386.

35. Institute for Safe Medication Practices. Oral dosage forms that should not be crushed, 2016. http://www.ismp.org/tools/DoNotCrush.pdf. Accessed November 20, 2017.

36. Salmon D, Pont E, Chevallard H, et al. Pharmaceutical and safety considerations of tablet crushing in patients undergoing enteral intubation. *Int J Pharmaceut.* 2013;443:146–153.

37. Jew RK, Soo-Hoo W, Erush SC. *Extemporaneous Formulations for Pediatric, Geriatric, and Special Needs Patients.* 2nd ed. Bethesda, MD: American Society of Health-System Pharmacists; 2010.

38. Allen LV, ed. *The Art, Science, and Technology of Pharmaceutical Compounding.* 4th ed. Washington, DC: American Pharmacists Association; 2012.

39. Trissel LA. *Trissel's Stability of Compounded Formulations.* 5th ed. Washington, DC: American Pharmacists Association; 2012.

40. Nahata MC, Pai VB, eds. *Pediatric Drug Formulations.* 6th ed. Cincinnati, OH: Harvey Whitney Books; 2014.

41. White R, Bradnam V. *Handbook of Drug Administration via Enteral Feeding Tubes.* 3rd ed. London, UK: Pharmaceutical Press; 2015.

42. Glass BD, Haywood A. Stability considerations in liquid dosage forms extemporaneously prepared from commercially available products. *J Pharm Pharmaceut Sci.* 2006;9:398–426.

43. Haywood A, Glass BD. Liquid dosage forms extemporaneously prepared from commercially available products—considering new evidence on stability. *J Pharm Pharmaceut Sci.* 2013;16:441–455.

44. United States Pharmacopeia. USP <795> Pharmaceutical compounding—nonsterile preparations. http://www.usp.org.

45. United States Pharmacopeia. USP <800> Hazardous drugs—handling in healthcare settings. http://www.usp.org.

46. United States Pharmacopeia. USP <1231> Water for pharmaceutical purposes. http://www.usp.org.

47. Crawford SY, Anaizi NH, Swenson C, Tam YK, Pereira CM. Tap water should not be used [letter]. *Am J Hosp Pharm.* 1993;50:1579.

48. Cacek AT, DeVito JM, Koonce JR. In vitro evaluation of nasogastric administration methods for phenytoin. *Am J Hosp Pharm.* 1986;43:689–692.

49. Clark-Schmidt AL. Loss of carbamazepine suspension through nasogastric tubes. *Am J Hosp Pharm.* 1990;47:2034–2037.

50. Dodds Ashley ES, Varkey JB, Krishna G, et al. Pharmacokinetics of posaconazole administration orally or by nasogastric tube in healthy volunteers. *Antimicrob Agents Chemother.* 2009;53:2960–2964.

51. Störzinger D, Borghorst S, Hofer S, et al. Plasma concentrations of posaconazole administered via nasogastric tube in patients in a surgical intensive care unit. *Antimicrob Agents Chemother.* 2012;56:4468–4470.

52. Holtz L, Milton J, Sturek JK. Compatibility of medications with enteral feedings. *JPEN J Parenter Enteral Nutr.* 1987;11:183–186.

53. Burns PE, McCall L, Wirsching R. Physical compatibility of enteral formulas with various common medications. *J Am Diet Assoc.* 1988;88: 1094–1096.

54. Strom JG, Miller SW. Stability of drugs with enteral nutrient formulas. *Drug Intell Clin Pharm.* 1990;24:130–134.

55. Williams NT. Medication administration though enteral feeding tubes. *Am J Health-Syst Pharm.* 2008;65:2347–2357.

56. Wohlt PD, Zheng L, Gunderson S, et al. Recommendations for the use of medications with continuous enteral nutrition. *Am J Health-Syst Pharm.* 2009;66:1458–1467.

57. McElvoy GK, ed. *AHFS Drug Information.* Bethesda, MD: American Society of Health-System Pharmacists; 2016.

58. Brayfield A, ed. *Martindale: The Complete Drug Reference.* 38th ed. London, UK: Pharmaceutical Press; 2014.

59. O'Neil MJ, ed. *The Merck Index.* 15th ed. Cambridge, UK: Royal Society of Chemistry; 2017.

60. Kararli TT. Comparison of the gastrointestinal anatomy, physiology, and biochemistry of humans and commonly used laboratory animals. *Biopharm Drug Dispos.* 1995;16:351–380.

61. Dahlgren D, Roos C, Lundqvist A, et al. Regional intestinal permeability of three model drugs in human. *Molec Pharmaceut.* 2016;13:3013–3021.

62. McIntyre CM, Monk HM. Medication absorption considerations in patients with postpyloric enteral feeding tubes. *Am J Health-Syst Pharm.* 2014;71:549–556.

PART

II

Drug Monographs

Monograph Abbreviations

6MNA	6-methoxy-2-naphthylacetic acid
9-CMMG	9-carboxymethoxymethylguanine
aka	also known as
ALT	alanine aminotransferase
AST	aspartate aminotransferase
BCRP	breast cancer resistance protein
BCS	Biopharmaceutics Classification System
BDDCS	Biopharmaceutics Drug Disposition Classification System
BHT	butylated hydroxytoluene
BMI	body mass index
BUD	beyond-use date
BUN	blood urea nitrogen
calc	calculated
CK	creatine kinase
Cl	clearance
CNS	central nervous system
CR	controlled-release
CYP	cytochrome P450
DHA	docosahexaenoic acid
EAD	enteral access device
ECMO	extracorporeal membrane oxygenation
EDTA	ethylenediaminetetraacetic acid
EN	enteral nutrition
GC	gas chromatography
GC-MS	gas chromatography–mass spectrometry
GI	gastrointestinal
GST	glutathione-S-transferases
HbA1c	glycated hemoglobin
HPLC	high-performance liquid chromatography
INR	international normalized ratio
IR	immediate-release

IV	intravenous
J-tube	jejunostomy tube
LC	liquid chromatography
LCT	long-chain triglyceride
LDL	low-density lipoprotein
LFT	liver function test
MATE	multidrug and toxin extrusion (transporter)
MCT	medium-chain triglyceride
MIC	minimum inhibitory concentration
MR	modified-release
MRP	multidrug resistance-associated protein
MS	mass spectrometry
n/a	not available
Na	sodium
NMS	neuroleptic malignant syndrome
OAT	organic anion transporter
OATP	organic-anion-transporting polypeptide
OCT	organic cation transporter
ODT	orally disintegrating tablet
OTC	over-the-counter
PEG	polyethylene glycol
PEPT1	peptide transporter 1
RBC	red blood cell
SIADH	syndrome of inappropriate antidiuretic hormone secretion
SULT	sulfotransferase
t_{max}	time to maximum drug concentration
UDP	uridine diphosphate
UGT	uridine diphosphate glucuronosyltransferase
UV	ultraviolet
V_d	volume of distribution
XR	extended-release

Abacavir Sulfate

Product Availability

Solid	• Tablet: 300 mg (base) (Ziagen® [ViiV Healthcare]; others)
Liquid	• Oral solution: 20 mg/mL (base) (Ziagen® [ViiV Healthcare]; others)

Physicochemical (drug)

Molecular weight: • 286.34 (salt 670.75)	Permeability: • LogP 1.20 • LogD 1.20 (pH 7.4)	Water solubility: • 77 mg/mL (25°C)
pKa: • 5.1	Classification: • BCS Class 3, BDDCS Class 1	

Pharmaceutical (product)

Solid	Immediate-release tablet is film-coated; may not crush easily or disperse in water.
Liquid	Oral solution: • pH n/a • Osmolality n/a • Viscosity n/a • May contain propylene glycol, saccharin, and sorbitol; strawberry-banana-flavored aqueous vehicle • Do not freeze. Can store at room temperature or under refrigeration.
Note	Tablets and oral solution are considered bioequivalent.

Pharmacokinetic (patient)

Absorption	• Specific site not known; t_{max} ~1 hour after oral dose (tablet) • Bioavailability ~83%
Transport	• Nonfacilitated diffusion • Substrate for P-glycoprotein and BCRP efflux • Plasma protein binding ~50% • V_d ~0.86 L/kg
Metabolism	• This prodrug is metabolized to the active carbovir triphosphate intracellularly; it is then further metabolized to a similar extent by alcohol dehydrogenase and a UGT, with most excretion in urine and the rest in feces. • Cl ~50 L/h

Enteral Administration and Nutrition Considerations

Compatibility, Stability, and Bioavailability Considerations
- No known stability concerns with crushing the tablet and diluting with water just prior to administration.
- Administration through gastrostomy tube resulted in adequate circulating drug concentrations.[1]
- A case report describes successful drug administration through a J-tube.[2]

Drug-Nutrition Interactions
- Drug may influence nutrition status directly or indirectly.
  - Body fat accumulation (central and dorsocervical) or redistribution, with facial and peripheral wasting.
  - CNS: malaise, fatigue, depression
  - GI: stomatitis; nausea, vomiting, abdominal pain, and diarrhea (can occur as part of hypersensitivity reaction in the absence of rash); hepatic steatosis; pancreatitis (rare)
  - Metabolic: anemia, hyperglycemia, lactic acidosis
  - Other: musculoskeletal pain, elevated CK, muscle weakness, peripheral neuropathy
- No data on the influence of malnutrition or obesity on drug disposition.
- Influence of food on oral absorption or bioavailability:
  - Food is reported to reduce the oral bioavailability by ~5%: a high-fat meal may reduce oral bioavailability by nearly 20%.[3,4]

Recommendations

Gastric	• Dilute the oral liquid with water (at least 1:1) prior to administration. • Consider holding EN beyond the time required to flush-administer-flush.
Postpyloric	• As above. • Monitor for any unexpected change in effect.

References
1. King JR, Yogev R, Aldrovandi G, et al. Pharmacokinetics of antiretrovirals administered to HIV-infected children via gastrostomy tube. *HIV Clin Trials.* 2004;5:288–293.
2. Kamimura M, Watanabe K, Kobayakawa M, et al. Successful absorption of antiretroviral drugs after gastrojejunal bypass surgery following failure of therapy through a jejunal tube. *Intern Med.* 2009;48:1103–1104.
3. Marier JF, Borges M, Plante G, et al. Bioequivalence of abacavir generic and innovator formulations under fasting and fed conditions. *Int J Clin Pharmacol Ther.* 2006;44:284–291.
4. Yuen GJ, Weller S, Pakes GE. A review of the pharmacokinetics of abacavir. *Clin Pharmacokinet.* 2008;47:351–371.

Acetaminophen (Paracetamol)

Product Availability

Solid	• Tablet:
	    ○ Immediate-release: 325 mg, 500 mg (Tylenol® [McNeil]; others)
	    ○ Oral dissolving tablet: 80 mg, 160 mg (Tylenol® Meltaways [McNeil])
	    ○ Chewable: 160 mg (Children's Tylenol® [McNeil])
	    ○ Extended-release: 650 mg (Tylenol® [McNeil]; others)
	• Capsule: 500 mg (Tylenol® [McNeil]; others)

Liquid	• Solution: 167 mg/5 mL (Tylenol® Adult [McNeil]; others) • Suspension: 160 mg/5 mL (Tylenol® Oral Suspension Children's [McNeil]; others)

Physicochemical (drug)

Molecular weight: • 151.2	Permeability: • LogP 0.20 • LogD 0.40 (pH 7.4)	Water solubility: • 14 mg/mL (warm water)
pKa: • 9.51	Classification: • BCS Class 1 or 4; BDDCS Class 1	

Pharmaceutical (product)

Solid	• Immediate-release tablet may disperse in water (20 mL) within 2 minutes. • Oral dissolving and chewable tablets may contain dextrose and sucralose. • Modified-release tablet should not be crushed, chewed, or dissolved in liquid. • Capsules are gel-coated.

Liquid	Solution:
	• pH 3.8–6.1
	• Osmolality:
	    ○ 5400 mOsm/kg (a previously available 325 mg/5 mL elixir)[1]
	    ○ 4035 mOsm/kg (calculated based on measurement of 1:5 dilution with sterile water)[2]
	• Viscosity n/a
	• Maintain at controlled room temperature (avoid freezing).
	Suspension:
	• pH 4–6.9
	• Osmolality 6425 mOsm/kg (calculated based on measurement of 1:5 dilution with sterile water)[1]
	• Viscosity ~350 mPa·s
	• May contain glycerin, high-fructose corn syrup, propylene glycol, and sorbitol
	• Maintain at controlled room temperature (avoid freezing).

Pharmacokinetic (patient)

Absorption	• Specific site not known; t_{max} within 30–60 minutes after oral dose (immediate-release) • Bioavailability ~79%–87%
Transport	• Substrate for P-glycoprotein efflux • Plasma protein binding ~10%–25% • V_d 0.76 L/kg
Metabolism	• Metabolized by conjugation (80%–85%) with glucuronic acid (via UGT1 family) more than with sulfuric acid (via SULT). • Toxic metabolite formed via CYP2E1, is cleared by subsequent conjugation with glutathione via GSTs • Cl 0.7 L/h/kg

Enteral Administration and Nutrition Considerations

Compatibility, Stability, and Bioavailability Considerations

- No known stability concerns with crushing the tablet and diluting with water prior to administration; stability in aqueous solution best at pH ~5–7.
- Jejunal administration yields similar blood concentrations.[3]
- Duodenal administration may increase bioavailability.[4]
- Rate of drug absorption reaches adult levels by about 1 week after birth.[5]
- An effervescent tablet (1000 mg) dissolved in a small volume of water and administered through a nasogastric tube (8 Fr, 120 cm, polyurethane) resulted in peak concentrations and bioavailability similar to those of oral administration in a crossover study.[6]
- The solution (10 mL) seemed physically compatible (no phase separation) when added to varying volumes (15–240 mL) of EN products (Ensure, Ensure HN, Ensure Plus, Ensure Plus HN, Osmolite, Osmolite HN, Vital).[7,8]
- The suspension (15 mL) seemed physically compatible when mixed with 10 mL of EN products (Enrich, TwoCal HN, Vivonex T.E.N.).[9]
- A dose of solution admixed with 200 mL of an EN product (Precitene) appeared physically compatible (no phase separation or particle growth).[10]
- Commercial drug solution combined (1:1) with Osmolite 1.2, under simulated clinical conditions, would result in clogging of an 8 Fr and a 20 Fr feeding tube.[2]
- Commercial drug suspension combined (1:1) with Osmolite 1.2, under simulated clinical conditions, would result in clogging of an 8 Fr and a 20 Fr feeding tube.[2]

Drug-Nutrition Interactions
- Drug may influence nutrition status directly or indirectly:
  - CNS: fatigue
  - GI: nausea, vomiting, abdominal pain, diarrhea, elevated LFTs, acute hepatotoxicity with or without encephalopathy
  - Metabolic: hypokalemia, hypomagnesemia, hypophosphatemia
  - Other: peripheral edema, hypervolemia
- Data on the influence of malnutrition on drug disposition:
  - Protein-energy malnutrition increases the risk for drug hepatotoxicity requiring dose reduction or discontinuation.
  - The body weight–normalized volume of distribution (L/kg) is lower in obesity, while drug clearance (L/h) is increased.
- Influence of food on oral absorption or bioavailability:
  - Food may slightly delay absorption but without influencing oral bioavailability, however, because rapid onset of analgesic action is clinically important, administration in the fasted state may be preferred.[11]

Recommendations

Gastric	• Disperse an immediate-release tablet in water prior to administration. • Alternative: Dilute oral liquid in water (at least 1:1) prior to administration. • No need to hold EN beyond the time required to flush-administer-flush.
Postpyloric	• As above. • Monitor for any unexpected change in effect.

References

1. Dickerson RN, Melnik G. Osmolality of oral drug solutions and suspensions. *Am J Hosp Pharm.* 1988;45:832–834.
2. Klang M, McLymont V, Ng N. Osmolality, pH, and compatibility of selected oral liquid medications with an enteral nutrition product. *JPEN J Parenter Enteral Nutr.* 2013;37:689–694.
3. Adams D. Administration of drugs through a jejunostomy tube. *Br J Intens Care.* 1994;4:10–17.
4. Reix N, Guhmann P, Bietiger W, et al. Duodenum-specific drug delivery: in vivo assessment of a pharmaceutically developed enteric-coated capsule for a broad applicability in rat studies. *Int J Pharm.* 2012;422:338–340.
5. Somani AA, Thelen K, Zheng S, et al. Evaluation of changes in oral drug absorption in preterm and term neonates for Biopharmaceutics Classification System (BCS) class I and II compounds. *Br J Clin Pharmacol.* 2015;81:137–147.
6. Podilsky G, Berger-Gryllaki M, Testa B, et al. The bioavailability of bromazepam, omeprazole and paracetamol given by nasogastric feeding tube. *Eur J Clin Pharmacol.* 2009;65:435–442.
7. Cutie AJ, Altman E, Lenkel L. Compatibility of enteral products with commonly employed drug additives. *JPEN J Parenter Enteral Nutr.* 1983;7:186–191.

8. Altman E, Cutie AJ. Compatibility of enteral products with commonly employed drug additives. *Nutr Supp Serv.* 1984;4:8–17.
9. Burns PE, McCall L, Wirsching R. Physical compatibility of enteral formulas with various common medications. *J Am Diet Assoc.* 1988;88:1094–1096.
10. Ortega de la Cruz C, Fernández Gallardo LC, Damas Fernández-Figares M, García Martínez E. Compatibilidad físico-química de medicamentos con nutrición enteral. *Nutr Hosp.* 1993;8:105–108.
11. Moore RA, Derry S, Wiffen PJ, Straube S. Effects of food on pharmacokinetics of immediate release oral formulations of aspirin, dipyrone, paracetamol and NSAIDs: a systematic review. *Br J Clin Pharmacol.* 2015;80:381–388.

Acyclovir

Product Availability

Solid	• Tablet: 400 mg, 800 mg (Zovirax® [Mylan]; others)
	• Capsule: 200 mg (Zovirax® [Mylan]; others)
Liquid	• Oral suspension: 200 mg/5 mL (Zovirax® [Mylan]; others)

Physicochemical (drug)

Molecular weight:	Permeability:	Water solubility:
• 225.21	• LogP –1.56	• Base 2.5 mg/mL (37°C)
	• LogD –1.76 (pH 7.4)	• Na-salt 100 mg/mL
pKa:	Classification:	
• 2.27, 9.25	• BCS Class 3 or 4; BDDCS Class 4	

Pharmaceutical (product)

Solid	• Tablets disperse in water (20 mL) within 2 minutes
Liquid	• Suspension:
	o pH 6.2
	o Osmolality: 874 mOsm/kg (measured 1:4 dilution with sterile water); 4205 mOsm/kg (calculated based on measurement of 1:5 dilution with sterile water)[1]
	o Viscosity 282 mPa·s
	o May contain glycerin and sorbitol
	o Maintain at controlled room temperature (do not refrigerate).
Note	• Capsules and oral suspension are considered bioequivalent.

Pharmacokinetic (patient)

Absorption	• Specific site not known; t_{max} within 2 hours after oral dose
	• Bioavailability ~10%–30% (variable, incomplete).
Transport	• Substrate for MATE1 efflux; OAT1 and OCT1 uptake
	• Plasma protein binding ~9%–33%
	• V_d ~0.69 L/kg
Metabolism	• Minimal hepatic metabolism to 9-CMMG and 8-hydroxy-acyclovir
	• Most is eliminated unchanged in urine.
	• Cl ~327 mL/min/1.73 m^2

Enteral Administration and Nutrition Considerations

Compatibility, Stability, and Bioavailability Considerations
- Tablet contents are absorbed when administered into duodenum.[2]
- Specific excipients (sodium lauryl sulfate and/or sodium caprate) can act as permeability enhancers for acyclovir, when included.[3]
- Acyclovir is unstable (HPLC analysis) in sucrose/maltitol or fructose/glucose solutions.[4]

- Commercial suspension combined (1:1) with Osmolite 1.2, under simulated clinical conditions, would result in clogging an 8 Fr, but not a 20 Fr, feeding tube.[1]
- Solid dispersions of acyclovir with multiple hydrophilic carriers resulted in enhanced dissolution and permeability.[5]
- Several amino acid ester prodrugs of acyclovir (eg, valine → valacyclovir) improve bioavailability by enhancing transport.[6]

Drug-Nutrition Interactions
- Drug may influence nutrition status directly or indirectly:
  - CNS: headache, encephalopathy, confusion, ataxia, paresthesia
  - GI: nausea, vomiting, diarrhea, elevated LFTs
  - Metabolic: hemolysis, anemia, transient elevation of BUN
  - Other: peripheral edema, myalgia
- Influence of malnutrition or obesity on drug disposition:
  - The body weight–normalized volume of distribution (L/kg) is much smaller in obesity and suggests that the drug is best dosed based on a lean body weight.[7]
- No known influence of food on oral absorption or bioavailability.

Recommendations

Gastric	<ul><li>Disperse tablet in water (20 mL) prior to administration.</li><li>Avoid using the suspension for enteral access device administration.</li><li>No need to hold EN beyond the time required to flush-administer-flush.</li></ul>
Postpyloric	<ul><li>As above.</li><li>Monitor for any unexpected change in effect.</li></ul>
Other	<ul><li>As with all antimicrobials, consider parenteral alternative for acutely ill patients to ensure therapeutic concentrations.</li></ul>

References

1. Klang M, McLymont V, Ng N. Osmolality, pH, and compatibility of selected oral liquid medications with an enteral nutrition product. *JPEN J Parenter Enteral Nutr.* 2013;37: 689–694.
2. Lewis LD, Fowle AS, Bittiner SB, et al. Human gastrointestinal absorption of acyclovir from tablet duodenal infusion and sipped solution. *Br J Clin Pharmacol.* 1986;21:459–462.
3. Ates M, Kaynak MS, Sahin S. Effect of permeability enhancers on paracellular permeability of acyclovir. *J Pharm Pharmacol.* 2016;68:781–790.
4. Desai D, Rao V, Guo H, et al. Stability of low concentrations of guanine-based antivirals in sucrose or maltitol solutions. *Int J Pharm.* 2007;34:87–94.
5. Nart V, França MT, Anzilaggo D, et al. Ball-milled solid dispersions of BCS Class IV drugs: impact on the dissolution rate and intestinal permeability of acyclovir. *Mater Sci Eng C Mater Biol Appl.* 2015;53:229–238.
6. Katragadda S, Jain R, Kwatra D, et al. Pharmacokinetics of amino acid ester prodrugs of acyclovir after oral administration: interaction with the transporters on Cac-2 cells. *Int J Pharm.* 2008;362:93–101.
7. Boullata JI. Drug disposition in obesity and protein-energy malnutrition. *Proceed Nutr Soc.* 2010;69:543–550.

Alendronate Sodium

Product Availability

Solid	• Tablet:
	○ Immediate-release: 5 mg, 10 mg, 35 mg, 40 mg, 70 mg (base) (Fosamax® [Merck]; others)
	○ Effervescent: 70 mg (base) (Binosto® [Mission Pharmacal])
Liquid	• Solution: 70 mg/75 mL (base) (various)

Physicochemical (drug)

Molecular weight:	Permeability:	Water solubility:
• 249.10 (salt 272.09)	• LogP −5.64 (calc)	• 39.1 mg/mL (sodium salt)
	• LogD n/a	
pKa:	**Classification:**	
• 2.7, 8.7, 10.5, 11.6	• BCS Class 3; BDDCS Class 3	

Pharmaceutical (product)

Solid	• Do not crush tablets (mucosal irritant).
	• Effervescent tablet is intended to be diluted in 120 mL water prior to oral administration.
Liquid	Solution:
	• pH n/a
	• Osmolality n/a
	• Viscosity n/a
	• May contain saccharin; raspberry-flavored
	• Store at room temperature.
Note	Tablets and solution are considered bioequivalent.

Pharmacokinetic (patient)

Absorption	• Specific site is not known, but better absorbed from jejunum than duodenum.
	• Bioavailability <2%
Transport	• Redistributed to bone
	• Plasma protein binding ~70%, mostly to albumin
	• V_d ~0.44 L/kg
Metabolism	• Does not undergo metabolism, but what is not deposited in bone is excreted in urine
	• Cl ~12 L/h

Enteral Administration and Nutrition Considerations

Compatibility, Stability, and Bioavailability Considerations
- A 1% aqueous solution of the sodium salt is expected to have a pH ~4–5.
- Bioavailability improves at GI pH >6.

- Alendronate tablet (70 mg) disperses in 10 mL water within 5 minutes, yielding fine particles that remain effective when administered via enteral feeding tube.[1]
- The inclusion of sodium lauryl sulfate as an excipient may significantly enhance bioavailability between products.[2]
- A drinkable solution (70 mg/100 mL) was found to be bioequivalent to the tablet (70 mg) in healthy male volunteers in a single-dose crossover study.[3]

Drug-Nutrition Interactions
- Drug may influence nutrition status directly or indirectly:
  - GI: oral, pharyngeal, esophageal, gastric, duodenal irritation, erosion, or ulceration
  - Other: bone, joint, and/or muscle pain
- No data on the influence of malnutrition or obesity on drug disposition.
- Influence of food on oral absorption or bioavailability:
  - Food and beverages taken within 30 minutes of medication administration reduce oral bioavailability.

Recommendations

Gastric	• Use the once-weekly tablet dispersed in at least 60 mL (up to 240 mL) of mineral-free water prior to administration. • Avoid EN for at least 30 minutes before and after drug administration; patient should be in an upright position to prevent esophageal damage if medication is refluxed.
Postpyloric	• As above. • Monitor for any unexpected change in effect.
Other	• Correct patient hypocalcemia or vitamin D deficiency prior to therapy with alendronate; maintain adequate calcium and vitamin D status.

References

1. Tanner S, Taylor HM. Feeding tube administration of bisphosphonates for treating osteoporosis in institutionalized patients with developmental disabilities. *Bone*. 2004; 34(Suppl 1):S97–S98.
2. García-Arita A. Interactions between active pharmaceutical ingredients and excipients affecting bioavailability: impact on bioequivalence. *Eur J Pharm Sci*. 2014;65:89–97.
3. Acotto CG, Antonelli C, Flynn D, et al. Upper gastrointestinal tract transit times of tablet and drinkable solution formulations of alendronate: a bioequivalence and a quantitative, randomized study using video deglutition. *Calcif Tissue Int*. 2012;91: 325–334.

Allopurinol

Product Availability

Solid	• Tablet: 100 mg, 300 mg (Zyloprim® [Casper Pharma]; others)

Physicochemical (drug)

Molecular weight: • 136.11	Permeability: • LogP –0.55 • LogD –0.55 (pH 7.4)	Water solubility: • 0.48 mg/mL (25°C)
pKa: • 9.4	Classification: • BCS Class 4; BDDCS Class 2	

Pharmaceutical (product)

Solid	• Some brands of tablet may disperse in water better than others. • Dispersion in 20 mL water within 5 minutes.

Pharmacokinetic (patient)

Absorption	• Specific site not known; t_{max} ~2–6 hours after oral dose • Bioavailability ~80%
Transport	• Neither allopurinol nor its metabolite (oxypurinol) are bound to plasma proteins. • V_d ~0.87 L/kg
Metabolism	• Allopurinol and oxypurinol are conjugated to form ribonucleosides. • Cl ~9.9 mL/min/kg

Enteral Administration and Nutrition Considerations

Compatibility, Stability, and Bioavailability Considerations

- The official USP formulation for compounding an oral suspension (20 mg/mL) is expected to have a pH of ~6.5–7.5 and can be given a BUD of 60 days stored at room temperature.
- The maximum stability of allopurinol in aqueous solution occurs at pH 3.1–3.4.
- An extemporaneous preparation (20 mg/mL) made from crushed tablets in either simple syrup/cherry syrup (2:1) or in OraSweet/OraPlus (1:1) remained stable (HPLC analysis) for several weeks in amber bottles when refrigerated or at room temperature.[1,2]
- A complex extemporaneous oral suspension (20 mg/mL) prepared from tablets and several components, stored in amber glass prescription bottles, remained stable (HPLC analysis) even at elevated temperatures.[3]
- An extemporaneous oral suspension prepared from pure drug powder in SyrSpend SF, stored in prescription bottles at refrigerator or room temperature, remained stable (HPLC analysis) for 90 days.[4]

Drug-Nutrition Interactions
- Drug may influence nutrition status directly or indirectly:
  - Weight loss
  - CNS: altered mental status, malaise
  - GI: anorexia, altered taste, stomatitis, mucositis, nausea, vomiting, dyspepsia, abdominal pain, constipation, flatulence, diarrhea, transient LFT abnormalities
  - Metabolic: hyperphosphatemia, hypomagnesemia, hypercalcemia, hyperferremia, hyper- or hyponatremia, hyper- or hypokalemia, bone marrow suppression
  - Other: alopecia, peripheral neuropathy; hypersensitivity reactions may manifest with fever, arthralgia, nausea, vomiting, and rash
- Data on the influence of malnutrition or obesity on drug disposition:
  - Protein-energy malnutrition increases the half-life of oxypurinol, which may increase the risk for toxicity.
- No known influence of food on oral absorption or bioavailability.

Recommendations

Gastric	• Disperse tablet in water. • Alternative: Consider a stable extemporaneous liquid preparation if using a larger bore tube and dilute in water (at least 1:1). • No need to hold EN beyond the time required to flush-administer-flush; for patient receiving intermittent EN, administer allopurinol after feed.
Postpyloric	• As above. • Monitor for any unexpected change in effect.

References

1. Dressman JB, Poust RI. Stability of allopurinol and of five antineoplastics in suspension. *Am J Hosp Pharm.* 1983;40:616–618.
2. Allen LV, Erickson MA. Stability of acetazolamide, allopurinol, azathioprine, clonazepam and flucytosine in extemporaneously compounded oral liquids. *Am J Health-Syst Pharm.* 1996;53:1944–1949.
3. Alexander KS, Davar N, Parker GA. Stability of allopurinol suspension compounded from tablets. *Int J Pharm Compd.* 1997;1:128–131.
4. Polonini HC, Loures S, de Araujo EP, et al. Stability of allopurinol, amitriptyline hydrochloride, carbamazepine, domperidone, isoniazid, ketoconazole, lisinopril, naproxen, paracetamol (acetaminophen), and sertraline hydrochloride in SyrSpend SF PH4 oral suspensions. *Int J Pharm Compd.* 2016;20:426–434.

Alprazolam

Product Availability

Solid	• Tablet:
	   ○ Immediate-release: 0.25 mg, 0.5 mg, 1 mg, 2 mg (Xanax® [Pfizer]; others)
	   ○ Extended-release: 0.5 mg, 1 mg, 2 mg, 3 mg (Xanax® XR [Pfizer]; others)

Liquid	• Oral solution: 1 mg/mL (various)

Physicochemical (drug)

Molecular weight: • 308.77	Permeability: • LogP 2.12 • LogD 1.26 (pH 7.4)	Water solubility: • 0.08 mg/mL
pKa: • 5.1	Classification: • BCS Class 1; BDDCS Class 1	

Pharmaceutical (product)

Solid	• Tablets disperse in water within 1 minute. • Avoid inhalation or skin exposure to alprazolam particles. • Do not crush the extended-release product. • Orally dissolving tablet (Niravam® [recently off-market]) disintegrated rapidly in the presence of any moisture.
Liquid	Oral solution: • pH 4.8 • Osmolality n/a • Viscosity is high. • May contain a sugar alcohol • This concentrated solution requires dilution in at least 30 mL prior to oral administration.

Pharmacokinetic (patient)

Absorption	• Specific site not known; t_{max} ~2.5 hours after an oral dose (fasted) • Bioavailability ~88%
Transport	• Plasma protein binding ~71% • V_d ~0.72 L/kg
Metabolism	• Hydroxylation (CYP3A4) to an inactive metabolite • Cl ~0.74 mL/min/kg

Enteral Administration and Nutrition Considerations

Compatibility/Stability Considerations

- The official USP formulation for compounding an oral suspension (1 mg/mL) is expected to have a pH of ~4–5 and be given a 60-day BUD when stored at room temperature or in refrigeration.
- Extemporaneous oral liquid preparations (1 mg/mL) made from tablets (2 mg) in either OraSweet/OraPlus (1:1), OraSweet SF/OraPlus (1:1), or cherry syrup concentrate/simple syrup (1:4), stored in amber polyethylene terephthalate bottles, remained stable (HPLC analysis) for 60 days in the dark at 5°C and 25°C.[1]

Drug-Nutrition Interactions

- Drug may influence nutrition status directly or indirectly:
  - CNS: fatigue, confusion, weakness, ataxia, anterograde amnesia, paradoxical CNS stimulation
  - GI: anorexia, bitter or metallic taste, dry mouth, nausea
  - Other: visual disturbances (diplopia, nystagmus, blurred vision)
- Data on the influence of malnutrition or obesity on drug disposition:
  - Obesity increases the sedative effects.
- Influence of food on oral absorption or bioavailability:
  - Food may reduce rate of drug absorption but with no influence on oral bioavailability; a high-fat meal reduces the rate of absorption of the orally dissolving tablet but without influence on oral bioavailability.[2]
  - Grapefruit juice may increase oral bioavailability, but this effect is less likely than with other CNS-active drugs.[3]

Recommendations

Gastric	• Disperse tablet in water just prior to administration. • Alternative: Consider concentrated solution if patient can tolerate volume (at least 30 mL) required for dilution. • No need to hold EN beyond the time required to flush-administer-flush.
Postpyloric	• As above. • Monitor for any unexpected change in effect.

References

1. Allen LV, Erickson MA. Stability of alprazolam, chloroquine phosphate, cisapride, enalapril maleate, and hydralazine hydrochloride in extemporaneously compounded oral liquids. *Am J Health-Syst Pharm.* 1998;55:1915–1920.
2. Erdman K, Stypinski D, Combs M, et al. Absence of food effect on the extent of alprazolam absorption from an orally disintegrating tablet. *Pharmacotherapy.* 2007;27: 1120–1124.
3. Yasui N, Kondo T, Furukori H, et al. Effects of repeated ingestion of grapefruit juice on the single and multiple oral-dose pharmacokinetics and pharmacodynamics of alprazolam. *Psychopharmacology.* 2000;150:185–190.

Amlodipine Besylate

Product Availability

Solid	• Tablet: 2.5 mg, 5 mg, 10 mg (base) (Norvasc® [Pfizer]; others)

Physicochemical (drug)

Molecular weight: • 408.89 (salt 567.05)	Permeability: • LogP 3.00 • LogD 1.68 (pH 7.4)	Water solubility: • 2.22 mg/mL
pKa: • 9.5	Classification: • BCS Class 1; BDDCS Class 1	

Pharmaceutical (product)

Solid	• Tablet disperses in water. • Solid and liquid (previously available) products considered bioequivalent.

Pharmacokinetic (patient)

Absorption	• Specific site not known; t_{max} 6–12 hours following oral dose • Bioavailability ~64%–90%
Transport	• Plasma protein binding ~93% • V_d ~16 L/kg
Metabolism	• Extensively metabolized by CYP3A4 to inactive pyridine derivatives • Cl ~5.9 mL/min/kg

Enteral Administration and Nutrition Considerations

Compatibility, Stability, and Bioavailability Considerations
- The official USP formulation for compounding an oral suspension is expected to have a pH of ~4–5, and be given a BUD of 60 days (room temperature) or 90 days (refrigerated).
- Most tablet products quickly disperse in water for enteral feeding tube administration without significant drug loss.
- Crushing and mixing drug with thickened water (pH 5.6, viscosity 767 mPa·s) to aid swallowing significantly delayed drug dissolution compared with whole tablets or crushed tablets in water (pH 6.7, viscosity 0.8 mPa·s).[1]
- The stability (HPLC analysis) of an extemporaneously compounded oral suspension (1 mg/mL) is better in OraPlus/OraSweet than in simple syrup/1% methylcellulose.[2]
- Extemporaneous suspensions (1 mg/mL) prepared either from tablets or pure drug powder, stored in amber glass bottles or plastic syringes at 5°C or 25°C (60% relative humidity), remained stable (HPLC analysis)

for 90 days in glass under refrigeration; in contrast, suspensions at room temperature remained stable for 60 days from powder (in glass or plastic), 60 days from tablets (in glass), and 14 days from tablets (in plastic).[3]

- An extemporaneous suspension (1 mg/mL) prepared from pure drug powder in SyrSpend SF, stored in prescription bottles at refrigeration or room temperature, remained stable (HPLC analysis) for 90 days at 2°C–8°C and 20°C–25°C.[4]

- An extemporaneous solution (0.5 mg/mL) prepared from pure drug powder diluted in methylparaben 15% solution, with simple syrup and purified water, remained stable for 12 months when stored in amber polyethylene terephthalate containers at 4°C and 25°C.[5]

- Although not a stability study, the bioavailability of amlodipine following oral administration with 240 mL water was similar to the bioavailability of an amlodipine tablet dispersed in a teaspoonful of applesauce for 5 minutes prior to administration in healthy subjects.[6]

Drug-Nutrition Interactions

- Drug may influence nutrition status directly or indirectly:
  - CNS: fatigue
  - GI: nausea, abdominal pain
  - Other: peripheral edema
- No data on the influence of malnutrition or obesity on drug disposition.
- Influence of food on oral absorption or bioavailability:
  - Food has no influence on the rate of drug absorption or oral bioavailability.[7]
  - Grapefruit juice does not seem to enhance drug bioavailability, which is unlike the influence of grapefruit juice on other drugs in this class.[8]

Recommendations

Gastric	• Disperse tablet in water just prior to administration. • Alternative: Consider oral solution if available. • No need to hold EN beyond the time required to flush-administer-flush.
Postpyloric	• As above. • Monitor for any unexpected change in effect.

References

1. Manrique YJ, Lee DJ, Islam F, et al. Crushed tablets: does the administration of food vehicles and thickened fluids to aid medication swallowing alter drug release? *J Pharm Pharm Sci*. 2014;17:207–219.
2. Nahata MC, Morosco RS, Hipple TF. Stability of amlodipine besylate in two liquid dosage forms. *J Am Pharm Assoc (Wash)*. 1999;39:375–377.
3. Friciu M, Zaraa S, LeClair G. Stability of extemporaneously compounded amlodipine besylate oral suspension. *Can J Hosp Pharm*. 2016;69:327–329.
4. Ferreira AO, Polonini HC, Silva SL, et al. Feasibility of amlodipine besylate, chloroquine phosphate, dapsone, phenytoin, pyridoxine hydrochloride, sulfadiazine, sulfasalazine,

tetracycline hydrochloride, trimethoprim and zonisamide in SyrSPend(®) SF PH4 oral suspensions. *J Pharm Biomed Anal.* 2016;118:105–112.

5. van der Vossen AC, van der Velde I, Smeets OSNM, et al. Design and stability study of an oral solution of amlodipine besylate for pediatric patients. *Eur J Pharm Sci.* 2016; 92:220–223.
6. Chung M, Garza D, Gaffney M, Glue P. Bioavailability of amlodipine besylate following oral administration as a tablet dispersed in applesauce. *J Clin Pharmacol.* 2005;45:695–698.
7. Sunkara G, Jiang X, Reynolds C, et al. Effect of food on the oral bioavailability of amlodipine/valsartan and amlodipine/valsartan/hydrochlorothiazide fixed dose combination tablets in healthy subjects. *Clin Pharmacol Drug Dev.* 2014;3:487–492.
8. Vincent J, Harris SI, Foulds G, et al. Lack of effect of grapefruit juice on the pharmacokinetics and pharmacodynamics of amlodipine. *Br J Clin Pharmacol.* 2000; 50:455–463.

Amoxicillin Trihydrate

Product Availability

Solid	• Tablet:
	  ○ Film-coated: 500 mg, 875 mg (anhydrous) (various)
	  ○ Chewable: 125 mg, 200 mg, 250 mg, 400 mg (anhydrous) (various)
	  ○ Extended-release: 775 mg (anhydrous) (Moxatag® [Vernalis Therapeutics])
	• Capsule: 250 mg, 500 mg (anhydrous) (various)

Liquid	• Powder for reconstitution:
	  ○ 125 mg/5 mL, 200 mg/5 mL, 250 mg/5 mL, 400 mg/5 mL (Amoxil® [GSK]; others)
	  ○ 50 mg/mL (Amoxil® Pediatric Drops [GSK])

Physicochemical (drug)

Molecular weight: • 365.41	Permeability: • LogP 0.87 • LogD −5.73 (pH 6.5), −1.52 or −6.63 (pH 7.4)	Water solubility: • 2.7–4 mg/mL
pKa: • 2.63, 7.55, 9.64	Classification: • BCS Class 3 or 4; BDDCS Class 3	

Pharmaceutical (product)

Solid	• Chewable tablets may contain aspartame. • Avoid crushing any sustained-release product.

Liquid	Suspension (reconstituted powder):
	• pH 5.0–7.5
	  ○ pH 5.14 (a 250 mg/5 mL sususpension product)
	• Osmolality:
	  ○ May vary by product depending on the sweeteners used
	  ○ 1775 mOsm/kg and 2250 mOsm/kg (for 2 different 250 mg/5 mL suspension products)[1,2]
	  ○ 1044 mOsm/kg in another product[3]
	  ○ 1541 mOsm/L (125 mg/5 mL)[4]
	  ○ Two additional products (100 mg/mL) from the same manufacturer:[5] 1548 mOsm/L and pH 4.6; 1717 mOsm/L and pH 5.6
	• Viscosity is moderate.
	• Store at refrigerator temperature for up to 14 days from preparation.
	• Shake well prior to measuring dose.

Pharmacokinetic (patient)

Absorption	• Proximal small intestine; t_{max} 1–2 hours following oral dose • Bioavailability ~74%–92%
Transport	• Plasma protein binding 15%–20% • V_d ~0.27–0.32 L/kg
Metabolism	• Metabolized by hydrolysis of the β-lactam ring to inactive penicilloic acid(s); otherwise eliminated renally unchanged • Cl ~0.28 L/min

Enteral Administration and Nutrition Considerations

Compatibility, Stability, and Bioavailability Considerations
- A 0.2% aqueous solution has a pH ~3.5–6
- The optimum stability in aqueous solutions is at pH 5.8–6.5.[6]
- Amoxicillin (as the trihydrate) is susceptible to degradation (hydrolysis and dimerization) in warm or alkaline solution or if solutions are frozen.[7]
- Effective absorption following administration into duodenum or jejunum.[8]
- The suspension (5 mL) seemed physically compatible (no phase separation) when added to varying volumes (15–240 mL) of EN products (Ensure, Ensure Plus, Osmolite).[9]
- The suspension (10 mL) seemed physically compatible when mixed with 10 mL of EN products (Enrich, TwoCal HN, Vivonex T.E.N.).[10]
- A dose of solution admixed with 200 mL of an EN product (Precitene) appeared physically compatible (no phase separation or particle growth).[11]

Drug-Nutrition Interactions
- Drug may influence nutrition status directly or indirectly:
  - GI: glossitis, stomatitis, anorexia, nausea, gastric distress, vomiting, diarrhea, enterocolitis with severe abdominal pain (± *Clostridium difficile*), LFT abnormalities
- Influence of malnutrition or obesity on drug disposition:
  - Expected to have a larger volume of distribution in obesity, with lower drug exposure using a standard dose.
- Influence of food on oral absorption or bioavailability:
  - Food may increase drug absorption and reduce GI complaints (especially from the combination product that includes clavulanate).

Recommendations

Gastric	• Use the suspension (reconstituted powder) and consider further dilution (1:1) just prior to administration, especially if via a lengthy small-bore enteral access device. • No need to hold EN beyond the time required to flush-administer-flush.

Postpyloric	• As above.
	• Monitor for any unexpected change in effect.
Other	• As with all antimicrobials, consider parenteral alternative for acutely ill patients to ensure therapeutic concentrations.

References

1. Niemiec PW, Vanderveen TW, Morrison JI, et al. Gastrointestinal disorders caused by medication and electrolyte solution osmolality during enteral nutrition. *JPEN J Parenter Enteral Nutr.* 1983;7:387–389.
2. Dickerson RN, Melnik G. Osmolality of oral drug solutions and suspensions. *Am J Hosp Pharm.* 1988;45:832–834.
3. Fernández Polo A, Cabañas Poy MJ, Clemente Bautista S, et al. Osmolality of oral liquid dosage forms to be administered to newborns in a hospital. *Farm Hosp.* 2007;31:311–314.
4. Beckwith MC, Feddema SS, Barton RG, Graves C. A guide to drug therapy in patients with enteral feeding tubes: dosage form selection and administration methods. *Hosp Pharm.* 2004;39:225–237.
5. Obladen M, Mutz A. Orale medikation bei frühgeborenen? *Monatsschr Kinderheilkd.* 1985;133:669–674.
6. Zia H, Shalchian N, Borhanian F. Kinetics of amoxicillin degradation in aqueous solutions. *Can J Pharm Sci.* 1977;12:80–83.
7. Vahdat L, Sunderland VB. Kinetics of amoxicillin and clavulanate degradation alone and in combination in aqueous solution under frozen conditions. *Int J Pharm.* 2007;342:95–104.
8. Barr WH, Zola EM, Candler EL, et al. Differential absorption of amoxicillin from the human small and large intestine. *Clin Pharmacol Ther.* 1994;56:279–285.
9. Cutie AJ, Altman E, Lenkel L. Compatibility of enteral products with commonly employed drug additives. *JPEN J Parenter Enteral Nutr.* 1983;7:186–191.
10. Burns PE, McCall L, Wirsching R. Physical compatibility of enteral formulas with various common medications. *J Am Diet Assoc.* 1988;88:1094–1096.
11. Ortega de la Cruz C, Fernández Gallardo LC, Damas Fernández-Figares M, García Martínez E. Compatibilidad físico-química de medicamentos con nutrición enteral. *Nutr Hosp.* 1993;8:105–108.

Aripiprazole

Product Availability

Solid	• Tablet: ○ Immediate-release: 2 mg, 5 mg, 10 mg, 15 mg, 20 mg, 30 mg (Abilify® [Otsuka]; others) ○ Orally dissolving: 10 mg, 15 mg (various)
Liquid	• Oral solution: 5 mg/5 mL (various)

Physicochemical (drug)

Molecular weight: • 448.40	Permeability: • LogP 5.21 • LogD 3.20 (pH 7.4)	Water solubility: • 0.001 mg/mL
pKa: • 7.5, 13.5	Classification: • BCS Class 2; BDDCS Class 2	

Pharmaceutical (product)

Solid	Orally dissolving tablet contains aspartame.
Liquid	Solution: • pH n/a • Osmolality n/a • Viscosity n/a • May contain fructose, glycerin, propylene glycol, and sucrose • Store at 2°C–8°C and keep no longer than 6 months after opening.

Pharmacokinetic (patient)

Absorption	• Specific site not known; t_{max} ~3–5 hours following oral dose • Bioavailability ~87% (tablet); solution has slightly greater bioavailability
Transport	• Plasma protein binding ~99%, primarily to albumin • V_d ~4.9 L/kg
Metabolism	• Extensive metabolism (dehydrogenation, hydroxylation, N-dealkylation) via CYP3A and CYP2D6 (may need to dose adjust based on CYP2D6 status) • Cl ~0.83 mL/min/kg

Enteral Administration and Nutrition Considerations

Compatibility, Stability, and Bioavailability Considerations
- Drug solubility is pH-dependent.
- Extemporaneous formulations (1 mg/mL) prepared in either OraPlus/OraSweet (1:1) or methylcellulose 1%/simple syrup (1:1) and stored at 4°C remained stable at 91 days or 67 days, respectively.[1]

- Decreasing particle size in a nanosuspension preparation increased drug solubility and dissolution to improve bioavailability.[2]

Drug-Nutrition Interactions
- Drug may influence nutrition status directly or indirectly:
  - Weight gain
  - CNS: somnolence, headache, restlessness, abnormal involuntary movements (eg, tardive dyskinesia), rare impulse-control abnormality (eg, binge eating)
  - GI: esophageal dysmotility, nausea, vomiting, constipation
  - Metabolic: hyperglycemia; dyslipidemia (less likely than hyperglycemia)
- No data on the influence of malnutrition or obesity on drug disposition.
- No known influence of food on oral absorption or bioavailability.

Recommendations

Gastric	• Crush and disperse tablet in water just prior to administration. • No need to hold EN beyond the time required to flush-administer-flush.
Postpyloric	• As above. • Monitor for any unexpected change in effect.

References
1. Pramann LA, Davidow LW, van Haandel L, Funk RS. Development of extemporaneously compounded aripiprazole oral suspensions for use in children. *Int J Pharm Compd.* 2016;20:257–261.
2. Xu Y, Liu X, Lian R, et al. Enhanced dissolution and oral bioavailability of aripiprazole nanosuspensions prepared by nanoprecipitation/homogenization based on acid-base neutralization. *Int J Pharm.* 2012;438:287–295.

Atenolol

Product Availability

Solid	• Tablet: 25 mg, 50 mg, 100 mg (Tenormin® [Alvogen Malta]; others)

Physicochemical (drug)

Molecular weight:	Permeability:	Water solubility:

• 266.34	• LogP 0.16
	• LogD −3.21 (pH 6.5 calc);
	  −2.31 (pH 7.4 calc);
	  −1.03 (pH 7.4 measured)
		• 26.5 mg/mL (37°C)

pKa: • 9.6	Classification: • BCS Class 3; BDDCS Class n/a	

Pharmaceutical (product)

Solid	• Tablet products are often film-coated. • Tablet may disperse in water (20 mL) within 5 minutes.

Pharmacokinetic (patient)

Absorption	• Specific site not known; t_{max} ~2–4 hours following oral dose • Bioavailability ~50%–60%
Transport	• Substrate for P-glycoprotein efflux • Substrate for OATP uptake • Plasma protein binding is limited (~6%–16%). • V_d ~1.3 L/kg
Metabolism	• Minimal metabolic clearance; most eliminated unchanged in the urine • Cl ~2.4 mL/min/kg

Enteral Administration and Nutrition Considerations

Compatibility, Stability, and Bioavailability Considerations

- The official USP oral liquid preparation (2 mg/mL) is expected to have pH 9.1–10.1 with a BUD of 60 days.
- Avoid using a sucrose-containing vehicle.[1]
- Atenolol is incompatible mixed with ascorbic acid or citric acid.[2]
- An extemporaneous preparation (2 mg/mL) made with tablets (50 mg) mixed in a diluent that included ethanol and PEG 8000 remained stable (HPLC analysis) when stored in amber glass vials at 5°C or 25°C for 40 days; however, microbial growth was evident in some samples.[3]
- An extemporaneous preparation (10 mg/mL) of atenolol in simple syrup, stored in glass containers (clear or amber) at 4°C or 25°C, remained stable (HPLC analysis) for up to 7–9 days.[4]

- Extemporaneous suspensions (1 mg/mL, 5 mg/mL) prepared from pure drug powder in SyrSpend-SF and stored in prescription bottles at room temperature or refrigerated, while protected from light, remained stable for 60 days (1 mg/mL) or 90 days (5 mg/mL).[5]
- Crushing and mixing the drug with thickened water (pH 5.6, viscosity 767 mPa·s) to aid swallowing significantly delayed drug dissolution compared with whole tablets or crushed tablets in water (pH 6.7, viscosity 0.8 mPa·s).[6]
- Jejunal administration yields similar bioavailability.[7]
- Tablets crushed and suspended in 50 mL water (type not specified), administered by nasogastric tube, followed by 50 mL water flush, in postoperative patients receiving various doses (25–200 mg), the bioavailability was lower (~16%) on postoperative day 2 compared with preoperative doses taken by mouth.[8]

Drug-Nutrition Interactions
- Drug may influence nutrition status directly or indirectly:
  - ○ CNS: fatigue, drowsiness, lightheadedness
  - ○ GI: dry mouth, nausea, diarrhea, elevated LFTs
  - ○ Metabolic: glucose intolerance
  - ○ Other: visual disturbances
- No data on the influence of malnutrition or obesity on drug disposition.
- Influence of food on oral absorption or bioavailability:
  - ○ Orange juice may decrease oral bioavailability (by ~40%) when consumed with or within 4 hours of drug administration.[9]

Recommendations

Gastric	• Crush and/or disperse tablet in water (20 mL) prior to administration. • No need to hold EN beyond the time required to flush-administer-flush.
Postpyloric	• As above. • Monitor for any unexpected change in effect.

References
1. Patel D, Doshi DH, Desai D. Short-term stability of atenolol in oral liquid formulations. *Int J Pharm Compd.* 1997;1:437–439.
2. Kumar V, Shah RP, Malik S, et al. Compatibility of atenolol with excipients: LC-MS/TOF characterization of degradation/interaction products, and mechanisms of their formation. *J Pharm Biomed Anal.* 2009;49:880–888.
3. Garner SS, Wiest DB, Reynolds ER. Stability of atenolol in an extemporaneously compounded oral liquid. *Am J Hosp Pharm.* 1994;51:508–511.
4. Foppa T, Murakami FS, Silva MA. Development, validation and stability study of pediatric atenolol syrup. *Pharmazie.* 2007;62:519–521.
5. Polonini HC, Loures S, Lima LC, et al. Stability of atenolol, clonazepam, dexamethasone, diclofenac sodium, diltiazem, enalapril maleate, ketoprofen, lamotrigine,

penicillamine-D and thiamine in SyrSpend SF PH4 oral suspensions. *Int J Pharm Compd.* 2016;20:167–174.

6. Manrique YJ, Lee DJ, Islam F, et al. Crushed tablets: does the administration of food vehicles and thickened fluids to aid medication swallowing alter drug release? *J Pharm Sci.* 2014;17:207–219.
7. Adams D. Administration of drugs through a jejunostomy tube. *Br J Intens Care.* 1994; 4:10–17.
8. Gosgnach M, Aymard G, Huraux C, et al. Atenolol administration via nasogastric tube after abdominal surgery: an unreliable route. *Anesth Analg.* 2005;100:137–140.
9. Lilja JJ, Raaska K, Neuvonen PJ. Effects of orange juice on the pharmacokinetics of atenolol. *Eur J Clin Pharmacol.* 2005;61:337–340.

Atomoxetine Hydrochloride

Product Availability

Solid	• Capsule: 10 mg, 18 mg, 25 mg, 40 mg, 60 mg, 80 mg, 100 mg (base) (Strattera® [Eli Lilly]; others)

Physicochemical (drug)

Molecular weight: • 255.36 (salt 291.82)	Permeability: • LogP 3.9 • LogD n/a	Water solubility: • 27.8 mg/mL
pKa: • 10.1	Classification: • BCS Class n/a; BDDCS Class 1	

Pharmaceutical (product)

Solid	Do not open capsule as contents are an ocular irritant.

Pharmacokinetic (patient)

Absorption	• Specific site not known; t_{max} ~2 hours after an oral dose • Readily absorbed, with bioavailability varying by CY2D6 phenotype (~63% in extensive metabolizers, 94% in poor metabolizers)
Transport	• Plasma protein binding ~98%, mostly to albumin • V_d ~0.85 L/kg
Metabolism	• Metabolized by oxidation (CYP2D6) with subsequent glucuronidation and excretion predominantly in urine • Cl ~0.35 L/h/kg (extensive) or ~0.03 L/h/kg (poor)

Enteral Administration and Nutrition Considerations

Compatibility, Stability, and Bioavailability Considerations
 • No data are available.

Drug-Nutrition Interactions
 • Drug may influence nutrition status directly or indirectly:
   ○ CNS: fatigue, insomnia
   ○ GI: reduced appetite, dry mouth, nausea, vomiting, abdominal pain, constipation
   ○ Metabolic: slowed growth velocity in pediatrics
 • No data on the influence of malnutrition or obesity on drug disposition.
 • Influence of food on oral absorption or bioavailability:
   ○ A high-fat meal can reduce the rate of absorption but without significant effect on oral bioavailability.

Recommendations

Gastric	• Avoid administration through an enteral access device in favor of a therapeutic alternative.
Postpyloric	• As above.

Atorvastatin Calcium

Product Availability

Solid	• Tablet: 10 mg, 20 mg, 40 mg, 80 mg (base) (Lipitor® [Pfizer]; others)

Physicochemical (drug)

Molecular weight: • 558.66 (salt 1155.36)	Permeability: • LogP 5.7 • LogD n/a	Water solubility: • 0.02–0.15 mg/mL
pKa: • 4.3, 14.9	Classification: • BCS Class 2; BDDCS Class 2	

Pharmaceutical (product)

Solid	• Tablet products are often film-coated, but they can otherwise disperse in water with or without crushing.

Pharmacokinetic (patient)

Absorption	• Specific site not known; t_{max} ~1–2 hours following oral dose • Bioavailability ~14%
Transport	• Substrate for P-glycoprotein and BCRP efflux • Substrate for OATP1B1 uptake • Plasma protein binding ~98% • V_d ~ 5.4 L/kg
Metabolism	• Metabolized (CYP3A4) to active metabolites and eliminated through bile without enterohepatic recirculation • Cl ~29 mL/min/kg

Enteral Administration and Nutrition Considerations

Compatibility, Stability, and Bioavailability Considerations
- Atorvastatin is insoluble in aqueous solutions at pH ≤4.
- Several techniques have been attempted commercially to improve solubility, dissolution, and bioavailability.[1]
  - A nanoparticle preparation of atorvastatin helped to enhance bioavailability.[2]
  - Preparation of a nanostructured lipid carrier for the drug allowed increased oral bioavailability in an animal model.[3]
  - An amorphous solid dispersion to create an orally disintegrating tablet improved gastric solubility, dissolution, and bioavailability.[4]
- Significant interpatient variability exists in the altered oral bioavailability (up to ~twofold increase or decrease) following gastric bypass.[5,6]

Drug-Nutrition Interactions
- Drug may influence nutrition status directly or indirectly:
  - CNS: cognitive impairment

- ○ GI: pharyngeal-laryngeal discomfort, nausea, dyspepsia, diarrhea, elevated aminotransferases (AST, ALT), and rare hepatic failure
- ○ Metabolic: glucose intolerance, elevated HbA1c
- ○ Other: myopathy, including immune-mediated and necrotizing forms
- No data on the influence of malnutrition or obesity on drug disposition.
- Influence of food on oral absorption or bioavailability:
  - ○ Food may reduce rate of absorption and oral bioavailability (by ~13%) but without influencing drug activity, so may be taken without regard to meals.
  - ○ Grapefruit juice may increase oral bioavailability by at least 1.8-fold.[7]

Recommendations

Gastric	• Disperse tablet in at least 10 mL of water prior to administration. • No need to hold EN beyond the time required to flush-administer-flush.
Postpyloric	• As above. • Monitor for any unexpected change in effect.

References

1. Prabhu P, Patravale V. Dissolution enhancement of atorvastatin calcium by co-grinding technique. *Drug Deliv Transl Res.* 2016;6:380–391.
2. Shilpi D, Kushwah V, Agrawal AK, Jain S. Improved stability and enhanced oral bioavailability of atorvastatin loaded stearic acid modified gelatin nanoparticles. *Pharm Res.* 2017;34:1505–1516.
3. Elmowafy M, Ibrahim HM, Ahmed MA, et al. Atorvastatin-loaded nanostructured lipid carriers (NLCs): strategy to overcome delivery drawbacks. *Drug Deliv.* 2017;24:932–941.
4. Salmani JMM, Lv H, Asghar S, Zhou J. Amorphous solid dispersion with increased gastric solubility in tandem with oral disintegrating tablets: a successful approach to improve the bioavailability of atorvastatin. *Pharm Dev Technol.* 2015;20:465–472.
5. Skottheim IB, Stormark K, Christensen H, et al. Significantly altered systemic exposure to atorvastatin acid following gastric bypass surgery in morbidly obese patients. *Clin Pharmacol Ther.* 2009;86:311–318.
6. Jakobsen GS, Skottheim IB, Sandbu R, et al. Long-term effects of gastric bypass and duodenal switch on systemic exposure of atorvastatin. *Surg Endoscop.* 2013;27: 2094–2102.
7. Ando H, Tsuruoka S, Yanagihara H, et al. Effects of grapefruit juice on the pharmacokinetics of pitavastatin and atorvastatin. *Br J Clin Pharmacol.* 2005;60: 494–497.

Azithromycin Dihydrate

Product Availability

Solid	• Tablet: 250 mg, 500 mg, 600 mg (anhydrous base) (Zithromax® [Pfizer]; others)
Liquid	• Powder for oral suspension: 100 mg/5 mL, 200 mg/5 mL, 1000 mg/packet (anhydrous base) (Zithromax® [Pfizer]; others) • Extended-release microspheres for oral suspension: 2000 mg/packet (anhydrous base) (Zmax® [Pfizer])

Physicochemical (drug)

Molecular weight: • 749.00 (dehydrate 785.03)	Permeability: • LogP 4.02 • LogD n/a	Water solubility: • 39 mg/mL (37°C, pH 7.4)
pKa: • 9.16, 9.37	Classification: • BCS Class 2 or 3; BDDCS Class 3	

Pharmaceutical (product)

Solid	• Tablet products are often film-coated.

Liquid	• Suspension (reconstituted, 200 mg/5 mL):
	  o pH 9.48; expected to be 8.5–11.0
	  o Osmolality 3950 mOsm/kg (calculated based on measurement of 1:5 dilution with sterile water)[1]
	  o Viscosity n/a
	  o May contain sucrose; cherry-banana-flavored
	  o Reconstituted powder for oral suspension should be stored at 5°C–30°C for up to 10 days.
	• Consider avoiding extended-release powder as it is not bioequivalent with other oral dosage forms and is to be taken on an empty stomach (at least 1 hour before or 2 hours after feeding).

Pharmacokinetic (patient)

Absorption	• Specific site not known, but assumed to be duodenum/jejunum; t_{max} ~2 hours following oral dose • Bioavailability ~34%–52%
Transport	• Substrate for P-glycoprotein efflux and MRP2 efflux • OATP may be involved in cell (including intestinal) uptake. • Plasma protein binding is modest (≤51%), varying with circulating drug concentration. • V_d ~31–33 L/kg

Metabolism	• Some metabolism (N-demethylation, O-demethylation, and hydrolysis) to about 10 inactive metabolites, but predominantly eliminated unchanged through the bile • Cl ~630 mL/min

Enteral Administration and Nutrition Considerations

Compatibility, Stability, and Bioavailability Considerations
- Resistant to acid degradation.
- Reconstituted suspension (200 mg/5 mL) combined (1:1) with Osmolite 1.2, under simulated clinical conditions, would result in no clogging of an 8 Fr or 20 Fr feeding tube.[1]
- A commercially prepared amorphous form of the drug has better solubility, dissolution rate, and permeability compared with the commercially available crystalline azithromycin dihydrate.[2]
- Oral bioavailability was reduced by one-third in patients following gastric bypass compared with controls.[3]

Drug-Nutrition Interactions
- Drug may influence nutrition status directly or indirectly:
  - CNS: headache, dizziness, somnolence, fatigue
  - GI: altered taste (and smell), nausea, vomiting, dyspepsia, diarrhea, abdominal pain, LFT elevations, hepatitis (rare), and pancreatitis (rare)
  - Metabolic: hyperkalemia, hyperphosphatemia
- Data on the influence of malnutrition on drug disposition:
  - No expected difference in drug disposition in obesity.[4,5]
- Influence of food on oral absorption or bioavailability:
  - Although a high-fat meal may increase the rate of oral absorption, it has no influence on oral bioavailability.
  - Although bioequivalent in the fasted state, capsule products exhibited 39%–52% lower oral bioavailability in the fed state compared with the tablet, most likely because of slower disintegration with greater gastric degradation.[6]

Recommendations

Gastric	• If there is no therapeutic alternative, dilute the reconstituted suspension with water (at least 1:1) just prior to administration. • No need to hold EN beyond the time required to flush-administer-flush, but administration in close proximity to EN may improve drug tolerance.
Postpyloric	• As above. • Monitor for any unexpected change in effect.
Other	• As with all antimicrobials, consider parenteral alternative for acutely ill patients to ensure therapeutic concentrations.

References

1. Klang M, McLymont V, Ng N. Osmolality, pH, and compatibility of selected oral liquid medications with an enteral nutrition product. *JPEN J Parenter Enteral Nutr.* 2013;37: 689–694.
2. Aucamp M, Odendaal R, Liebenberg W, Hamman J. Amorphous azithromycin with improved aqueous solubility and intestinal permeability. *Drug Dev Indust Pharm.* 2015; 41:1100–1108.
3. Padwal RS, Ben-Eltriki M, Wang X, et al. Effect of gastric bypass surgery on azithromycin oral bioavailability. *J Antimicrob Chemother.* 2012;67:2203–2206.
4. Wurtz R, Itokazu G, Rodvold K. Antimicrobial dosing in obese patients. *Clin Infect Dis.* 1997;25:112–118.
5. Ben-Eltriki M, Somayaji V, Padwall RS, Brocks DR. A liquid chromatography-mass spectrometric method for the quantification of azithromycin in human plasma. *Biomed Chromatogr.* 2013;27:1012–1017.
6. Curatolo W, Liu P, Johnson BA, et al. Effects of food on a gastrically degraded drug: azithromycin fast-dissolving gelatin capsules and HPMC capsules. *Pharm Res.* 2011; 28:1531–1539.

Baclofen

Product Availability

Solid	Tablet: 5 mg, 10 mg, 20 mg (various)

Physicochemical (drug)

Molecular weight:	Permeability:	Water solubility:
• 213.67	• LogP –0.96	• 5 mg/mL
	• LogD –0.96 (pH 7.4)	
pKa:	Classification:	
• 5.4, 9.5	• BCS Class n/a; BDDCS Class 3	

Pharmaceutical (product)

Solid	• Scored tablets; tablets do not disperse in water.

Pharmacokinetic (patient)

Absorption	• In proximal small intestine; t_{max} within 2 hours following oral dose
	• Bioavailability ~70%–85%
Transport	• Substrate for several amino acid transporters
	• Plasma protein binding ~30%, varying with circulating drug concentration
	• V_d ~0.81 L/kg
Metabolism	• Some metabolism (~15%) by deamination
	• Otherwise eliminated unchanged mostly in urine
	• Cl ~17 L/h

Enteral Administration and Nutrition Considerations

Compatibility, Stability, and Bioavailability Considerations

- The official USP formulation for compounding an oral suspension (5 mg/mL) is expected to have a pH of 4.2–5.2; should be stored at refrigeration and provided a BUD of no more than 35 days.
- An extemporaneously compounded oral liquid (10 mg/mL) had a pH of 4.57.
- An extemporaneously compounded oral liquid (5 mg/mL) prepared from tablets (20 mg) in glycerin and simple syrup, or from pure drug powder in simple syrup, stored in 60 mL amber glass bottles at 4°C, remained stable (HPLC analysis) at 35 days.[1]
- Extemporaneously compounded oral suspensions (10 mg/mL) prepared from tablets (10 mg) in one of three vehicles—OraSweet/OraPlus (1:1), OraSweet SF/OraPlus (1:1), or cherry syrup/simple syrup (1:4)—stored in amber polyethylene terephthalate bottles at 5°C and 25°C in the dark, remained stable (HPLC analysis) for 60 days at each temperature.[2]

- An extemporaneously compounded oral elixir (2 mg/5 mL) prepared from tablets (10 mg) in ethanol, carboxymethylcellulose, parabens, and water, as recommended by the manufacturer, can be given a 2-week BUD if stored at controlled room temperature and protected from light, although no stability data were reported.[3]

Drug-Nutrition Interactions

- Drug may influence nutrition status directly or indirectly:
  - Weight gain
  - CNS: drowsiness, dizziness, fatigue, but also tremor, rigidity, dystonia and ataxia; psychiatric disturbances (eg, confusion, depression)
  - GI: dry mouth, altered taste, anorexia, nausea, vomiting, diarrhea (or constipation), abdominal pain, increased AST and alkaline phosphatase
  - Metabolic: glucose intolerance
- No data on the influence of malnutrition or obesity on drug disposition.
- Influence of food on oral absorption or bioavailability:
  - The branched-chain amino acid leucine, found in significant concentrations in whey protein, may reduce baclofen bioavailability.[4]

Recommendations

Gastric	• Crush and disperse tablet in water (at least 10 mL) prior to administration.
	• Alternative: Prepare an oral liquid with known stability, then dilute the dose with water (at least 1:1) just prior to administration.
	• No need to hold EN beyond the time required to flush-administer-flush, but administration in close proximity to EN may reduce GI side effects.
Postpyloric	• As above.
	• Monitor for any unexpected change in effect.

References

1. Johnson CE, Hart SM. Stability of an extemporaneously compounded baclofen oral liquid. *Am J Hosp Pharm*. 1993;50:2353–2355.
2. Allen LV, Erickson MA. Stability of baclofen, captopril, diltiazem hydrochloride, dipyridamole, and flecainide acetate in extemporaneously compounded oral liquids. *Am J Health-Syst Pharm*. 1996;53:2179–2184.
3. Woods DJ. *Formulation in Pharmacy Practice*. Dunedin, New Zealand: Healthcare Otago; 1993:1–104.
4. Cercós-Fortea T, Polache A, Nácher A, et al. Influence of leucine on intestinal baclofen absorption as a model compound of neutral α-amino acids. *Biopharm Drug Disp*. 1995; 16:563–577.

Benazepril Hydrochloride

Product Availability

Solid	• Tablet: 5 mg, 10 mg, 20 mg, 40 mg (Lotensin® [US Pharms]; others)

Physicochemical (drug)

Molecular weight: • 424.50 (salt 460.96)	Permeability: • LogP 1.82 (calc) • LogD 1.10 (pH 7.4)	Water solubility: • 128 mg/mL
pKa: • 3.5, 5.4	Classification: • BCS Class 1; BDDCS Class 1	

Pharmaceutical (product)

Solid	• Tablet products are often film-coated. • Some tablet products may be dispersible in water.

Pharmacokinetic (patient)

Absorption	• Specific site not known; t_{max} ~0.5–2 hours following oral dose (fasted) • Bioavailability >37%
Transport	• May be a substrate for the peptide uptake transporter PEPT1 • Plasma protein binding ~95%–96% • V_d ~0.7 L/kg
Metabolism	• This prodrug is hydrolyzed to the active form (benazeprilat), which undergoes glucuronic acid conjugation prior to excretion. • Cl ~0.13 L/h/kg

Enteral Administration and Nutrition Considerations

Compatibility, Stability, and Bioavailability Considerations
- Tablets (20 mg) do not need to be crushed; may be combined with the diluent OraPlus and shaken further (1:1) with OraSweet to make a 2 mg/mL dispersion.[1]
- According to the manufacturer, such an extemporaneous suspension (2 mg/mL) made from fifteen 20 mg tablets shaken in 75 mL of a vehicle (OraPlus) and then diluted further with 75 mL of OraSweet, stored in an amber polyethylene terephthalate bottle, was stable for 30 days at 2°C–8°C.

Drug-Nutrition Interactions
- Drug may influence nutrition status directly or indirectly:
  - CNS: headache, dizziness, fatigue
  - GI: intestinal angioedema manifest as abdominal pain, cholestasis
  - Metabolic: hyperkalemia

- No data on the influence of malnutrition or obesity on drug disposition.
- Influence of food on oral absorption or bioavailability:
  - Food does not influence the rate or extent of oral absorption.

Recommendations

Gastric	• Crush and/or disperse tablet in water prior to administration. • Alternative: Prepare an oral liquid with known stability, then dilute the dose with water (at least 1:1) just prior to administration. • No need to hold EN beyond the time required to flush-administer-flush.
Postpyloric	• As above. • Monitor for any unexpected change in effect.

Reference

1. Allen LV. Benazepril 2-mg/mL oral liquid. *Int J Pharm Compd*. 2007;11:247.

Benzonatate

Product Availability

Solid	• Capsule: 100 mg, 200 mg (Tessalon® [Pfizer]; others)

Physicochemical (drug)

Molecular weight: • 603.75	Permeability: • LogP 2.45 • LogD n/a	Water solubility: • 0.001 mg/mL
pKa: • 3.4	Classification: • BCS Class n/a; BDDCS Class 2	

Pharmaceutical (product)

Solid	Capsule: • Capsules are liquid-filled ("perles"). • Do not alter (break, cut, chew) integrity of dosage form; local mucosal irritant and anesthetic.

Pharmacokinetic (patient)

Absorption	• Specific site not known; t_{max} within 1 hour following oral dose • Bioavailability not well described
Transport	• Plasma protein binding n/a • V_d n/a
Metabolism	• Hydrolyzed by plasma esterases to para-aminobenzoic acid • Cl n/a

Enteral Administration and Nutrition Considerations

Compatibility, Stability, and Bioavailability Considerations
• No data are available.

Drug-Nutrition Interactions
• Drug may influence nutrition status directly or indirectly:
  o CNS: sedation, headache, dizziness, confusion
  o GI: nausea, constipation
• No data on the influence of malnutrition or obesity on drug disposition.
• No known influence of food on oral absorption or bioavailability.

Recommendations

Gastric	• Avoid administration by enteral access device.
Postpyloric	• As above.

Benztropine Mesylate

Product Availability

Solid	• Tablet: 0.5 mg, 1 mg, 2 mg (various)

Physicochemical (drug)

Molecular weight: • 424.50 (mesylate 403.54)	Permeability: • LogP 4.3 • LogD n/a	Water solubility: • 0.24 mg/mL
pKa: • 9.5	Classification: • BCS Class n/a; BDDCS Class 1	

Pharmaceutical (product)

Solid	• Tablets disperse in water (20 mL) within 2 minutes.

Pharmacokinetic (patient)

Absorption	• Specific site not known; t_{max} ~2 hours following oral dose • Bioavailability not well described
Transport	• Plasma protein binding ~95% • V_d n/a
Metabolism	• Metabolized in part by CYP2C19 • Cl n/a

Enteral Administration and Nutrition Considerations

Compatibility, Stability, and Bioavailability Considerations
  • The drug is most stable at pH 5–8.

Drug-Nutrition Interactions
  • Drug may influence nutrition status directly or indirectly:
    o CNS: blurred vision
    o GI: dry mouth, vomiting, constipation, paralytic ileus
    o Other: muscle weakness
  • No data on the influence of malnutrition or obesity on drug disposition.
  • No known influence of food on oral absorption or bioavailability.

Recommendations

Gastric	• Disperse tablet in water (20 mL) prior to administration. • No need to hold EN beyond the time required to flush-administer-flush.
Postpyloric	• As above. • Monitor for any unexpected change in effect.

Bisoprolol Fumarate

Product Availability

Solid	Tablet: 5 mg, 10 mg (various)

Physicochemical (drug)

Molecular weight: • 325.45 (fumarate 766.97)	Permeability: • LogP 1.87 • LogD –0.23 (pH 7.4)	Water solubility: • 831 mg/mL
pKa: • 9.57	Classification: • BCS Class 1; BDDCS Class 3	

Pharmaceutical (product)

Solid	• Tablet products are often film-coated. • Do not crush; may disperse in water.

Pharmacokinetic (patient)

Absorption	• Specific site not known; t_{max} ~1–3 hours following oral dose • Bioavailability ~80%–90%
Transport	• Saturable, pH-dependent (alkaline) intestinal uptake • Plasma protein binding ~30% • V_d ~2.6–3.5 L/kg
Metabolism	• First-pass hepatic metabolism by CYP3A4, with remainder of drug excreted unchanged in urine • Cl ~15 L/h

Enteral Administration and Nutrition Considerations

Compatibility, Stability, and Bioavailability Considerations
- Aqueous solubility improves at pH >6.5.
- Three different preparation methods were compared: (a) open crushing with mortar and pestle followed by suspension in water; (b) closed crushing in a commercial tablet crusher then open suspension in water; or (c) closed crushing and confined suspension in water in a different commercial device). Although similar in the efficiency of preparation, the fully closed method prevented particle aerosolization.[1]
- An extemporaneously compounded oral liquid (0.25 mg/mL) in a phosphate buffer of pH 7.4 remained stable (HPLC analysis) even at temperatures of up to 90°C in 84 hours.[2]
- The oral bioavailability can be quite variable between individuals.[3]

Drug-Nutrition Interactions
- Drug may influence nutrition status directly or indirectly:
  - CNS: dizziness, headache, depression
  - GI: dry mouth, nausea, vomiting, epigastric pain, diarrhea or constipation

o Metabolic: peripheral edema
o Other: arthralgia
- Influence of malnutrition or obesity on drug disposition:
  o The body weight–normalized volume of distribution is lower in obesity.
- No known influence of food on oral absorption or bioavailability.

Recommendations

Gastric	• Disperse tablet in water (at least 10 mL) prior to administration. • No need to hold EN beyond the time required to flush-administer-flush.
Postpyloric	• As above. • Monitor for any unexpected change in effect.

References

1. Salmon D, Pont E, Chevallard H, et al. Pharmaceutical and safety considerations of tablet crushing in patients undergoing enteral intubation. *Int J Pharm.* 2013;443:146–153.
2. Modamio P, Lastra CF, Montejo O, et al. Development and validation of liquid chromatography methods for the quantitation of propranolol, metoprolol, atenolol, and bisoprolol: application in solution stability studies. *Int J Pharm.* 1996;130:137–140.
3. Ishida K, Horie A, Nishimura M, et al. Variability of bioavailability and intestinal absorption characteristics of bisoprolol. *Drug Metab Pharmacokinet.* 2013;28:491–496.

Budesonide

Product Availability

Solid	• Tablet: 9 mg (Uceris® [Salix Pharms]) • Capsule: 3 mg (Entocort® EC [Perrigo Pharma]; others)

Physicochemical (drug)

Molecular weight: • 430.55	Permeability: • LogP 1.90 or 2.42 • LogD 2.70 (pH 7.4)	Water solubility: • 0.011 mg/mL
pKa: • 2.9, 13.7	Classification: • BCS Class 1; BDDCS Class 1	

Pharmaceutical (product)

Solid	• Do not crush tablet, which is an extended-release formulation. • Capsules contain enteric-coated granules in an extended-release matrix; can open capsules but do not crush contents. • The products are formulated to release active drug at mid- to late small intestine.

Pharmacokinetic (patient)

Absorption	• Specific site not known; t_{max} ~3–5 hours following oral dose • Bioavailability ~15%–21%
Transport	• Substrate for P-glycoprotein efflux • Plasma protein binding ~85%–90% • V_d ~2.2–3.9 L/kg
Metabolism	• Extensive (80%–95%) metabolism via CYP3A4 to two inactive metabolites that are excreted in urine and feces • Cl ~0.9–1.8 L/min

Enteral Administration and Nutrition Considerations

Compatibility, Stability, and Bioavailability Considerations

- Enteric-coated granules found in capsules dissolve at pH >5.5, but the drug itself is subject to hydrolysis in alkaline solution.
- A nanosuspension formulation under development resulted in greater cell membrane permeability, compared with a saturated solution of micronized drug particles, and is expected to improve oral bioavailability.[1]

Drug-Nutrition Interactions

- Drug may influence nutrition status directly or indirectly:
  - CNS: headache, dizziness, fatigue
  - GI: nausea, vomiting, dyspepsia, abdominal pain, diarrhea

- o Metabolic: glucose intolerance; reduced bone mineral density with long-term systemic use
- o Other: arthralgia, myalgia
- No data on the influence of malnutrition or obesity on drug disposition.
- Influence of food on oral absorption or bioavailability:
  - o Although a high-fat meal may delay oral absorption, there is no significant change in oral bioavailability.
  - o Grapefruit juice may inhibit drug metabolism, resulting in a near doubling of bioavailability.

Recommendations

Gastric	Consider a therapeutic alternative.
Postpyloric	As above.

Reference

1. Lenhardt T, Vergnault G, Grenier P, Scherer D, Langguth P. Evaluation of nanosuspensions for absorption enhancement of poorly soluble drugs: in vitro transport studies across intestinal epithelial monolayers. *AAPS J*. 2008;10:435–438.

Buprenorphine Hydrochloride

Product Availability

Solid	Tablet (sublingual): 2 mg, 8 mg (anhydrous base) (various)

Physicochemical (drug)

Molecular weight: • 467.65 (salt 504.11)	Permeability: • LogP 4.98 • LogD n/a	Water solubility: • 17 mg/mL (pH 4.4, 25°C)
pKa: • 8.31	Classification: • BCS Class n/a; BDDCS Class 1	

Pharmaceutical (product)

Solid	Tablets are intended for sublingual administration.

Pharmacokinetic (patient)

Absorption	• Specific site not known; t_{max} within 2 hours following sublingual administration • Bioavailability ~55% (15%–95%) following sublingual administration • Swallowing the tablet reduces the bioavailability considerably.
Transport	• Significant plasma protein binding (~96%), to α- and β-globulins rather than to albumin • V_d ~4.8 L/kg
Metabolism	• Extensive metabolism via CYP3A4 (and CYP2C9) to norbuprenorphine, subsequently conjugated via UGT1A3 (and UGT1A1/2B7) to buprenorphine and norbuprenorphine glucuronides • Excretion predominantly through the biliary route with some enterohepatic recirculation • Cl ~1.28 L/min

Enteral Administration and Nutrition Considerations

Compatibility, Stability, and Bioavailability Considerations
- The drug is most stable in aqueous solution at pH 3.5–5.5, but it remains sensitive to light.
- An extemporaneously compounded liquid (75 µg/mL) intended for sublingual administration, prepared from the injectable product (0.3 mg/mL), ethanol and simple syrup, with a pH of ~5.4 and stored in amber glass bottles at 2.2°C–7.8°C and 20°C–25°C or in propylene oral syringes, remained stable (liquid chromatography-electrospray ionization analysis) at 30 days.[1]

Drug-Nutrition Interactions

- Drug may influence nutrition status directly or indirectly:
  - ○ CNS: sedation, depression (eg, altered level of consciousness), confusion, weakness, fatigue, visual abnormalities (eg, blurred vision, diplopia)
  - ○ GI: dry mouth, nausea, vomiting, abdominal cramps, constipation
  - ○ Metabolic: anemia, reduced total serum protein concentration
  - ○ Other: peripheral edema
- No data on the influence of malnutrition or obesity on drug disposition.
- Influence of food on oral absorption or bioavailability:
  - ○ Certain dietary components (eg, chrysin, curcumin, ginger extract, hesperitin, quercetin) may significantly reduce intestinal/hepatic metabolism to increase oral bioavailability.[2]

Recommendations

Gastric	• Consider a therapeutic alternative (eg, transdermal or parenteral route).
Postpyloric	• As above.

References

1. Anagnostis EA, Sadaka RE, Sailor LA, et al. Formulation of buprenorphine for sublingual use in neonates. *J Pediatr Pharmacol Ther*. 2011;16:281–284.
2. Maharao NV, Joshi AA, Gerk PM. Inhibition of glucuronidation and oxidative metabolism of buprenorphine using GRAS compounds or dietary constituents/supplements: in vitro proof of concept. *Biopharm Drug Disp*. 2017;38:139–154.

Bupropion Hydrochloride

Product Availability

Solid	• Tablet: o Immediate-release: 75 mg, 100 mg (various) o Extended-release: 100 mg, 150 mg, 200 mg, 300 mg, 450 mg (various)

Physicochemical (drug)

Molecular weight: • 239.75 (salt 276.21)	Permeability: • LogP 3.60 • LogD 3.27 (pH 7.4)	Water solubility: • 312 mg/mL
pKa: • 7.9	Classification: • BCS Class 1; BDDCS Class 1	

Pharmaceutical (product)

Solid	• Immediate-release tablet products may be film-coated. • Do not crush extended-release tablets.

Pharmacokinetic (patient)

Absorption	• Specific site not known; t_{max} ~2–3 hours following oral administration • Bioavailability ~5%–20% • Extended-release tablet considered bioequivalent with the immediate-release tablet
Transport	• Plasma protein binding ≥80% bound to albumin • V_d ~65 liters
Metabolism	• Extensive metabolism via CYP2B6 to several active metabolites; then conjugated and eliminated renally • Cl ~74 mL/min/kg

Enteral Administration and Nutrition Considerations

Compatibility, Stability, and Bioavailability Considerations
- The drug is not stable in an isotonic phosphate buffer solution (pH 7.4) at 32°C.[1]
- In aqueous solutions, the drug is most stable (HPLC analysis with ultraviolet and mass spectrometric detection) near pH 2.5, with degradation increasing as pH rises.[2]

Drug-Nutrition Interactions
- Drug may influence nutrition status directly or indirectly:
  - Weight loss more common than weight gain.
  - CNS: agitation, headache, dyskinesia, ataxia
  - GI: dry mouth, taste disturbance, dysphagia, anorexia, nausea, vomiting, constipation, abdominal pain, diarrhea

o Metabolic: dysglycemia, SIADH
o Other: peripheral edema, arthralgia, myalgia
* No data on the influence of malnutrition or obesity on drug disposition.
* No known influence of food on oral absorption or bioavailability.

Recommendations

Gastric	• If there is no therapeutic alternative, crush and disperse immediate-release tablet in water just prior to administration. • No need to hold EN beyond the time required to flush-administer-flush.
Postpyloric	• As above. • Monitor for any unexpected change in effect.

References

1. Kiptoo PK, Paudel KS, Hammell DC, et al. Transdermal delivery of bupropion and its active metabolite, hydroxybupropion: a prodrug strategy as an alternative approach. *J Pharm Sci.* 2009;98:583–594.
2. O'Byrne PM, Williams R, Walsh JJ, et al. The aqueous stability of bupropion. *J Pharm Biomed Anal.* 2010;53:376–381.

Buspirone Hydrochloride

Product Availability

Solid	Tablet: 5 mg, 7.5 mg, 10 mg, 15 mg, 30 mg (various)

Physicochemical (drug)

Molecular weight:	Permeability:	Water solubility:
• 385.51 (salt 421.97)	• LogP 2.63 • LogD 3.39 (pH 7.4)	• 865 mg/mL
pKa: • 4.12, 7.32	Classification: • BCS Class 1; BDDCS Class 2	

Pharmaceutical (product)

Solid	• Some tablet products may be film-coated. • Tablet may require crushing before dispersing in water.

Pharmacokinetic (patient)

Absorption	• Specific site not known; t_{max} ~30–90 minutes after an oral dose • Bioavailability <5%
Transport	• Plasma protein binding extensive (86%–95%), to albumin more than to α_1-acid glycoprotein • V_d ~5.3 L/kg
Metabolism	• Extensive first-pass metabolism via CYP3A4 to several compounds, including the active 1-(2-pyrimidinyl)-piperazine, with subsequent conjugation and renal elimination more than biliary elimination; limits systemic bioavailability • Cl ~28 mL/min/kg

Enteral Administration and Nutrition Considerations

Compatibility, Stability, and Bioavailability Considerations
- An extemporaneously compounded oral liquid (2.5 mg/mL) prepared from drug powder and diluted in OraSweet, and then stored at room or refrigeration temperature, remained stable (HPLC analysis) at 30 days.[1]
- When the liquid preparation described in the previous point was administered orally with water or apple juice (100 mL) after a breakfast meal, the bioavailability was within the expected range.[1]
- A commercially prepared lipid nanoparticle formulation significantly increased oral bioavailability.[2]

Drug-Nutrition Interactions
- Drug may influence nutrition status directly or indirectly:
  - Weight gain or weight loss
  - CNS: sedation, headache, fatigue

- o GI: dry mouth, altered taste/smell, nausea, vomiting, abdominal distress, diarrhea or constipation
- o Other: muscle aches, cramps, weakness
- No data on the influence of malnutrition or obesity on drug disposition.
- Influence of food on oral absorption or bioavailability:
  - o Food may increase oral bioavailability by 1.8 times.
  - o Grapefruit juice can significantly increase oral bioavailability (4.3–9.2 times).[3]
  - o In an animal model, pomegranate juice significantly increased the rate of drug absorption and its bioavailability.[4]

Recommendations

Gastric	• Crush and/or disperse tablet in water prior to administration. • Administer in close proximity to EN to optimize bioavailability.
Postpyloric	• As above. • Monitor for any unexpected change in effect.

References

1. Edwards DJ, Chugani DC, Chugani HT, et al. Pharmacokinetics of buspirone in autistic children. *J Clin Pharmacol.* 2006;46:508–514.
2. Varshosaz J, Tabbakhian M, Mohammadi MY. Formulation and optimization of solid lipid nanoparticles of buspirone HCl for enhancement of its oral bioavailability. *J Liposome Res.* 2010;20:286–296.
3. Lilja JJ, Kivisto KT, Backman JT, Lamberg TS, Neuvonen PJ. Grapefruit juice substantially increases plasma concentrations of buspirone. *Clin Pharmacol Ther.* 1998; 64:655–660.
4. Shravan KY, Adukondalu D, Bhargavi LA, et al. Effect of pomegranate pretreatment on the oral bioavailability of buspirone in male albino rabbits. *DARU J Pharm Sci.* 2011; 19:266–269.

Captopril

Product Availability

Solid	• Tablet: 12.5 mg, 25 mg, 50 mg, 100 mg (various)

Physicochemical (drug)

Molecular weight: • 217.29	Permeability: • LogP 0.34 • LogD −1.98 (pH 7.4)	Water solubility: • 160 mg/mL
pKa: • 3.7, 9.8	Classification: • BCS Class 3; BDDCS Class 3	

Pharmaceutical (product)

Solid	• Tablets disperse in water (20 mL) within 2 minutes. • Avoid exposure from crushing (in pregnancy).

Pharmacokinetic (patient)

Absorption	• Specific site not known; t_{max} ~1 hour following oral dose • Bioavailability ~60%–75%
Transport	• Possible substrate for peptide uptake transporter(s) • Plasma protein binding 25%–30%, mostly to albumin • V_d ~0.7 L/kg
Metabolism	• Rapid metabolism (~50%) to disulfides • Renal elimination of parent drug and metabolites • Cl ~0.8 L/h/kg

Enteral Administration and Nutrition Considerations

Compatibility, Stability, and Bioavailability Considerations

- An aqueous solution (2%) is expected to have a pH of 2.0–2.6.
- An extemporaneously compounded oral liquid (5 mg/mL) had a pH of 3.45.
- Oxidative degradation takes place in aqueous solution but is the least in acidic pH (2–4) at higher drug concentration.[1]
- The official USP formulation for oral solution has a final pH of 3.8–4.3, but it makes use of the pure drug powder (not crushed tablets) because the excipients may accelerate oxidation.
- A captopril solution (1 mg/mL) in glass, made from commercial tablets, is more stable in distilled water with sodium ascorbate (5 mg/mL) than in syrup or distilled water alone.[2]
- A captopril solution (0.75 mg/mL) in plastic, made from commercial tablets, was poorly stable in OraSweet/OraPlus, OraSweet SF/OraPlus, or cherry syrup/simple syrup.[1]

- Captopril solution (1 mg/mL) stability was better in distilled water than in tap water, with degradation in tap water at least twice the rate seen in distilled water or sterile water for irrigation.[3-5]
- An extemporaneously compounded oral liquid (1 mg/mL) prepared with InOrpha, stored in amber glass bottles at 4°C and 25°C, revealed better stability when EDTA was included (14 days at room temperature, 60 days refrigerated) than without (4 days room temperature, 14 days refrigerated).[6]
- Of 10 formulations evaluated, the most stable (HPLC analysis) used pure captopril powder dispersed in purified water (1 mg/mL) with edetate disodium to inactivate any trace metal ions, with pH ~3.4, when stored at 2°C–8°C for 2 years.[7]
- Another oral suspension (0.8 mg/mL) prepared from pure powder dispersed in SyrSpend SF, stored in low-actinic bottles at 2°C–8°C, exhibited ~5% drug loss (HPLC analysis) at 14 days but was unstable (~14% drug loss) at 32 days.[8]
- Extemporaneously compounded oral liquids (1 mg/mL and 5 mg/mL) prepared from drug powder in sterile water with sorbitol, edetate disodium, and sodium benzoate and kept to pH ~3.9, stored in amber glass bottles at 22°C, remained stable (HPLC analysis) for 12 months, although the higher-concentration preparation exhibited sulfur odor and taste.[9]
- An extemporaneously compounded oral solution (2 mg/mL) was reported to have an osmolality of 1177 mOsm/kg.[10]

Drug-Nutrition Interactions

- Drug may influence nutrition status directly or indirectly:
  - Weight loss, associated with taste impairment
  - Zinc deficiency (manifesting as alopecia, asteatosis, dysgeusia, and cutaneous eruptions)
  - GI: loss of or altered (metallic) taste, glossitis, oral cavity infections (associated with agranulocytosis/neutropenia), intestinal angioedema (manifest by abdominal pain, nausea and vomiting), hepatitis
  - Metabolic: hyperkalemia, hyponatremia, transient increases in BUN and creatinine, proteinuria
  - Other: muscle aches, cramps, weakness
- No data on the influence of malnutrition or obesity on drug disposition.
- Influence of food on oral absorption or bioavailability:
  - Food may reduce absorption by 30%–40%.[11]
  - Magnesium-containing antacids may reduce oral drug bioavailability; potassium-containing salt substitutes may increase the risk for hyperkalemia.

Recommendations

Gastric	• In the absence of a therapeutic alternative administered less frequently, disperse tablet in water (20 mL) prior to administration. • Consider holding EN 1 hour before and after drug administration.
Postpyloric	• As above. • Monitor for any unexpected change in effect.

References

1. Allen LV, Erickson MA. Stability of baclofen, captopril, diltiazem hydrochloride, dipyridamole, and flecainide acetate in extemporaneously compounded oral liquids. *Am J Health-Syst Pharm.* 1996;53:2179–2184.
2. Nahata M, Morosco R, Hipple T. Stability of captopril in three liquid dosage forms. *Am J Hosp Pharm.* 1994;51:95–96.
3. Anaizi NH, Swenson C. Instability of aqueous captopril solutions. *Am J Hosp Pharm.* 1993;50:486–488.
4. Sabol BJ, Kerr TM, Schroeder LA. Stability of captopril solution. *US Pharm.* 1996;21: HS-28,31,32,36.
5. Escribano Garcia MJ, Torrado Duran S, Torado Duran JJ. Stability study of an aqueous formulation of captopril at 1 mg/mL. *Farm Hosp.* 2005;29:30–36.
6. Lambert S, Millot-Lustig H, Aujoulat O. Stability of captopril with and without EDTA using a new vehicle: InOrpha. *Int J Clin Pharm.* 2013;35:886.
7. Berger-Gryllaki M, Podilsky G, Widmer N, et al. The development of a stable oral solution of captopril for paediatric patients. *Eur J Hosp Pharm Sci.* 2007;13:67–72.
8. Geiger CM, Sorenson B, Whaley PA. Stability of captopril in SyrSpend SF. *Int J Pharm Compound.* 2013;17:336–338.
9. Brustugun J, Lao YE, Fagernaes C, et al. Long-term stability of extemporaneously prepared captopril oral liquids in glass bottles. *Am J Health-Syst Pharm.* 2009;66: 1722–1725.
10. Fernández Polo A, Cabañas Poy MJ, Clemente Bautista S, et al. Osmolality of oral liquid dosage forms to be administered to newborns in a hospital. *Farm Hosp.* 2007;31: 311–314.
11. Nahata M, Morosco R, Hipple T. Stability of captopril in three liquid dosage forms. *Am J Hosp Pharm.* 1994;51:95–96.

Carbamazepine

Product Availability

Solid	• Tablet:
	   ○ Immediate-release: 200 mg (Tegretol® [Novartis]; others)
	   ○ Chewable: 100 mg (Tegretol® [Novartis]; others)
	   ○ Extended-release: 100 mg, 200 mg, 400 mg (Tegretol® XR [Novartis])
	• Capsule (extended-release): 100 mg, 200 mg, 300 mg (Carbatrol® [Shire]; Equetro® [Validus Pharms]; others)

Liquid	• Oral suspension: 100 mg/5 mL (Tegretol® [Novartis]; others)

Physicochemical (drug)

Molecular weight:
• 236.27
	Permeability:
	• LogP 2.45
	• LogD 2.60 (pH 6.5),
	  2.45 (pH 7.4),
	  2.38 (pH 7.4 calc)
		Water solubility:
		• 0.018 mg/mL

pKa: • 13.9	Classification: • BCS Class 2; BDDCS Class 2	

Pharmaceutical (product)

Solid	• Immediate-release tablets may disperse in water (20 mL) in about 1 minute. • Tablets may lose at least one-third of oral bioavailability if exposed to excessive moisture prior to administration by an influence on dissolution characteristics. • Do not break, chew, or crush extended-release tablets (coating is not "digested" and can appear in stool). • Do not chew or crush extended-release capsules (they contain 3 types of granules, each with a different release profile).

Liquid	Oral suspension:
	• pH 3.68
	• Osmolality:
	  ○ 1100 mOsm/L[1]
	  ○ 4225 mOsm/kg (calculated based on measurement of 1:5 dilution with sterile water)[2]
	• Viscosity n/a
	• May contain propylene glycol, sorbitol, and sucrose; orange-vanilla flavored
	• Store at controlled room temperature.
	• Shake well before measuring a dose.
	• Avoid administering the oral suspension with any other liquid preparation.

Pharmacokinetic (patient)

Absorption	• Specific site not known; t_{max} varies by formulation and form: ~2 hours (liquid), ~6 hours (chew tabs), and ~12 hours (tablets). • Bioavailability varies and is often incomplete. • Immediate-release tablets and oral suspension are considered bioequivalent.
Transport	• Substrate for P-glycoprotein efflux • Plasma protein binding ~75%–90% • V_d ~1.1 L/kg
Metabolism	• Metabolized to the active 10,11-epoxide via CYP3A4 and then to the 10,11-transdiol derivative; also metabolized to 2-hydroxy- and 3-hydroxy-carbamazepine via aromatic hydroxylation • Renal elimination of the metabolites • Cl ~0.73 mL/min/kg

Enteral Administration and Nutrition Considerations

Compatibility, Stability, and Bioavailability Considerations

- Under humid conditions, intact tablets may experience reduced bioavailability after carbamazepine dihydrate formation hardens the dosage form.
- Undiluted suspension (100 mg/5 mL) administered through a nasogastric tube (12 Fr) results in <90% of the dose delivered to the distal end despite flushing twice with 50 mL, compared with >90% delivery when first diluted (1:1) with sterile water, 0.9% sodium chloride, or 5% dextrose.[3]
- Dilution of the suspension is expected to improve absorption in patients.[4]
- Commercial suspension combined (1:1) with Osmolite 1.2, under simulated clinical conditions, would result in clogging of both an 8 Fr and a 20 Fr feeding tube.[2]
- Adsorption to fibers (ie, guar gum, xanthan gum, dextrin hydrate) used in enteral formulations with viscosity of ~0–4 Pa·s, was significant at 15%–67% of the drug dose, leading to reduced bioavailability.[5]
- Crushing and mixing drug with thickened water (to aid swallowing) significantly delayed dissolution.[6]
- An extemporaneously compounded oral suspension (200 mg/5 mL) was prepared from tablets (200 mg) using either sorbitol or simple syrup and stored in amber bottles at 4°C, 25°C, or 37°C or in syringes at 4°C. The sorbitol preparation froze at refrigeration, whereas the simple syrup preparation remained stable (enzyme-multiplied immunoassay analysis) but exhibited increased particle size.[7]

- Extemporaneously compounded oral suspensions (25 mg/mL, 50 mg/mL) prepared from bulk powder in OraSweet SF/OraPlus (1:1), stored in amber glass at 24°C–27°C, with a pH ~4.5, remained stable (HPLC analysis) for 6 months.[8]
- A similar oral suspension (25 mg/mL) prepared from pure drug powder in SyrSpend SF PH4, stored at refrigeration and room temperature, remained stable (HPLC analysis) for up to 90 days.[9]
- Amorphous and crystalline drug nanodispersions being studied may improve dissolution, permeability, and absorption.[10]

Drug-Nutrition Interactions
- Drug may influence nutrition status directly or indirectly:
  - Impairs biotin status, possibly by reduced absorption and/or increased catabolism.
  - CNS: dizziness, vertigo, drowsiness, fatigue, ataxia, confusion, headache, visual disturbances (nystagmus, blurred vision, transient diplopia), abnormal involuntary movements
  - GI: dry mouth, glossitis, stomatitis, anorexia, nausea, vomiting, GI distress, abdominal pain, diarrhea, constipation, abnormal LFTs, hepatitis, and rare hepatic failure
  - Metabolic: azotemia, hyponatremia, SIADH, hypocalcemia, albuminuria, glycosuria
  - Other: peripheral neuritis and paresthesia, arthralgia, myalgia
- Influence of malnutrition or obesity on drug disposition:
  - The body weight–normalized volume of distribution is lower in obesity, and clearance is slightly reduced, suggesting use of an appropriately adjusted body weight for initial dosing and close monitoring.[11,12]
- Food components may influence drug disposition:
  - A high-fat meal increases the rate of absorption from extended-release capsules without influencing the overall extent of absorption (ie, bioavailability).
  - Osmolite reduces carbamazepine (25 mL = 500 mg) bioavailability by 10% when administered together via nasogastric tube (10 Fr, 104 cm), followed by 60 mL flush, compared with administration in the fasted state.[13]
  - Crushing and mixing drug in yogurt (pH 4.5, viscosity 723 mPa·s) slowed dissolution compared with crushing/dispersing in water (pH 6.7, viscosity 0.8 mPa·s).[6]
  - Grapefruit juice can increase oral drug bioavailability.

Recommendations

Gastric	• Dilute the suspension with water (at least 1:1) just prior to administration. • No need to hold EN beyond the time required to flush-administer-flush.
Postpyloric	• As above. • Jejunal administration may be less effective. • Monitor for any unexpected change in effect.

References

1. Obladen M, Mutz A. Orale medikation bei frühgeborenen? *Monatsschr Kinderheilkd.* 1985;133:669–674.
2. Klang M, McLymont V, Ng N. Osmolality, pH, and compatibility of selected oral liquid medications with an enteral nutrition product. *JPEN J Parenter Enteral Nutr.* 2013;37: 689–694.
3. Clark-Schmidt AL, Garnett WR, Lowe DR, et al. Loss of carbamazepine suspension through nasogastric feeding tubes. *Am J Hosp Pharm.* 1990;47:2034–2037.
4. Williams NT. Medication administration through enteral feeding tubes. *Am J Health-Syst Pharm.* 2008;65:2347–2357.
5. Nagai K, Omotani S, Otani M, et al. In vitro and in vivo effects of fibers on the pharmacokinetics of orally administered carbamazepine: possible interaction between therapeutic drugs and semisolid nutrients. *Nutrition.* 2018;46:44–47.
6. Manrique YJ, Lee DJ, Islam F, et al. Crushed tablets: does the administration of food vehicles and thickened fluids to aid medication swallowing alter drug release? *J Pharm Pharmaceut Sci.* 2014;17:207–219.
7. Burckart GJ, Hammond RW, Akers MJ. Stability of extemporaneous suspensions of carbamazepine. *Am J Hosp Pharm.* 1981;38:1929–1931.
8. Jover Botella A, Marquez Peiró JF, González Loreiro MD, et al. Analysing the stability of two oral carbamazepine suspensions. *Farm Hosp.* 2011;35:28–31.
9. Polonini HC, Loures S, de Araujo EP, et al. Stability of allopurinol, amitriptyline hydrochloride, carbamazepine, domperidone, isoniazid, ketoconazole, lisinopril, naproxen, paracetamol (acetaminophen), and sertraline hydrochloride in SyrSpend SF PH4 oral suspensions. *Int J Pharm Compound.* 2016;20:426–434.
10. Warnken Z, Puppolo M, Hughey J, et al. In vitro-in vivo correlations of carbamazepine nanodispersions for application in formulation development. *J Pharm Sci.* 2018;107: 453–465.
11. Caracao Y, Zylber-Katz E, Berry EM, Levy M. Significant weight reduction in obese subjects enhances carbamazepine elimination. *Clin Pharmacol Ther.* 1992;51:501–506.
12. Caracao Y, Zylber-Katz E, Berry EM, Levy M. Carbamazepine pharmacokinetics in obese and lean subjects. *Ann Pharmacother.* 1995;29:843–847.
13. Bass DJ, Miles MV, Tennison MB, et al. Effects of enteral tube feeding on the absorption and pharmacokinetic profile of carbamazepine suspension. *Epilepsia.* 1989;30:364–369.

Carisoprodol

Product Availability

Solid	• Tablet: 250 mg, 350 mg (Soma® [Mylan]; others)

Physicochemical (drug)

Molecular weight: • 260.33	Permeability: • LogP 2.1 • LogD n/a	Water solubility: • 0.3 mg/mL
pKa: • 4.2	Classification: • BCS Class n/a; BDDCS Class 1	

Pharmaceutical (product)

Solid	• Tablet may disperse in water with or without crushing first.

Pharmacokinetic (patient)

Absorption	• Specific site not known; t_{max} ~1.5–2 hours after oral dose • Bioavailability is dose-proportional
Transport	• Plasma protein binding ~60% • V_d ~0.9–1.3 L/kg
Metabolism	• Extensively metabolized to meprobamate, hydroxyl-meprobamate, hydroxyl-carisoprodol via CYP2C19 • Cl ~0.4 L/h/kg (men) and ~0.7 L/h/kg (women)

Enteral Administration and Nutrition Considerations

Compatibility, Stability, and Bioavailability Considerations
• No data are available.

Drug-Nutrition Interactions
• Drug may influence nutrition status directly or indirectly:
  ○ CNS: drowsiness, dizziness, vertigo, ataxia, tremor, headache, syncope
  ○ GI: stomatitis (as part of severe hypersensitivity reactions), nausea, vomiting, epigastric distress
  ○ Other: peripheral edema
• No data on the influence of malnutrition or obesity on drug disposition.
• Influence of food on oral absorption or bioavailability:
  ○ No known influence of food, including high-fat meals, on oral bioavailability.

Recommendations

Gastric	• Crush and/or disperse tablet in water just prior to administration. • No need to hold EN beyond the time required to flush-administer-flush.
Postpyloric	• As above. • Monitor for any unexpected change in effect.

Carvedilol

Product Availability

Solid	• Tablet: 3.125 mg, 6.25 mg, 12.5 mg, 25 mg (Coreg® [GSK]; others) • Capsule: 10 mg, 20 mg, 40 mg, 80 mg (phosphate salt) (Coreg® CR [GSK]; others)

Physicochemical (drug)

Molecular weight: • 406.48 (phosphate 504.48)	Permeability: • LogP 4.19 • LogD n/a	Water solubility: • 0.013 mg/mL
pKa: • 7.8	Classification: • BCS Class 2; BDDCS Class 2	

Pharmaceutical (product)

Solid	• Immediate-release tablet products may be film-coated. • Do not open, chew, or crush extended-release capsules.

Pharmacokinetic (patient)

Absorption	• Proximal small bowel; t_{max} ~1 hour following oral dose • Bioavailability ~25%–35%
Transport	• Substrate for P-glycoprotein efflux • Plasma protein binding ~98%, primarily to albumin • V_d ~1.5 L/kg
Metabolism	• Extensive metabolism via demethylation (CYP2D6) and hydroxylation (CYP2C9) more so than via CYP3A4, -C19, -1A2, or -2E1 to several metabolites, including actives, followed by glucuronidation (UGT1A1, UGT2B7) for renal elimination • Cl ~500–700 mL/min

Enteral Administration and Nutrition Considerations

Compatibility, Stability, and Bioavailability Considerations
- Decomposition in aqueous solution occurs at alkaline pH.[1]
- An extemporaneously compounded oral solution (1 mg/mL) prepared in polyvinyl pyrrolidone and propylene glycol plus flavoring, stored in amber glass at 4°C, 25°C, and 40°C, remained stable for 56 days in acidic solutions (pH 4.2), but it was unstable in alkaline solutions (pH 8.2), especially at refrigeration.[2]
- An extemporaneously compounded oral liquid (0.625 mg/mL) prepared from tablets (25 mg) with deionized water and sorbitol was stored in amber polyethylene terephthalate bottles at 4°C–8°C and 22°C–26°C; the room-temperature preparations remained stable for up to 8 weeks.[3]

- Decreased absorption rate from jejunum to ileum.[4]
- Dissolution rate and bioavailability can be significantly improved by particle-size reduction (nanosuspensions are better than microsuspensions), according to recent research.[5]

Drug-Nutrition Interactions
- Drug may influence nutrition status directly or indirectly:
  o Weight gain
  o CNS: dizziness, headache, fatigue
  o GI: nausea, vomiting, diarrhea
  o Metabolic: elevated BUN, increased nonprotein nitrogen, hyperglycemia
  o Other: arthralgia, edema
- No data on the influence of malnutrition or obesity on drug disposition.
- Influence of food on oral absorption or bioavailability:
  o Food may reduce rate of oral drug absorption, but without an influence on oral bioavailability.
  o Food increases oral bioavailability of carvedilol phosphate.

Recommendations

Gastric	• Disperse tablets in water just prior to administration. • Administer after an intermittent feed; otherwise, there is no need to hold EN beyond the time required to flush-administer-flush.
Postpyloric	• As above. • Jejunal administration may be less effective. • Monitor for any unexpected change in effect.

References

1. Lanzanova FA, Argenta D, Arend MZ, et al. LC and LC-MS evaluation of stress degradation behavior of carvedilol. *J Liquid Chromatogr Rel Technol.* 2009;32:526–543.
2. Buontempo F, Bernabeu E, Glisoni RJ, et al. Carvedilol stability in paediatric oral liquid formulations. *Farm Hosp.* 2010;34:293–297.
3. Yamreudeewong W, Dolence EK, Pahl D. Stability of two extemporaneously prepared oral metoprolol and carvedilol liquids. *Hosp Pharm.* 2006;41:254–259.
4. Cheng J, Kamiya K, Kodama I. Carvedilol: molecular and cellular basis for its multifaceted therapeutic potential. *Cardiovasc Drug Rev.* 2001;19:152–171.
5. Liu D, Pan H, He F, et al. Effect of particle size on oral absorption of carvedilol nanosuspensions: in vitro and in vivo evaluation. *Int J Nanomed.* 2015;10:6425–6434.

Cefdinir

Product Availability

Solid	• Capsule: 300 mg (various)
Liquid	• Powder for oral suspension: 125 mg/5 mL, 250 mg/5 mL (various)

Physicochemical (drug)

Molecular weight: • 395.42	Permeability: • LogP −1.52 • LogD n/a	Water solubility: • 0.36 mg/mL
pKa: • 9.7	Classification: • BCS Class 4; BDDCS Class 4	

Pharmaceutical (product)

Solid	• Capsule contents may disperse in water
Liquid	• Suspension (reconstituted): ○ pH n/a ○ Osmolality n/a ○ Viscosity n/a ○ May contain sucrose (up to ~3 g/5 mL); color/flavor vary by manufacturer ○ Reconstituted oral suspension may be maintained at controlled room temperature and should be used within 10 days. ○ Shake well before drawing up dose for administration.
Note	Capsule and oral suspension are not bioequivalent.

Pharmacokinetic (patient)

Absorption	• Specific site not known; t_{max} 2–4 hours after an oral dose • Bioavailability is dose-dependent, varying by dosage form: ~15%–20% (capsules) and 25% (suspension).
Transport	• Substrate for PEPT1 and OAT uptake • Plasma protein binding ~60%–70% independent of drug concentration • V_d ~0.35 L/kg
Metabolism	• Minimal metabolism with renal elimination • Cl ~12–16 mL/min/kg

Enteral Administration and Nutrition Considerations

Compatibility, Stability, and Bioavailability Considerations
- A cefdinir granule formulation is considered to be bioequivalent with the capsule in healthy subjects when administered in the fasted state.[1]
- Commercially prepared cefdinir solid dispersions exhibited greater solubility, dissolution, and potential bioavailability than the suspension formulation.[2]

Drug-Nutrition Interactions
- Drug may influence nutrition status directly or indirectly:
  - CNS: headache, malaise, fatigue
  - GI: anorexia, glossitis, nausea, vomiting, diarrhea (including *Clostridium difficile*–associated), transient increases in LFTs
  - Metabolic: dysglycemia
  - Other: arthralgia and edema (as part of a severe hypersensitivity reaction)
- No data on the influence of malnutrition or obesity on drug disposition.
- Influence of food on oral absorption or bioavailability:
  - A high-fat meal may reduce oral bioavailability by ~10% (capsules) or ~30% (suspension).
  - Iron-containing and magnesium-containing preparations may reduce oral bioavailability, requiring a separation of 2 hours before and after drug administration.

Recommendations

Gastric	• Disperse capsule contents in water just prior to administration. • Alternative: Dilute reconstituted suspension in water (1:1) just prior to administration. • Consider holding EN at least 1 hour before and after drug administration.
Postpyloric	• As above. • Monitor for any unexpected change in effect.
Other	• As with all antimicrobials, consider parenteral alternative for acutely ill patients to ensure therapeutic concentrations.

References
1. Chen J, Jiang B, Lou H, et al. Bioequivalence evaluation of cefdinir in healthy fasting subjects. *Arzneimitt.* 2012;62:9–13.
2. Cho H-J, Jee J-P, Kang J-Y, et al. Cefdinir solid dispersion composed of hydrophilic polymers with enhanced solubility, dissolution, and bioavailability in rats. *Molecules.* 2017;22:E280. doi: 10.3390/molecules22020280.

Cefuroxime Axetil

Product Availability

Solid	• Tablet: 125 mg, 250 mg, 500 mg (base) (Ceftin® [GSK]; others)
Liquid	• Powder for oral suspension: 125 mg/5 mL, 250 mg/5 mL (base) (Ceftin® [GSK]; others)

Physicochemical (drug)

Molecular weight: • 424.39 (axetil 510.47)	Permeability: • Log P –0.16 • Log D –1.91 (pH 7.4)	Water solubility: • 200 mg/mL
pKa: • 2.45	Classification: • BCS Class 4; BDDCS Class 3	

Pharmaceutical (product)

Solid	• Tablet products may be film-coated but may disperse in water (20 mL) in about 1 minute. • Do not crush (risk of sensitization, and taste is unacceptable for oral administration).
Liquid	• Oral suspension (reconstituted): o pH n/a o Osmolality n/a o Viscosity n/a o May contain acesulfame potassium, aspartame, and sucrose o Store reconstituted oral suspension at 2°C–8°C; use within 10 days. o Shake well before drawing up dose for administration.
Note	• Tablet and oral suspension are not bioequivalent.

Pharmacokinetic (patient)

Absorption	• Specific site not known, but mainly in proximal small intestine; t_{max} 2–3 hours after an oral dose (fed state) • Bioavailability of tablet ~37% (fasted) and ~52% (fed); suspension bioavailability ~90% of tablet bioavailability
Transport	• Uptake transport (intestinal, renal tubular) is a saturable process. • Plasma protein binding ~33%–50% • V_d ~9.3–15.8 L/1.73 m^2
Metabolism	• Cefuroxime axetil (prodrug) is hydrolyzed to cefuroxime (active) by esterases in the gut mucosa and blood. • Cefuroxime is eliminated renally unchanged. • Cl ~0.6 mL/min/kg

Enteral Administration and Nutrition Considerations

Compatibility, Stability, and Bioavailability Considerations

- For oral administration, tablets (125 mg or 250 mg) dispersed in 40 mL of cold (5°C) apple juice (Gerber, Mott's Natural, and Tropicana) remained stable (HPLC analysis) for up to 24 hours at room temperature; pH and osmolality of the beverages were not reported.[1]
- For oral administration, tablets (125 mg or 250 mg) dispersed in 40 mL orange juice (Tropicana), grape juice (Welch's) or chocolate milk (Nestle's) remained stable (HPLC analysis) at 2 hours; pH and osmolality of the beverages were not reported.[2]
- Extemporaneously compounded oral suspensions (125 mg/5 mL, 250 mg/5 mL) prepared from tablets in OraPlus, OraSweet and peppermint oil, stored in amber plastic bottles and polypropylene syringes at 5°C and 25°C, remained stable (HPLC analysis) for 7 days (room temperature) and 17 days (refrigerated).[3]
- An extemporaneously compounded oral suspension (10 mg/mL) prepared from tablets in simple syrup (three different formulations ranging in pH from 3.3 to 6.8) and stored in amber bottles at 4°C–6°C remained stable (HPLC analysis) for 28 days.[4]
- Commercially prepared nanoparticles improved the dissolution and bioavailability of cefuroxime.[5]

Drug-Nutrition Interactions

- Drug may influence nutrition status directly or indirectly:
  - CNS: headache, somnolence, dizziness
  - GI: anorexia, glossitis, nausea, vomiting, epigastric burning, GI bleeding, abdominal pain, diarrhea (including *Clostridium difficile*–associated), transient increases in LFTs
  - Other: muscle cramps/stiffness, weakness, arthralgia
- Influence of malnutrition or obesity on drug disposition:
  - An animal model of malnutrition revealed significant decreases in drug bioavailability: ~20%–35% relative reduction depending on the degree of energy or protein deficits.[6]
- Influence of food on oral absorption or bioavailability:
  - Food increases the absolute oral bioavailability by ~10%–15%.[7,8]
    - Administer tablets after food.
    - Administer suspension with food.

Recommendations

Gastric	• Disperse tablet in water (20 mL) prior to administration. • Alternative: Dilute reconstituted suspension with water (1:1) just prior to administration via a tube ≥12 Fr. • No need to separate from continuous enteral feeds beyond the time required to flush-administer-flush; administer tablets just after an intermittent feed.
Postpyloric	• Disperse tablet in water (20 mL) prior to administration. • Monitor for any unexpected change in effect.
Other	• As with all antimicrobials, consider parenteral alternative for acutely ill patients to ensure therapeutic concentrations.

References

1. St. Claire RL, Wilbourne DK, Caudill WL. Stability of cefuroxime axetil in apple juice. *Pediatr Infect Dis J.* 1988;7:744.
2. St. Claire RL, Caudill WL. Stability of cefuroxime axetil in beverages. *Am J Hosp Pharm.* 1989;46:256.
3. Farrington EA, Bawdon RA, Fox JL. Stability of cefuroxime axetil suspensions. *ASHP Midyr Clin Meet.* 1991:580E.
4. Pramar Y, Gupta VD, Bethea C, et al. Stability of cefuroxime axetil in suspensions. *J Clin Pharm Ther.* 1991;16:341–344.
5. Dhumal RS, Biradar SV, Yamamura S, et al. Preparation of amorphous cefuroxime axetil nanoparticles by sonoprecipitation for enhancement of bioavailability. *Eur J Pharm Biopharm.* 2008;70:109–115.
6. González-Hernández I, Jung-Cook H, Sotelo A. Effect of malnutrition on the pharmacokinetics of cefuroxime axetil in young rats. *J Pharm Pharmaceut Sci.* 2008;11:9–21.
7. Harding SM. The absolute bioavailability of oral cefuroxime axetil in male and female volunteers after fasting and after food. *J Antimicrob Chemother.* 1984;13:191–196.
8. Finn A, Straughn A, Meyer M, Chubb J. Effect of dose and food on the bioavailability of cefuroxime axetil. *Biopharm Drug Dispos.* 1987;8:519–526.

Celecoxib

Product Availability

Solid	Capsule: 50 mg, 100 mg, 200 mg, 400 mg (Celebrex® [GD Searle]; others)

Physicochemical (drug)

Molecular weight: • 381.38	Permeability: • LogP 4.37 (calc) • Log D 3.00 (pH 7) (calc)	Water solubility: • ≤0.01 mg/mL
pKa: • 11.1	Classification: • BCS Class 2; BDDCS Class 2	

Pharmaceutical (product)

Solid	• Capsule may be opened, with contents dispersed in water.

Pharmacokinetic (patient)

Absorption	• Specific site not known, but drug is likely absorbed throughout the GI tract; t_{max} ~2–3 hours after an oral dose • Bioavailability ~22%–40%
Transport	• Plasma protein binding ~97%, mostly to albumin • V_d ~7.14 L/kg
Metabolism	• Metabolized by CYP2C9 to inactives, including a carboxylic acid that itself may be conjugated (with glucuronic acid) before elimination in feces and urine • Cl ~500 mL/min

Enteral Administration and Nutrition Considerations

Compatibility, Stability, and Bioavailability Considerations

- An extemporaneously compounded oral suspension (10 mg/mL) prepared from capsules in OraBlend, stored in amber polyvinyl chloride plastic bottles at 5°C and 23°C, had a pH of ~4.4–4.5 and remained stable (HPLC analysis) for 93 days.[1]
- When administered as a solution, oral bioavailability may be considerably higher than the intact capsule.[2]
- An oral solution being developed had a shorter time to peak and an oral bioavailability 140% of the similarly dosed intact capsule in healthy subjects.[3]
- An amorphous nanoparticle formulation of celecoxib as a dry powder, administered as an aqueous suspension, can improve oral bioavailability compared with commercial capsules.[4]
- Another attempt to control the crystallinity of the drug molecule also resulted in improved dissolution and oral bioavailability in an animal model.[5]

- Capsule contents mixed with apple sauce (3 brands tested, pH 3.3–4.0) were stable for 6 hours at refrigeration, although with slightly reduced bioavailability, when administered orally in healthy subjects.[6]

Drug-Nutrition Interactions
- Drug may influence nutrition status directly or indirectly:
  - Weight gain
  - CNS: headache, dizziness, insomnia, neuropathy, blurred vision
  - GI: anorexia, nausea, dry mouth, altered taste, stomatitis, esophagitis, gastritis, dyspepsia, abdominal pain, diarrhea, melena, rare intestinal obstruction, perforation, and pancreatitis and hepatitis
  - Metabolic: anemia, albuminuria, azotemia, hyponatremia, hyperglycemia, hypercholesterolemia, hypokalemia
  - Other: peripheral edema, arthralgia, myalgia, leg cramps, CK elevation
- Influence of malnutrition or obesity on drug disposition:
  - Lower body weight, as seen in older adults, is associated with higher bioavailability.
- Influence of food on oral absorption or bioavailability:
  - A high-fat meal (24 g) increased oral bioavailability (10%–20%) compared with a meal containing 8 g fat or fasting.
  - The influence of a meal on oral bioavailability may not be clinically significant.[2]
  - Incorporating results of dissolution tests (in simulated GI fluids) into physiologically based pharmacokinetic modeling adequately predicts food effect, including a 1.3-fold increase in oral bioavailability.[7]

Recommendations

Gastric	• If no therapeutic alternative is available, disperse capsule contents in water prior to administration. • No need to hold EN beyond the time required to flush-administer-flush.
Postpyloric	• Not recommended.

References

1. Donnelly RF, Pascuet E, Ma C, et al. Stability of celecoxib oral suspension. *Can J Hosp Pharm*. 2009;62:464–468.
2. Paulson SK, Vaughn MB, Jessen SM, et al. Pharmacokinetics of celecoxib after oral administration in dogs and humans: effect of food and site of absorption. *J Pharmacol Exp Ther*. 2001;297:638–645.
3. Pal A, Shenoy S, Gautam A, et al. Pharmacokinetics of DFN-15, a novel oral solution of celecoxib, versus celecoxib 400-mg capsules: a randomized crossover study in fasting healthy volunteers. *Clin Drug Investig*. 2017;37:937–946.
4. Morgen M, Bloom C, Beyerinck R, et al. Polymeric nanoparticles for increases oral bioavailability and rapid absorption using celecoxib as a model of a low-solubility, high-permeability drug. *Pharm Res*. 2012;29:427–440.

5. Zhu W, Zhao Q, Sun C, et al. Mesoporous carbon with spherical pores as a carrier for celecoxib with needle-like crystallinity: improve dissolution rate and bioavailability. *Mater Sci Engineer C Mater Biol Appl.* 2014;39:13–20.
6. Data on file (141, 142) with Pfizer, Inc; 2016.
7. Shono Y, Jantratid E, Janssen N, et al. Prediction of food effects on the absorption of celecoxib based on biorelevant dissolution testing coupled with physiologically based pharmacokinetic modeling. *Eur J Pharm Biopharm.* 2009;73:107–114.

Cephalexin

Product Availability

Solid	• Tablet: 250 mg, 500 mg (various) • Capsule: 250 mg, 500 mg, 750 mg (Keflex® [Pragma Pharms]; others)
Liquid	• Powder for oral suspension: 125 mg/5 mL, 250 mg/5 mL (various)

Physicochemical (drug)

Molecular weight: • 347.40	Permeability: • LogP –0.67 • LogD –5.67 (pH 6.5), –6.57 or –2.40 (pH 7.4)	Water solubility: • 1–2 mg/mL
pKa: • 5.2, 7.3	Classification: • BCS Class n/a; BDDCS Class 3	

Pharmaceutical (product)

Solid	• Tablet products are often film-coated. • Do not crush tablet or manipulate capsule contents (risk of sensitization).

Liquid	• Suspension (reconstituted):
	• pH 3.0–5.5 (250 mg/5 mL)[1]
	• Osmolality:
	  ○ Reported as 1950 mOsm/kg or 2445 mOsm/kg (250 mg/5 mL products)[2,3]
	  ○ 2220 mOsm/L (105.2 mg/mL product)[4]
	• Viscosity n/a
	• May contain sorbitol and saccharin; strawberry-flavored
	• Reconstituted oral suspension should be refrigerated and used within 10 days.
	• Shake well before drawing up dose for administration.

Pharmacokinetic (patient)

Absorption	• Likely absorbed in duodenum (ie, narrow absorption window); t_{max} ~1 hour after an oral dose • Bioavailability ~83%–90%
Transport	• Substrate for peptide transporter(s) (eg, PEPT1) uptake and MRP2 efflux • Plasma protein binding ~10%–15% • V_d ~0.26 L/kg
Metabolism	• Unmetabolized, the drug is eliminated renally unchanged. • Cl ~4.3 mL/min/kg

Enteral Administration and Nutrition Considerations

Compatibility, Stability, and Bioavailability Considerations
- The drug is acid-stable but degrades at intestinal conditions (pH 6.5).
- Expect ~25% loss of drug within 24 hours in an alkaline (pH 7–8) solution.[5]
- Altering drug excipients to prolong the time in stomach (ie, "gastro-floating" delivery system) may increase oral bioavailability but is intended for oral administration.[6]
- Admixtures of the oral suspension (5 mL) with EN formulations (15–240 mL of Ensure, Ensure HN, Ensure Plus, Ensure Plus HN, Osmolite, or Osmolite HN) appeared physically compatible (no granulation or phase separation).[1,7]
- Admixtures of the oral suspension (10 mL) with EN formulations (10 mL of Enrich, TwoCal HN, or Vivonex T.E.N.) appeared physically compatible (no granulation or phase separation).[8]
- The admixture of capsule contents (250 mg) or oral suspension (250 mg/5 mL), first dispersed in deionized water (10 mL), then with 240 mL of EN formulations (Isocal [8.1 g protein, 10.5 g fat, 31.5 g carbohydrate], Sustacal [14.5 g protein, 5.5 g fat, 33.1 g carbohydrate], or Sustacal HC [14.4 g protein, 13.6 g fat, 45.0 g carbohydrate]), indicated drug stability (HPLC analysis) for up to 24 hours at 24°C in all three formulas (using capsule contents) but in only two for the suspension (which was not stable in Sustacal HC).[9]

Drug-Nutrition Interactions
- Drug may influence nutrition status directly or indirectly:
  - CNS: headache, somnolence, dizziness
  - GI: anorexia, glossitis, nausea, vomiting, epigastric burning, GI bleeding, abdominal pain, diarrhea (including *Clostridium difficile*–associated), transient increases in LFTs
  - Other: muscle cramps/stiffness, weakness, arthralgia
- No data on the influence of malnutrition or obesity on drug disposition.
- Influence of food on oral absorption or bioavailability:
  - Food may decrease rate of absorption but has no significant influence on oral bioavailability.
  - The concurrent administration of zinc 56 mg (as sulfate) reduced oral bioavailability (~27%) and the time that drug concentration remained above the MIC (~22%), compared with cephalexin alone; the findings were similar when zinc was administered 3 hours before the drug.[10]

Recommendations

Gastric	• Dilute reconstituted oral suspension with water (at least 1:1) prior to administration. • No need to hold EN beyond the time required to flush-administer-flush.
Postpyloric	• As above. • Jejunal administration risks decreased absorption. • Monitor for any unexpected change in effect.
Other	• As with all antimicrobials, consider parenteral alternative for acutely ill patients to ensure therapeutic concentrations.

References

1. Cutie AJ, Altman E, Lenkel L. Compatibility of enteral products with commonly employed drug additives. *JPEN J Parenter Enteral Nutr.* 1983;7:186–191.
2. Niemiec PW, Vanderveen TW, Morrison JI, et al. Gastrointestinal disorders caused by medication and electrolyte solution osmolality during enteral nutrition. *JPEN J Parenter Enteral Nutr.* 1983;7:387–389.
3. Dickerson RN, Melnik G. Osmolality of oral drug solutions and suspensions. *Am J Hosp Pharm.* 1988;45:832–834.
4. Obladen M, Mutz A. Orale medikation bei frühgeborenen? *Monatsschr Kinderheilkd.* 1985;133:669–674.
5. Puigdellivol E, Carral ME, Dalmau JM. Comparative study of cefadroxil and cephalexin in solid form and in solution. *Afinidad.* 1981;38:337–342.
6. Yin L, Qin C, Chen K, et al. Gastro-floating tablets of cephalexin: preparation and in vitro/in vivo evaluation. *Int J Pharm.* 2013;452:241–248.
7. Altman E, Cutie AJ. Compatibility of enteral products with commonly employed drug additives. *Nutr Supp Serv.* 1984;4:8–17.
8. Burns PE, McCall L, Wirsching R. Physical compatibility of enteral formulas with various common medications. *J Am Diet Assoc.* 1988;88:1094–1096.
9. Strom JG, Miller SW. Stability of drugs with enteral nutrition formulas. *DICP Ann Pharmacother.* 1990;24:130–134.
10. Ding Y, Jia YY, Li F, et al. The effect of staggered administration of zinc sulfate on the pharmacokinetics of oral cephalexin. *Br J Clin Pharmacol.* 2011;73:422–427.

Cetirizine Hydrochloride

Product Availability

Solid	• Tablet: o Immediate-release: 5 mg, 10 mg (Zyrtec® [J&J Consumer]; others) o Chewable: 5 mg, 10 mg (various) o Orally disintegrating: 10 mg (various)
Liquid	• Oral solution: 5 mg/5 mL (various)

Physicochemical (drug)

Molecular weight: • 388.90 (salt 461.81)	Permeability: • LogP 1.70 • LogD –0.31 (pH 7.4)	Water solubility: • 0.1 mg/mL
pKa: • 2.70, 3.57, 7.56	Classification: • BCS Class 1; BDDCS Class 3	

Pharmaceutical (product)

Solid	• Tablet products may disperse in water.
Liquid	• Oral solution: o pH 4–5 o Osmolality n/a o Viscosity n/a, but less than isotonic EN o May contain propylene glycol, sorbitol, and sucralose o May be stored at refrigeration or room temperature
Note	• Solid and liquid products are considered to be bioequivalent.

Pharmacokinetic (patient)

Absorption	• Proximal intestine; t_{max} within 1 hour after an oral dose • Bioavailability ~90%
Transport	• Plasma protein-binding ~93% • V_d ~0.39–0.6 L/kg
Metabolism	• Most of the drug is eliminated renally unchanged, although some may undergo metabolism (oxidative dealkylation). • Cl ~53 mL/min

Enteral Administration and Nutrition Considerations

Compatibility, Stability, and Bioavailability Considerations
• The orally disintegrating tablet formulations, which are meant to rapidly form a suspension in saliva, disintegrate in 16–22 seconds in 10 mL of aqueous buffer (pH 6.28, 37°C).[1]

Drug-Nutrition Interactions

- Drug may influence nutrition status directly or indirectly:
  - CNS: somnolence, fatigue, dizziness
  - GI: dry mouth, nausea, vomiting, abdominal pain, diarrhea
- No data on the influence of malnutrition or obesity on drug disposition.
- Influence of food on oral absorption or bioavailability:
  - Food may slow the rate of drug absorption but without a significant influence on oral bioavailability.

Recommendations

Gastric	• Dilute oral solution in water (1:1) prior to administration. • No need to hold EN beyond the time required to flush-administer-flush.
Postpyloric	• As above. • Monitor for any unexpected change in effect.

Reference

1. Subramanian S, Sankar V, Manakadan AA, et al. Formulation and evaluation of cetirizine dihydrochloride orodispersible tablet. *Pak J Pharm Sci.* 2010;23:232–235.

Ciprofloxacin Anhydrous or Hydrochloride

Product Availability

Solid	• Tablet (HCl): 100 mg, 250 mg, 500 mg, 750 mg (base) (Cipro® [Bayer]; others) • Tablet extended-release (HCl + anhydrous): 500 mg, 1000 mg (various)
Liquid	• Microcapsules for oral suspension (anhydrous): 250 mg/5 mL, 500 mg/5 mL (base) (Cipro® [Bayer]; others)

Physicochemical (drug)

Molecular weight: • 331.35 (salt 367.81)	Permeability: • LogP 0.28, –0.94 (37°C), –1.70 (25°C) • LogD –1.21 (pH 7.4)	Water solubility: • 0.15 mg/mL (base, neutral pH, 37°C) • 36 mg/mL (base, acidic pH, 25°C)
pKa: • 6.09, 8.74	Classification: • BCS Class 4; BDDCS Class 4	

Pharmaceutical (product)

Solid	• Tablet products are film-coated; they require crushing to disperse in water. • Do not split, chew, or crush extended-release tablet.

Liquid	• Oral suspension:
	   ○ Microcapsules for oral suspension should not be chewed/crushed.
	   ○ Not intended for enteral administration
	   ○ pH n/a
	   ○ Osmolality n/a
	   ○ Viscosity n/a
	   ○ Suspension diluent may contain MCTs and sucrose; strawberry-flavored
	   ○ Store reconstituted oral suspension at 25°C; use within 14 days.
	   ○ Do not add water to the oral suspension.

Note	• Extended-release tablet is not interchangeable with immediate-release tablet or oral suspension.

Pharmacokinetic (patient)

Absorption	• Duodenum; t_{max} ~1 hour after an oral dose • Bioavailability ~50%–85%
Transport	• Substrate for BCRP efflux (at jejunum) and possibly also an MRP efflux transporter[1] • Plasma protein binding ~16%–43% • V_d ~2–3.5 L/kg

Metabolism	• Partially metabolized (liver) to 4 or more metabolites with limited antimicrobial activity; subsequent elimination of metabolites and parent drug in urine and feces • Cl ~7.6 mL/min/kg

Enteral Administration and Nutrition Considerations

Compatibility, Stability, and Bioavailability Considerations

- A 2.5% aqueous solution is expected to have a pH of 3.0–4.5 while remaining sensitive to light.
- Solubility and dissolution are limited in aqueous environments with intestinal pH; as a zwitterion, solubility is best at pH<5 and pH>10.[2]
- Altered drug morphology (eg, ciprofloxacin saccharinate) can improve dissolution rate and bioavailability.[3]
- Extemporaneously compounded oral suspensions (50 mg/mL) prepared from tablets (750 mg) in OraPlus and simple syrup (1:1), stored in amber, plastic bottles and at 24°C–26°C or 3°C–5°C, remained stable (HPLC analysis) for 56 days; the suspension pH remained ~4.5 throughout.[4,5]
- Crushed ciprofloxacin tablets are most stable in water, compared with other common foods/beverages.[6]
- Tablets, including the 750 mg strength, can be crushed and/or dispersed in water (50 mL).
- The admixture of a crushed tablet (500 mg) with an EN product (Ensure, 240 mL) was incompatible, decreasing drug availability (83%); this did not occur when the drug was admixed in water or water containing calcium and/or magnesium and regardless of temperature (5°C–37°C).[7]
- When a 750 mg tablet was administered orally with 240 mL of EN (Resource), there was a 25% reduction in drug absorption.[8]
- The administration of EN (Ensure), 120 mL every 30 minutes for 5 doses, including a 750 mg tablet crushed and mixed into the second aliquot, resulted in a 28% relative decrease in oral bioavailability.[9]
- Administration of 750 mg tablets every 12 hours by nasogastric tube required crushing and diluting in 50 mL sterile water (with an additional 30 mL sterile water flush) in acutely ill patients who received EN (Pulmocare) continuously; drug absorption was noted to be reduced.[10]
- Another group of acutely ill patients receiving continuous EN (Normo-Réal Fibers) through a nasogastric tube (8 Fr, 110 cm) received 750 mg tablets crushed and suspended in 20 mL water before administration, followed by 40 mL water flush; this resulted in lower drug bioavailability.[11]

Drug-Nutrition Interactions
- Drug may influence nutrition status directly or indirectly:
  - CNS: agitation, anxiety, insomnia, confusion, depression, blurred vision
  - GI: anorexia, bad taste, oral pain, nausea, vomiting, abdominal discomfort, diarrhea (including *Clostridium difficile*–associated), abnormal LFTs, rare hepatotoxicity
  - Metabolic: hyperamylasemia, hypoglycemia, crystalluria
  - Other: peripheral neuropathy (sensory or sensorimotor), weakness, arthralgia, tendonitis
- Influence of malnutrition or obesity on drug disposition:
  - The body weight–normalized volume of distribution is slightly lower in obesity (distributing into only ~45% of the excess body weight), while drug clearance is increased, suggesting that dosing may be based on an appropriately adjusted body weight.[12,13]
- Influence of food on oral absorption or bioavailability:
  - No known influence of food on oral drug bioavailability.
  - Dairy products (eg, milk, yogurt) or calcium-fortified products (eg, orange juice) can significantly reduce oral drug bioavailability (by at least 30%).
  - Divalent- and trivalent-containing mineral supplements or antacids can reduce oral drug bioavailability.
  - Drug administration with a viscous soup (500–5000 mPa·s) reduced drug dissolution but was not expected to alter oral bioavailability.[14]
  - Increasing the enteral dose may not overcome the interaction with EN nor result in equivalent therapeutic outcomes as a parenteral dose.[15]
  - Orange juice (~350 mL) may reduce oral bioavailability (~22%) when administered with or within 4 hours of drug administration.[16]

Recommendations

Gastric	• Crush and/or disperse tablet in water (25–50 mL) just prior to administration. • Consider holding continuous EN by 1–2 hours before and after drug administration; separate drug administration by 2 hours from intermittent EN and any other products containing 500 mg or more calcium.
Postpyloric	• As above. • Significant risks for lower absorption. • Monitor for any unexpected change in effect.
Other	• As with all antimicrobials, consider parenteral alternative for acutely ill patients to ensure therapeutic concentrations.

References

1. Haslam IS, Wright JA, O'Reilly DA, et al. Intestinal ciprofloxacin efflux: the role of breast cancer resistance protein (ABCG2). *Drug Metab Disp.* 2011;39:2321–2328.
2. Olivera ME, Manzo RH, Junginger HE, et al. Biowaiver monographs for immediate release solid oral dosage forms: ciprofloxacin hydrochloride. *J Pharm Sci.* 2011;100:22–33.
3. Singh P, Chadha R. A new polymorph of ciprofloxacin saccharinate: structural characterization and pharmaceutical profile. *J Pharm Biomed Anal.* 2017;146:7–14.
4. Johnson CE, Wong DV, Hoppe HL, Bhatt-Mehta V. Stability of ciprofloxacin in an extemporaneous oral liquid dosage form. *Int J Pharm Compd.* 1998;2:314–317.
5. Nahata MC, Morosco RS, Hipple TF, et al. Development of stable oral suspensions of ciprofloxacin. *J Appl Ther Res.* 2000;3:61–65.
6. Sadrieh N, Brower J, Yu L, et al. Stability, dose uniformity, and palatability of three counterterrorism drugs: human subject and electronic tongue studies. *Pharm Res.* 2005; 22:1747–1756.
7. Wright DH, Pietz SL, Konstantinides FN, Rotschafer JC. Decreased in vitro fluoroquinolone concentrations after admixture with an enteral feeding formulation. *JPEN J Parenter Enteral Nutr.* 2000;24:42–48.
8. Piccolo ML, Toossi Z, Goldman M. Effect of coadministration of a nutritional supplement on ciprofloxacin absorption. *Am J Hosp Pharm.* 1994;51:2697–2699.
9. Mueller BA, Brierton DG, Abel SR, et al. Effects of enteral feeding with Ensure on oral bioavailabilies of ofloxacin and ciprofloxacin. *Antimicrob Agents Chemother.* 1994;38: 2101–2105.
10. Cohn SM, Sawyer MD, Burns GA, et al. Enteric absorption of ciprofloxacin during tube feeding in the critically ill. *J Antimicrob Chemother.* 1996;38:871–876.
11. Mimoz O, Binter V, Jacolot A, et al. Pharmacokinetics and absolute bioavailability of ciprofloxacin administered through a nasogastric tube with continuous enteral feeding to critically ill patients. *Intensive Care Med.* 1998;24:1047–1051.
12. Allard S, Kinzig M, Boivin G, Sorgel F, LeBel M. Intravenous ciprofloxacin disposition in obesity. *Clin Pharmacol Ther.* 1993;54:368–373.
13. Caldwell JB, Nilsen AK. Intravenous ciprofloxacin dosing in a morbidly obese patient. *Ann Pharmacother.* 1994;28:806.
14. Radwan A, Zaid AN, Jaradat N, Odeh Y. Food effect: the combined effect of media pH and viscosity on the gastrointestinal absorption of ciprofloxacin tablet. *Eur J Pharm Sci.* 2017;101:100–106.
15. Chui D, Cheng L, Tejani AM. Clinical equivalency of ciprofloxacin 750 mg enterally and 400 mg intravenously for patients receiving enteral feeding: systematic review. *Can J Hosp Pharm.* 2009;62:127–134.
16. Bailey DG. Fruit juice inhibition of uptake transport: a new type of food-drug interaction. *Br J Clin Pharmacol.* 2010;70:645–655.

Citalopram Hydrobromide

Product Availability

Solid	• Tablet: 10 mg, 20 mg, 40 mg (base) (Celexa® [Allergan]; others)
Liquid	• Oral solution: 10 mg/5 mL (base) (various)

Physicochemical (drug)

Molecular weight: • 324.40 (salt 405.31) • Racemic mixture (50:50) of R- and S-enantiomers	Permeability: • LogP 3.41 • LogD 0.74 (pH 7.4)	Water solubility: • 0.03 mg/mL
pKa: • 9.5	Classification: • BCS Class 1; BDDCS Class 2	

Pharmaceutical (product)

Solid	• Tablet products are often film-coated.

Liquid	• Solution:
	   o pH n/a
	   o Osmolality n/a
	   o Viscosity n/a
	   o Clear, colorless with paraben preservatives
	   o May contain sorbitol and propylene glycol; peppermint-flavored
	   o Store at controlled room temperature.

Note	• Tablet and solution are considered bioequivalent.

Pharmacokinetic (patient)

Absorption	• Specific site not known; t_{max} ~2–4 hours after an oral dose • Bioavailability ~80% (slightly higher for liquid)
Transport	• Substrate for P-glycoprotein efflux • Plasma protein binding ~80% • V_d ~12 L/kg
Metabolism	• Metabolized to ≥3 metabolites (via CYP3A4 and CYP2C19), one of which (demethylcitalopram) is further metabolized by CYP2D6, with some parent drug eliminated unchanged • Cl ~330 mL/min

Enteral Administration and Nutrition Considerations

Compatibility, Stability, and Bioavailability Considerations
• No data are available.

Drug-Nutrition Interactions
- Drug may influence nutrition status directly or indirectly:
  - Weight loss or gain
  - CNS: somnolence, insomnia, anxiety, fatigue, tremor, abnormal gait
  - GI: dry mouth, anorexia, nausea, vomiting, dyspepsia, abdominal pain, diarrhea
  - Metabolic: abnormal glucose tolerance, hyponatremia, SIADH
  - Other: arthralgia, myalgia
- No data on the influence of malnutrition or obesity on drug disposition.
- Influence of food on oral absorption or bioavailability:
  - No significant influence of food on oral bioavailability.

Recommendations

Gastric	• Disperse non-film-coated tablet in water (10–20 mL) prior to administration. • No need to hold EN beyond the time required to flush-administer-flush.
Postpyloric	• As above. • Monitor for any unexpected change in effect.
Other	• Correct hypokalemia and hypomagnesemia prior to administration.

Clarithromycin

Product Availability

Solid	• Tablet: 250 mg, 500 mg (Biaxin® Filmtab [Abbvie]; others) • Tablet (extended-release, film-coated): 500 mg, 1000 mg (Biaxin® XL Filmtab [Abbott]; others)
Liquid	• Granules for oral suspension: 125 mg/5 mL, 250 mg/5 mL (Biaxin® Granules [Abbvie]; others)

Physicochemical (drug)

Molecular weight: • 747.96	Permeability: • LogP 3.16 • LogD n/a	Water solubility: • ≤2 mg/mL
pKa: • 8.99	Classification: • BCS Class 2; BDDCS Class 3	

Pharmaceutical (product)

Solid	• Tablet products are film-coated and are unlikely to disperse well in water even after crushing. • Do not crush extended-release tablets.

Liquid	• Oral suspension (reconstituted):
	    o pH n/a
	    o Osmolality n/a
	    o Viscosity is greater than EN formulations and expected to occlude small-bore enteral access devices.
	    o May contain maltodextrin and sucrose; fruit punch–flavored
	    o Maintain reconstituted suspension at controlled room temperature (do not refrigerate) and use within 14 days.

Pharmacokinetic (patient)

Absorption	• Small bowel (jejunum); t_{max} ~2–3 hours after an oral dose (immediate-release) • Bioavailability ~50%–55%
Transport	• Substrate for P-glycoprotein and possibly MRP efflux • At usual serum concentrations, plasma protein binding ~42%–50% • V_d ~2.6 L/kg
Metabolism	• Rapidly metabolized to the active 14-hydroxy-clarithromycin (via N-demethylation and hydroxylation), with additional minor metabolites reported, followed by both renal and non-renal elimination • Cl ~1 L/min (lower capacity at single doses ≥1.2 g)

Enteral Administration and Nutrition Considerations

Compatibility, Stability, and Bioavailability Considerations

- Drug solubility is pH-dependent with improved solubility at lower (acidic) pH; however, chemical stability is worse under acidic conditions.
- Undiluted suspension (500 mg dose) was administered via nasogastric tube followed by 30 mL water flush without clinical problems when EN and other medications were avoided from 4 hours before to 2 hours following drug administration.[1]
- Available suspension product has been shown to have comparative bioavailability to the reference product.[2]
- Ideally, bioavailability evaluations (fed or fasted conditions) would include the active metabolite (14-hydroxy-clarithromycin) as well.[3]
- An amorphous solid dispersion formulation may improve drug stability.[4]
- Differing excipients can alter dissolution and increase potential oral bioavailability.[5]
- Altering drug excipients to prolong the time in the stomach (ie, "gastro-floating" delivery system) may increase oral bioavailability, but it is intended for oral administration.[6]

Drug-Nutrition Interactions

- Drug may influence nutrition status directly or indirectly:
  - CNS: headache, behavioral change and confusion, tremor
  - GI: abnormal taste, stomatitis, glossitis, anorexia, nausea, dyspepsia, abdominal discomfort, diarrhea, pancreatitis, abnormal LFT elevations
  - Metabolic: transient elevation of BUN with or without elevation of serum creatinine
- Influence of malnutrition or obesity on drug disposition:
  - A higher systemic drug exposure, despite no change in volume of distribution but based on a lower drug clearance, may occur in protein-energy malnutrition.
- Influence of food on oral absorption or bioavailability:
  - Food may delay oral absorption but does not significantly influence oral bioavailability.
  - Extended-release tablets benefit from administration with food.
  - Grapefruit juice is not expected to influence oral bioavailability.

Recommendations

Gastric	• Dilute suspension with water (at least 1:1) just prior to administration. • No need to hold EN beyond the time required to flush-administer-flush.
Postpyloric	• As above. • Monitor for any unexpected change in effect.
Other	• As with all antimicrobials, consider parenteral alternative for acutely ill patients to ensure therapeutic concentrations.

References

1. Fish DN, Abraham E. Pharmacokinetics of a clarithromycin suspension administered via nasogastric tube to seriously ill patients. *Antimicrob Agents Chemother.* 1999;43: 1277–1280.
2. Zakeri-Milani P, Valizadeh H, Ghanbarzadeh S, Nemati M. Pharmacokinetics and comparative bioavailability study of two clarithromycin suspensions following administration of a single oral dose to healthy volunteers. *Arzneimittelforschung.* 2009; 59:429–432.
3. Benninger P, Cooper A, Moisan R, et al. A comparative clarithromycin bioavailability study: determination of clarithromycin and 14-(R)-hydroxyclarithromycin under fasting and fed conditions. *Int J Clin Pharmacol Ther.* 2004;42:342–349.
4. Pereira JM, Mejia-Ariza R, Ilevbare GA, et al. Interplay of degradation, dissolution and stabilization of clarithromycin and its amorphous solid dispersions. *Mol Pharm.* 2013;10: 4640–4653.
5. Ullah S, Shah MR, Shoaib M, et al. Development of a biocompatible creatinine-based niosomal delivery system for enhanced oral bioavailability of clarithromycin. *Drug Deliv.* 2016;23:3480–3491.
6. Reddy AB, Reddy ND. Development of multiple-unit floating drug delivery system of clarithromycin: formulation, in vitro dissolution by modified dissolution apparatus, in vivo radiographic studies in human volunteers. *Drug Res.* 2017;67:412–418.

Clindamycin Hydrochloride or Palmitate Hydrochloride

Product Availability

Solid	• Capsules (hydrochloride): 75 mg, 150 mg, 300 mg (base) (Cleocin HCl® [Pharmacia & Upjohn]; others)
Liquid	• Granules for oral solution (palmitate hydrochloride): 75 mg/ 5 mL (base) (Cleocin Pediatric® [Pharmacia & Upjohn]; others)

Physicochemical (drug)

Molecular weight: • 424.99 o hydrochloride 461.45 o palmitate hydrochloride 699.85	Permeability: • LogP 2.16 • LogD n/a	Water solubility: • 40–400 mg/mL (25°C)
pKa: • 7.6	Classification: • BCS Class n/a; BDDCS Class 1	

Pharmaceutical (product)

Solid	• Avoid inhalation of (or cross-contamination with) capsule contents.
Liquid	• Oral solution (reconstituted): o pH 3.0–5.5 o Osmolality n/a o Viscosity n/a o May contain sucrose; cherry-flavored o Store reconstituted oral solution at controlled room temperature; do not refrigerate; use within 14 days.

Pharmacokinetic (patient)

Absorption	• Specific site not known; t_{max} within 1 hour after oral dose • Bioavailability approaches 90%.
Transport	• Plasma protein binding ~93% • V_d ~0.8–1.1 L/kg
Metabolism	• Partially metabolized to several metabolites (eg, N-demethyl-clindamycin, clindamycin sulfoxide) • Parent and metabolites eliminated through urine and feces • Cl ~0.3 L/h/kg

Enteral Administration and Nutrition Considerations

Compatibility, Stability, and Bioavailability Considerations
- Maximal solution stability occurs at pH 4, which avoids hydrolytic decomposition that can occur at pH <3 and pH >5.
- To avoid thickening, do not refrigerate oral solution after reconstitution of granules.[1]

Drug-Nutrition Interactions
- Drug may influence nutrition status directly or indirectly:
  - Weight loss
  - GI: anorexia, nausea, vomiting, abdominal bloating and pain, diarrhea (including *Clostridium difficile*–associated), tenesmus, transient LFT elevations
  - Metabolic: rare proteinuria
  - Other: polyarthritis
- Influence of malnutrition or obesity on drug disposition:
  - Use of a standard dose may result in therapeutic failure in obesity based on an increased drug clearance.[2,3]
- Influence of food on oral absorption or bioavailability:
  - Food may delay oral absorption but does not significantly influence oral bioavailability.

Recommendations

Gastric	• Disperse capsule contents in water just prior to administration. • No need to hold EN beyond the time required to flush-administer-flush.
Postpyloric	• As above. • Monitor for any unexpected change in effect.
Other	• As with all antimicrobials, consider parenteral alternative for acutely ill patients to ensure therapeutic concentrations.

References

1. Riebe KW, Oesterling TO. Parenteral development of clindamycin-2-phosphate. *Bull Parenter Drug Assoc.* 1972;26:139–145.
2. Bouazza N, Pestre V, Jullien V, et al. Population pharmacokinetics of clindamycin orally and intravenously administered in patients with osteomyelitis. *Br J Clin Pharmacol.* 2012;74:971–977.
3. Halilovic J, Heintz BH, Brown J. Risk factors for clinical failure in patients hospitalized with cellulitis and cutaneous abscess. *J Infect.* 2012;65:128–134.

Clonazepam

Product Availability

Solid	• Tablet:
	    ◦ Immediate-release: 0.5 mg, 1 mg, 2 mg (Klonopin® [Roche]; others)
	    ◦ Orally disintegrating: 0.125 mg, 0.25 mg, 0.5 mg, 1 mg, 2 mg (various)

Physicochemical (drug)

Molecular weight: • 315.72	Permeability: • LogP 2.41 • LogD 2.4 (pH 7.4)	Water solubility: • 0.1 mg/mL (25°C)
pKa: • 1.5, 10.5	Classification: • BCS Class n/a; BDDCS Class 1	

Pharmaceutical (product)

Solid	• Immediate-release tablet disperses in water (20 mL) within 2 minutes.

Pharmacokinetic (patient)

Absorption	• Specific site not known; t_{max} ~1–4 hours after oral dose • Bioavailability ~90%
Transport	• Plasma protein binding ~85% • V_d ~2.6 L/kg
Metabolism	• Extensively metabolized to several metabolites, subsequently conjugated (glucuronic acid, sulfate) and eliminated renally • Cl ~0.8 mL/min/kg

Enteral Administration and Nutrition Considerations

Compatibility, Stability, and Bioavailability Considerations
- The Official USP formulation for clonazepam suspension (0.1 mg/mL) from tablets will have a pH of 3.6–4.6 and provided a BUD of 60 days.
- A clonazepam solution (2.5 mg/mL) commercially available outside of the United States was reported to have pH 4.9 and osmolarity 14,500 mOsm/L.[1]
- An extemporaneously compounded oral suspension (0.1 mg/mL) prepared from tablets (2 mg) and diluted in OraSweet/OraPlus (1:1), OraSweet SF/OraPlus (1:1), or cherry syrup/simple syrup (1:4), stored in amber polyethylene terephthalate plastic bottles at 5°C and 25°C and protected from light, remained stable (HPLC analysis) at 60 days.[2]

- An extemporaneously compounded oral suspension (0.1 mg/mL) prepared from tablets (0.5 mg) using a 1% methylcellulose suspension and simple syrup (7:3), stored in amber polyvinyl chloride bottles at 4°C, remained stable (HPLC analysis) for 60 days.[3]
- A suspension (0.2 mg/mL) made from pure drug powder in SyrSpend SF PH4, stored in bottles at 2°C–8°C or 20°C–25°C, remained stable for 90 days.[4]

Drug-Nutrition Interactions
- Drug may influence nutrition status directly or indirectly:
  - Change in appetite and weight loss or gain possible
  - CNS: sedation, ataxia, diplopia, tremor
  - GI: dry mouth, nausea, gastritis, constipation
  - Metabolic: dehydration
- No data on the influence of malnutrition or obesity on drug disposition.
- No known influence of food on oral absorption or bioavailability.

Recommendations

Gastric	• Disperse tablet in water (20 mL) just prior to administration. • No need to hold EN beyond the time required to flush-administer-flush.
Postpyloric	• As above. • Monitor for any unexpected change in effect.

References

1. Obladen M, Mutz A. Orale medikation bei frühgeborenen? *Monatsschr Kinderheilkd.* 1985;133:669–674.
2. Allen LV, Erickson MA. Stability of acetazolamide, allopurinol, azathioprine, clonazepam and flucytosine in extemporaneously compounded oral liquids. *Am J Health-Syst Pharm.* 1996;53:1944–1949.
3. Roy JJ, Besner JG. Stability of clonazepam suspension in HSC vehicle. *Int J Pharm Compd.* 1997;1:440–441.
4. Polonini HC, Loures S, Lima LC, et al. Stability of atenolol, clonazepam, dexamethasone, diclofenac sodium, diltiazem, enalapril maleate, ketoprofen, lamotrigine, penicillamine-D and thiamine in SyrSpend SF PH4 oral suspensions. *Int J Pharm Compd.* 2016;20:167–174.

Clonidine Hydrochloride

Product Availability

Solid	• Tablet: o Immediate-release: 0.1 mg, 0.2 mg, 0.3 mg (Catapres® [Boehringer-Ingelheim]; others) o Extended-release: 0.1 mg (Kapvay® [Concordia]; others)

Physicochemical (drug)

Molecular weight: • 230.10 (salt 266.56)	Permeability: • LogP 1.43 • LogD 0.83 (pH 7.4)	Water solubility: • 77 mg/mL (20°C)
pKa: • 8.2	Classification: • BCS Class 3; BDDCS Class 1	

Pharmaceutical (product)

Solid	• Immediate-release tablet may disperse in water (20 mL) within 5 minutes. • Do not crush any sustained-release product.

Pharmacokinetic (patient)

Absorption	• Specific site not known; t_{max} ~3 hours after oral dose (immediate-release) • Bioavailability ~70%–80%
Transport	• Plasma protein binding ~20%–40%, mostly to albumin • V_d ~2.1 L/kg
Metabolism	• Metabolized to 4 metabolites, with about half of the drug appearing unchanged in the urine • Cl ~3.1 mL/min/kg

Enteral Administration and Nutrition Considerations

Compatibility, Stability, and Bioavailability Considerations
- Liquid formulations may prolong time to effect, including when administered by nasogastric tube.[1]
- An extemporaneously compounded solution (20 µg/mL) prepared from tablets (0.1 mg) in simple syrup had a pH of 4.4–4.5 and an osmolality of 3180 mOsm/kg; when stored in amber plastic bottles at 2°C–8°C, it remained stable (HPLC analysis) for 35 days.[2]
- An extemporaneous oral liquid (0.1 mg/mL) prepared from tablets (0.2 mg) in water and simple syrup, stored in amber glass bottles and refrigerated (4°C) for 28 days, remained stable (HPLC analysis) with 6%–8% drug loss in that time.[3]

- An extemporaneously compounded suspension (10 μg/mL) prepared from tablets (0.1 mg) in OraBlend, stored in 5 mL plastic syringes at 4°C and 25°C, remained stable (HPLC with UV detection analysis) for 91 days.[4]
- An extemporaneously compounded suspension (10 μg/mL) prepared from tablets (0.1 mg) in Oral Mix and Oral Mix SF, stored in amber glass and polyethylene terephthalate bottles and plastic syringes at 4°C and 25°C, remained stable (HPLC analysis) for 91 days.[5]

Drug-Nutrition Interactions
- Drug may influence nutrition status directly or indirectly:
  o Weight gain possible
  o CNS: dizziness, drowsiness, fatigue, weakness
  o GI: dry mouth, anorexia, nausea, vomiting, constipation
  o Other: myalgia, leg cramps
- No data on the influence of malnutrition or obesity on drug disposition.
- No known influence of food on oral absorption or bioavailability.

Recommendations

Gastric	• Disperse immediate-release tablet in water (20 mL) just prior to administration. • No need to hold EN beyond the time required to flush-administer-flush.
Postpyloric	• As above. • Monitor for any unexpected change in effect.

References

1. Hanning SM, Gul MO, Toni I, et al. A mini-review of non-parenteral clonidine preparations for paediatric sedation. *J Pharm Pharmacol.* 2017;69:398–405.
2. Sauberan JB, Phuong P, Ilog ND, et al. Stability and osmolality of extemporaneously prepared clonidine oral liquid for neonates. *Ann Pharmacother.* 2016;50:243–244.
3. Levinson ML, Johnson CE. Stability of an extemporaneously compounded clonidine hydrochloride oral liquid. *Am J Hosp Pharm.* 1992;49:122–125.
4. Ma C, Décarie D, Ensom MHH. Stability of clonidine suspension in oral plastic syringes. *Am J Health-Syst Pharm.* 2014;71:657–771.
5. Ensom MHH, Décarie D. Stability of extemporaneously compounded clonidine in glass and plastic bottles and plastic syringes. *Can J Hosp Pharm.* 2014;67:308–310.

Clopidogrel Bisulfate

Product Availability

Solid	• Tablet: 75 mg, 300 mg (base) (Plavix® [Sanofi-Aventis]; others)

Physicochemical (drug)

Molecular weight: • 321.83 (salt 419.91)	Permeability: • LogP 4.21 (calc) • LogD 4.30 (pH 7.4) (calc)	Water solubility: • 0.05 mg/mL
pKa: • 4.55	Classification: • BCS Class 2; BDDCS Class 2	

Pharmaceutical (product)

Solid	• Tablet products may be film-coated.

Pharmacokinetic (patient)

Absorption	• Specific site not known; t_{max} ~1 hour after oral dose (based on the main circulating metabolite) • Bioavailability ≥50%
Transport	• Substrate for P-glycoprotein efflux • Plasma protein binding ~98% • V_d ~40 liters
Metabolism	• The prodrug is activated to the thiol metabolite via CYP2C19 and, to a lesser extent, other isoenzymes (CYP3A, CYP2B6, CYP1A2); some metabolites may undergo glucuronidation (UGT2B7) prior to excretion (urine and feces). • Cl ~17 L/h

Enteral Administration and Nutrition Considerations

Compatibility, Stability, and Bioavailability Considerations
- Clopidogrel is soluble in an acidic (pH ~1) aqueous solution.
- Loading dose administration of tablets by nasogastric tube, after crushing and dispersing in 10 mL sterile water with a 20 mL flush, resulted in greater absorption (based on the carboxylic acid metabolite) compared with intact tablet administration in healthy subjects in the fasted state.[1]
- Altering excipients in a product can enhance dissolution, with a potential to improve stability.[2]
- Studies that evaluate bioavailability may need to address P-glycoprotein variants.[3,4]
- An extemporaneously compounded suspension (5 mg/mL) prepared from tablets in OraPlus/OraSweet (1:1) had a pH of 2.65; when stored in amber plastic bottles at 2°C–8°C and 23°C–25°C, it remained stable (HPLC analysis) for 60 days.[5]

- An extemporaneously compounded suspension (7.5 mg/mL) prepared from tablets in water or water/SF syrup and stored in bottles at 4°C–8°C or 23°C–25°C remained stable (HPLC analysis) for 28 days under all temperature conditions.[6]

Drug-Nutrition Interactions

- Drug may influence nutrition status directly or indirectly:
  - CNS: fatigue, weakness
  - GI: nausea, abdominal pain, diarrhea
  - Metabolic: edema, hypercholesterolemia
- Influence of malnutrition or obesity on drug disposition:
  - Although there is no reported change in drug volume of distribution or clearance with obesity, platelet inhibitory effects may be lower.[7]
- Influence of food on oral absorption or bioavailability:
  - A high-fat meal may significantly increase (up to ~9-fold) the oral bioavailability of clopidogrel compared with the fasted state, although no influence is seen on the appearance of the carboxylic acid metabolite in the circulation.[8–10]
  - Grapefruit juice may inhibit drug metabolism, resulting in greater oral bioavailability.

Recommendations

Gastric	• Crush and disperse non-film-coated tablet in water just prior to administration. • No need to hold EN beyond the time required to flush-administer-flush.
Postpyloric	• As above. • Monitor for any unexpected change in effect.

References

1. Zafar MU, Farkouh ME, Fuster V, Chesebro JH. Crushed clopidogrel administered via nasogastric tube has a faster and greater absorption than oral whole tablets. *J Interven Cardiol.* 2009;22:385–389.
2. Bali DE, Osman MA, El Maghraby GM. Enhancement of dissolution rate and intestinal stability of clopidogrel hydrogen sulfate. *Eur J Drug Metab Pharmacokinet.* 2016;41: 807–818.
3. Luo M, Li J, Xu X, Sun X, Sheng W. ABCB1 C3435T polymorphism and risk of adverse clinical events in clopidogrel treated patients: a meta-analysis. *Thromb Res.* 2012;129: 754–759.
4. Taubert D, von Beckerath N, Grimberg G, et al. Impact of P-glycoprotein on clopidogrel absorption. *Clin Pharmacol Ther.* 2006;80:486–501.
5. Skillman KL, Caruthers RL, Johnson CE. Stability of an extemporaneously prepared clopidogrel oral suspension. *Am J Health-Syst Pharm.* 2010;67:559–561.
6. Yamreudeewong W, Dolence EK, Teixeira MG. Stability of clopidogrel in three extemporaneously compounded oral liquid preparations. *Int J Pharm Compd.* 2011;15: 435–437.

7. Gremmel T, Steiner S, Seidinger D, et al. Obesity is associated with poor response to clopidogrel and an increased susceptibility to protease activated receptor-1 mediated platelet activation. *Transl Res.* 2013;1611:421–429.
8. McEwen J, Strauch G, Perles P, et al. Clopidogrel bioavailability: absence of influence of food or antacids. *Semin Thromb Hemost.* 1999;25:(Suppl 2):47–50.
9. Nirogi RV, Kandikere VN, Mudiginda K. Effect of food on bioavailability of a single oral dose of clopidogrel in healthy male subjects. *Arzneim Forsch (Drug Res).* 2006;56: 735–739.
10. Brvar N, LaChance S, Lévesque A, et al. Comparative bioavailability of two oral formulations of clopidogrel: determination of clopidogrel and its carboxylic acid metabolite (SR26334) under fasting and fed conditions in healthy subjects. *Acta Pharm.* 2014;64:45–62.

Codeine Sulfate or Phosphate

Product Availability

Solid	• Tablet: 15 mg, 30 mg, 60 mg (various)
Liquid	• Oral solution: 30 mg/5 mL (various)

Physicochemical (drug)

Molecular weight:	Permeability:	Water solubility:

• 299.37
  ○ sulfate 696.81
  ○ phosphate 397.36
	• LogP 1.19
	• LogD 0.21 (pH 7.4)
		• 33 mg/mL (sulfate)
		• 400–435 mg/mL
		  (phosphate)

pKa: • 8.20	Classification: • BCS Class 1 or 3; BDDCS Class 1	

Pharmaceutical (product)

Solid	• Tablet products may be film-coated.

Liquid	• Oral solution:
	  ○ pH ~3.3
	  ○ Osmolality n/a
	  ○ Viscosity may be significant.
	  ○ May contain sorbitol, glycerin, and sucralose; orange-flavored
	  ○ Store at controlled room temperature.

Pharmacokinetic (patient)

Absorption	• Specific site not known; t_{max} within 1 hour after an oral dose • Bioavailability ~50%
Transport	• Plasma protein binding <10% • V_d 3–7 L/kg
Metabolism	• Metabolized by demethylation through the action of CYP3A4 and CYP2D6 to norcodeine and morphine, with subsequent conjugation with glucuronic acid and renal elimination • Cl ~40–140 L/h

Enteral Administration and Nutrition Considerations

Compatibility, Stability, and Bioavailability Considerations
- A compounded aqueous formulation of codeine phosphate (3 mg/mL) using drug powder has good stability at pH 4.2.[1]
- An aqueous solution of codeine sulfate exhibits best stability when pH is between 3 and 8, and it remains stable much longer than codeine phosphate.[2]
- The official USP codeine phosphate oral suspension is expected to have a pH of 3.7–4.7, with a BUD of 90 days when stored at room temperature.

- A dose of drug solution admixed with 200 mL of an EN product (Precitene) appeared physically compatible (no phase separation or particle growth).[3]
- A codeine liquid formulation mixed (1:1) with EN products (Vital, Osmolite, Osmolite HN), appeared physically compatible (no granulation, thickening, or precipitation).[4]

Drug-Nutrition Interactions

- Drug may influence nutrition status directly or indirectly:
  - CNS: sedation, confusion
  - GI: constipation
- No data on the influence of malnutrition or obesity on drug disposition.
- No known influence of food on oral absorption or bioavailability.

Recommendations

Gastric	• Dilute liquid preparation with water (at least 1:1) just prior to administration. • No need to hold EN beyond the time required to flush-administer-flush.
Postpyloric	• As above. • Monitor for any unexpected change in effect.

References

1. Dentinger PJ, Swenson CF. Stability of codeine phosphate in an extemporaneously compounded syrup. *Am J Health-Syst Pharm.* 2007;64:2569–2573.
2. Powell MF. Enhanced stability of codeine sulfate: effect of pH, buffer, and temperature on the degradation of codeine in aqueous solution. *J Pharm Sci.* 1986;75:901–903.
3. Ortega de la Cruz C, Fernández Gallardo LC, Damas Fernández-Figares M, García Martínez E. Compatibilidad físico-química de medicamentos con nutrición enteral. *Nutr Hosp.* 1993;8:105–108.
4. Fagerman KE, Ballou AE. Drug compatibilities with enteral feeding solutions coadministered by tube. *Nutr Supp Serv.* 1988;8:31–32.

Colchicine

Product Availability

Solid	• Tablet: 0.6 mg (Colcrys® [Takeda]; others)
	• Capsule: 0.6 mg (Mitigare® [Hikma]; others)

Physicochemical (drug)

Molecular weight:	Permeability:	Water solubility:
• 399.45	• LogP 1.30	• 45 mg/mL
	• LogD 1.03 (pH 7.4)	
pKa:	Classification:	
• 12.4	• BCS Class 3; BDDCS Class 3	

Pharmaceutical (product)

Solid	• Tablets may disperse in water (20 mL) within 5 minutes.
	• Tablets can be crushed, but exposure should be avoided.

Pharmacokinetic (patient)

Absorption	• Jejunum and ileum; t_{max} ~1–2 hours after an oral dose
	• Bioavailability ~45%
Transport	• Substrate for P-glycoprotein efflux
	• Plasma protein binding ~39%, mostly to albumin
	• V_d ~5.3 L/kg
Metabolism	• Partial metabolism by demethylation through CYP3A4, with some enterohepatic recirculation of the parent drug; some unchanged drug excreted renally
	• Cl ~1.8 mL/min/kg

Enteral Administration and Nutrition Considerations

Compatibility, Stability, and Bioavailability Considerations

- Alterations in product formulation may enhance solubility and bioavailability.[1]
- A nanoemulsion formulation that included eugenol (a P-glycoprotein inhibitor) increased drug permeability and bioavailability.[2]

Drug-Nutrition Interactions

- Drug may influence nutrition status directly or indirectly:
  - GI: stomatitis, nausea, vomiting, abdominal discomfort, paralytic ileus, diarrhea
  - Metabolic: hypothyroid
  - Other: neuropathy, myopathy, rhabdomyolysis, hair loss
- No data on the influence of malnutrition or obesity on drug disposition.

- Influence of food on oral absorption or bioavailability:
  - Food can reduce oral bioavailability by ~15%.
  - Grapefruit juice may increase intestinal permeability based on an in situ animal perfusion model.[3]
  - Seville orange juice (240 mL twice daily for 4 days) decreased oral bioavailability by ~20% in healthy volunteers, while grapefruit juice had no effect.[4]

Recommendations

Gastric	• Disperse tablet in water (20 mL) prior to administration. • No need to hold EN beyond the time required to flush-administer-flush.
Postpyloric	• As above. • Monitor for any unexpected change in effect.

References

1. Chauhan R, Madan J, Kaushik D, et al. Inclusion complex of colchicine in hydroxypropyl-β-cyclodextrin tenders better solubility and improved pharmacokinetics. *Pharm Dev Tech.* 2013;18:313–322.
2. Shen Q, Wang Y, Zhang Y. Improvement of colchicine oral bioavailability by incorporating eugenol in the nanoemulsion as an oil excipient and enhancer. *Int J Nanomedicine.* 2011;6:1237–1243.
3. Dahan A, Amidon GL. Grapefruit juice and its constituents augment colchicine intestinal absorption: potential hazardous interaction and the role of P-glycoprotein. *Pharm Res.* 2009;26:883–892.
4. Wason S, Digiacinto JL, Davis MW. Effects of grapefruit and Seville orange juices on the pharmacokinetic properties of colchicine in healthy subjects. *Clin Ther.* 2012;34:2161–2173.

Cyclobenzaprine Hydrochloride

Product Availability

Solid	• Tablet: 5 mg, 7.5 mg, 10 mg (various)
	• Capsule, extended-release: 15 mg, 30 mg (Amrix® [ECR Pharma])

Physicochemical (drug)

Molecular weight: • 275.40 (salt 311.86)	Permeability: • LogP 5.10 (calc) • LogD n/a	Water solubility: • 200 mg/mL
pKa: • 8.47	Classification: • BCS Class 1; BDDCS Class 1	

Pharmaceutical (product)

Solid	• Some tablet products may be crushed.
	• Do not open or crush extended-release capsules.

Pharmacokinetic (patient)

Absorption	• Specific site not known; t_{max} ~4 hours after an oral dose (immediate-release, fasted) • Bioavailability ~33%–55%
Transport	• Plasma protein binding ~93% • V_d ~146 liters
Metabolism	• Extensive metabolism through CYP3A4, CYP1A2, and CYP2D6, with subsequent glucuronidation and renal elimination • Cl ~33 L/h

Enteral Administration and Nutrition Considerations

Compatibility, Stability, and Bioavailability Considerations
• No data are available.

Drug-Nutrition Interactions
• Drug may influence nutrition status directly or indirectly:
  ○ CNS: drowsiness, fatigue, headache, confusion, blurred vision
  ○ GI: dry mouth, altered taste, dyspepsia, abdominal pain, constipation
  ○ Other: local muscle twitching and weakness
• No data on the influence of malnutrition or obesity on drug disposition.
• Influence of food on oral absorption or bioavailability:
  ○ A high-fat meal (900 kcal, 50% fat) reduced oral bioavailability (~27% immediate-release; ~12% modified-release)[1]

Recommendations

Gastric	• If there is no therapeutic alternative, consider crushing and dispersing tablet in water prior to administration. • No need to hold EN beyond the time required to flush-administer-flush.
Postpyloric	• As above. • Monitor for any unexpected change in effect.

Reference

1. Gai MN, Costa E, Arancibia A. Bioavailability of a controlled-release cyclobenzaprine tablet and influence of a high fat meal on bioavailability. *Int J Clin Pharmacol Ther*. 2009;47:269–274.

Diazepam

Product Availability

Solid	• Tablet: 2 mg, 5 mg, 10 mg (Valium® [Roche]; others)
Liquid	• Solution: 5 mg/5 mL (various) • Solution, concentrate: 5 mg/mL (various)

Physicochemical (drug)

Molecular weight: • 284.74	Permeability: • LogP 2.82 • LogD 2.99 (pH 7.4)	Water solubility: • 3 mg/mL (25°C)
pKa: • 3.40	Classification: • BCS Class 2; BDDCS Class n/a	

Pharmaceutical (product)

Solid	• Lower dose tablets (≤5 mg) may disperse in water (20 mL) within 5 minutes.
Liquid	• Solution: ○ pH 5.2 (2 mg/mL product)[1] ○ Osmolality 4287 mOsm/L (2 mg/mL product), with pH 5.2;[1] 8258 mOsm/kg (2 mg/mL product)[2] ○ Viscosity n/a ○ Drug in solution may bind to tubing material. ○ The oral concentrate solution is intended to be further diluted before administration.

Pharmacokinetic (patient)

Absorption	• Specific site not known; t_{max} ~15–75 minutes after an oral dose • Bioavailability ~93%–100%
Transport	• Plasma protein binding ~98% • V_d ~0.8–1.1 L/kg
Metabolism	• Major metabolites via CYP2C19 include desmethyldiazepam, 3-hydroxydiazepam, and oxazepam, subsequently conjugated (glucuronic acid, sulfate) prior to elimination • Cl ~20–30 mL/min

Enteral Administration and Nutrition Considerations

Compatibility, Stability, and Bioavailability Considerations

- The maximal stability of diazepam in aqueous solution occurs at pH ~5, as hydrolysis is more likely at pH <3.[3,4]
- An extemporaneously compounded oral suspension (1 mg/mL) prepared from tablets (10 mg) in (a) simple syrup or (b) ethanol, propylene glycol,

and simple syrup, stored in amber glass at room temperature and in room lighting, did not remain stable (spectrophotometric analysis) for 14 days.[5]

- An extemporaneously compounded oral suspension (1 mg/mL) prepared from tablets (10 mg) in ethanol, propylene glycol, and a suspension vehicle adjusted to pH 4.2, stored in amber glass bottles at 5°C, 22°C, and 40°C for 60 days, remained stable (HPLC analysis) at room and refrigerator temperatures.[6]

- The admixture of tablet (10 mg) or oral liquid (5 mg/5 mL), first dispersed in deionized water (10 mL), then with 240 mL of an EN formulation (Isocal, Sustacal, Sustacal HC), was reported to be stable (HPLC analysis) and appeared physically compatible for up to 24 hours at 24°C in all three formulations.[7]

- Drug was adequately absorbed in a patient with multiple small bowel enterocutaneous fistulas.[8]

Drug-Nutrition Interactions
- Drug may influence nutrition status directly or indirectly:
  - Weight gain or weight loss
  - CNS: somnolence, drowsiness, fatigue, ataxia, confusion, anterograde amnesia, tremor
  - GI: buccal dyskinesia, dry mouth, bitter or metallic taste, anorexia, nausea, constipation
  - Metabolic: hyperprolactinemia, elevated testosterone
- Influence of malnutrition or obesity on drug disposition:
  - The body weight–normalized volume of distribution is significantly greater in obesity and associated with a longer duration of drug effect, suggesting less-frequent dosing based on a lean body weight.
- Influence of food on oral absorption or bioavailability:
  - A light meal (166 kcal, 37.8 g carbohydrate, 0.44 g fat, 2.7 g protein) may delay absorption of the tablet form but without a significant effect on oral bioavailability.[9]
  - Grapefruit juice may increase oral bioavailability.[10]

Recommendations

Gastric	• Crush and/or disperse tablet in water prior to administration. • No need to hold EN beyond the time required to flush-administer-flush.
Postpyloric	• As above. • Monitor for any unexpected change in effect.

References
1. Obladen M, Mutz A. Orale medikation bei frühgeborenen? *Monatsschr Kinderheilkd.* 1985;133:669–674.
2. Fernández Polo A, Cabañas Poy MJ, Clemente Bautista S, et al. Osmolality of oral liquid dosage forms to be administered to newborns in a hospital. *Farm Hosp.* 2007;31:311–314.

3. Allen LV. Diazepam oral suspension. *US Pharmacist.* 1989;14:64–65.
4. Newton DW, Driscoll DF, Goudreau JL, et al. Solubility characteristics of diazepam in aqueous admixture solutions: theory and practice. *Am J Hosp Pharm.* 1981;38:179–182.
5. Newton DW, Schulman SG, Becker CH. Limitations of compounding diazepam suspensions from tablets. *Am J Hosp Pharm.* 1976;33:450–452.
6. Strom JG, Kalu AU. Formulation and stability of diazepam suspension compounded from tablets. *Am J Hosp Pharm.* 1986;43:1489–1491.
7. Strom JG, Miller SW. Stability of drugs with enteral nutrition formulas. *DICP Ann Pharmacother.* 1990;24:130–134.
8. Viswesh VV. Unpredictable absorption of oral opioid medications in a quadriplegic patient with chronic enterocutaneous fistulas. *J Pain Palliat Care Pharmacother.* 2012;26: 254–256.
9. Yamazaki A, Kumagai Y, Fujita T, et al. Different effects of light food on pharmacokinetics and pharmacodynamics of three benzodiazepines, quazepam, nitrazepam and diazepam. *J Clin Pharm Ther.* 2007;32:31–39.
10. Ozedemir M, Aktan Y, Boydag BS, Cingi MI, Musmul A. Interaction between grapefruit juice and diazepam in humans. *Eur J Drug Metab Pharmacokinet.* 1998;23:55–59.

Diclofenac

Product Availability

Solid	• Tablet: o Immediate-release: 25 mg, 50 mg (potassium salt) (various) o Enteric-coated: 25 mg, 50 mg, 75 mg (sodium salt) (various) o Extended-release: 100 mg (sodium salt) (various) • Capsule: o 18 mg, 36 mg (free acid) (Zorvolex® [Iroko Pharms]) o 25 mg (potassium salt) (Zipsor® [Depomed])
Liquid	• Powder for oral solution: 50 mg/packet (potassium salt) (Cambia® [Depomed]; others)

Physicochemical (drug)

Molecular weight: • 296.15 o sodium salt 318.13 o potassium salt 334.24	Permeability: • LogP 4.51 • LogD 3.5 (pH 6.5), 1.13 (pH 7.4)	Water solubility: • 9 mg/mL
pKa: • 3.8	Classification: • BCS Class 2; BDDCS Class 2	

Pharmaceutical (product)

Solid	• Tablets do not disperse in water. • Do not crush modified-release tablets (enteric-coated, extended-release). • Do not interfere with the integrity of the liquid-filled (potassium salt) capsule.
Liquid	• Oral solution (reconstituted): o Intended to be diluted in water (30–60 mL) o pH n/a o Osmolality n/a o Viscosity n/a o May contain aspartame, glycerol, mannitol, and saccharin
Note	• Different dosage formulation products are not necessarily bioequivalent.

Pharmacokinetic (patient)

Absorption	• Specific site not known; t_{max} ~0.5–2 hours after an oral dose, depending on the formulation (immediate-release) • Bioavailability ~50%–60%
Transport	• Plasma protein binding reaches 99%, mostly to albumin • V_d ~1.3–1.4 L/kg

Metabolism	• Extensive first-pass metabolism by hydroxylation (CYP2C9) then conjugation (with glucuronic acid via UGT2B7, sulfate, taurine, others); excreted in urine and bile • Cl ~263–350 mL/min

Enteral Administration and Nutrition Considerations

Compatibility, Stability, and Bioavailability Considerations

- An extemporaneously compounded oral suspension (5 mg/mL) prepared from diclofenac sodium powder in SyrSpend SF PH4 and stored in bottles at 2°C–8°C or 20°C–25°C remained stable (HPLC analysis) for 90 days.[1]
- An extemporaneously compounded oral suspension (10 mg/mL) prepared from diclofenac sodium tablets in OraBlend, stored in amber polyvinyl chloride plastic bottles at 5°C or 23°C, remained stable (HPLC analysis) for 93 days.[2]
- A suspension form of the sodium salt under development contains microspheres (<100 μm) that act as a slow-release formulation.[3]
- Nanoparticle formulations under study vary in how well they may improve dissolution and bioavailability.[4]
- The oral solution results in quicker and higher plasma drug concentrations than tablets, especially under fasted conditions.[5,6]

Drug-Nutrition Interactions

- Drug may influence nutrition status directly or indirectly:
  - Weight gain (related to edema)
  - CNS: headache, dizziness, paresthesia, tremor, blurred vision
  - GI: glossitis, stomatitis, dry mouth, anorexia, nausea, dyspepsia, GI ulceration, bleeding, perforation, rare pancreatitis and hepatitis
  - Metabolic: edema, hyponatremia, hyperglycemia, proteinuria
- No data on the influence of malnutrition or obesity on drug disposition.
- Influence of food on oral absorption or bioavailability:
  - Food may delay the rate of absorption, with lower peak concentrations from immediate-release products, which may influence their acute analgesic effect.[5,7]
  - Otherwise, food has no significant influence on oral bioavailability.

Recommendations

Gastric	• If there is no therapeutic alternative, dilute the oral solution with water (1:1) just prior to administration. • Consider holding EN (~30 minutes) when the drug is administered for acute effect; otherwise, no need to hold EN beyond the time required to flush-administer-flush.
Postpyloric	• As above. • Monitor for any unexpected change in effect.

References

1. Polonini HC, Loures S, Lima LC, et al. Stability of atenolol, clonazepam, dexamethasone, diclofenac sodium, diltiazem, enalapril maleate, ketoprofen, lamotrigine, penicillamine-D and thiamine in SyrSpend SF PH4 oral suspensions. *Int J Pharm Compd.* 2016;20:167–174.
2. Donnelly RF, Pascuet E, Ma C, et al. Stability of diclofenac sodium oral suspensions packaged in amber polyvinyl chloride bottles. *Can J Hosp Pharm.* 2010;63:25–30.
3. Oz UC, Devrim B, Bozkir A, Canefe K. Development of reconstitutable suspensions containing diclofenac sodium-loaded microspheres for pediatric delivery. *J Microencapsul.* 2015;32:317–328.
4. Lai F, Sinico C, Ennas G, et al. Diclofenac nanosuspensions: influence of preparation procedure and crystal form on drug dissolution behavior. *Int J Pharm.* 2009;373:124–132.
5. Chen C, Bujanover S, Kareht S, Rapoport AM. Differential pharmacokinetics of diclofenac potassium for oral solution vs immediate-release tablets from a randomized trial: effect of fed and fasting conditions. *Headache.* 2015;55:265–275.
6. Bende G, Biswal S, Bhad P, et al. Relative bioavailability of diclofenac potassium from softgel capsule versus powder for oral solution and immediate-release tablet formulation. *Clin Pharmacol Drug Dev.* 2016;5:76–82.
7. Moore RA, Derry S, Wiffen PJ, Straube S. Effects of food on pharmacokinetics of immediate release oral formulations of aspirin, dipyrone, paracetamol and NSAIDs: a systematic review. *Br J Clin Pharmacol.* 2015;80:381–388.

Dicyclomine Hydrochloride

Product Availability

Solid	• Tablet: 20 mg (Bentyl® [Allergan]; others) • Capsule: 10 mg (Bentyl® [Allergan]; others)
Liquid	• Oral solution: 10 mg/5 mL (various)

Physicochemical (drug)

Molecular weight: • 309.49 (salt 345.95)	Permeability: • LogP n/a • LogD n/a	Water solubility: • 77 mg/mL
pKa: • 9.0	Classification: • BCS Class n/a; BDDCS Class n/a	

Pharmaceutical (product)

Solid	• Tablets do not disperse in water. • Capsule contents may disperse in water.

Liquid	• Oral solution (syrup):
	  o pH 4.5 (pH 3–5)
	  o Osmolality n/a
	  o Viscosity n/a
	  o May contain glucose, propylene glycol, saccharin
	  o Store at room temperature.

Note	• Solid and liquid dosage forms are considered bioequivalent.

Pharmacokinetic (patient)

Absorption	• Specific site not known; t_{max} ~1–1.5 hours after an oral dose • Bioavailability ~50%–67%
Transport	• Plasma protein binding ~99% • V_d ~3.65 L/kg
Metabolism	• Metabolic fate is unclear, but ~80% is eliminated renally. • Cl n/a

Enteral Administration and Nutrition Considerations

Compatibility, Stability, and Bioavailability Considerations
- The drug is unstable in alkaline solutions, with free base precipitate more likely at pH >7.
- Dicyclomine syrup (pH 4.5) admixed (1:1) with Osmolite, Osmolite-HN, or Vital was incompatible with the first two formulas, causing formula thickening that did not improve with agitation, but appeared compatible with Vital.[1]

Drug-Nutrition Interactions
- Drug may influence nutrition status directly or indirectly:
  o CNS: somnolence, dizziness, blurred vision
  o GI: dry mouth, anorexia, nausea, vomiting, abdominal distension
  o Metabolic: facial edema
- No data on the influence of malnutrition or obesity on drug disposition.
- No known influence of food on oral bioavailability.

Recommendations

Gastric	• Disperse capsule contents in water prior to administration. • Alternative: Dilute syrup with water (at least 1:1) just prior to administration. • No need to hold EN beyond the time required to flush-administer-flush.
Postpyloric	• As above. • Monitor for any unexpected change in effect.

Reference

1. Fagerman KE, Ballou AE. Drug compatibilities with enteral feeding solutions coadministered by tube. *Nutr Supp Serv.* 1988;8:31–32.

Digoxin

Product Availability

Solid	• Tablet: 62.5 μg, 125 μg, 187.5 μg, 250 μg (Lanoxin® [Concordia Pharms]; others)
Liquid	• Elixir: 50 μg/mL (various)

Physicochemical (drug)

Molecular weight: • 780.95	Permeability: • LogP 1.26 • LogD 1.4 (pH 6.5), 1.26 (pH 7.4)	Water solubility: • 0.08 mg/mL
pKa: • 7.2	Classification: • BCS Class 3; BDDCS Class 3	

Pharmaceutical (product)

Solid	• Tablets may disperse in water (20 mL) within 5 minutes.

Liquid	• Elixir:
	• pH 6.46–7.00[1–3]
	• Osmolality:
	  ○ 1350 mOsm/kg[4]
	  ○ 3583 mOsm/kg (1:9 dilution with sterile water → 360 mOsm/kg)[5]
	  ○ 3647 mOsm/L[2]
	  ○ 5950 mOsm/kg (calculated based on measurement of 1:5 dilution with sterile water)[3]
	• Viscosity n/a
	• May contain ethanol (10%), glycerin and sorbitol; lime-flavored
	• Store at room temperature and protect from light.

Note	• Tablet and elixir dosage forms are considered bioequivalent.

Pharmacokinetic (patient)

Absorption	• Proximal small intestine; t_{max} ~1.5 hours after an oral dose. • Bioavailability ~60%–85% (tablet, elixir) or higher (previously available liquid-filled capsule)
Transport	• Substrate for P-glycoprotein efflux • Plasma protein binding 20%–30%, primarily albumin • V_d ~7 L/kg
Metabolism	• Minimal metabolism (gut microbiota and hepatic) but varies by individual, forming numerous active and inactive metabolites following glycoside cleavage and lactone reduction • Parent and metabolites eliminated predominantly renally • Cl ~2.8 mL/min/kg

Enteral Administration and Nutrition Considerations

Compatibility, Stability, and Bioavailability Considerations
- An aqueous solution of digoxin is susceptible to hydrolysis at pH <3 but is stable at pH 5–8.[6-9]
- Commercial elixir combined (1:1) with Osmolite 1.2, under simulated clinical conditions, would result in no clogging of an 8 Fr or 20 Fr feeding tube.[3]
- A dose of oral liquid admixed with 200 mL of an EN product (Precitene) appeared physically incompatible (phase separation or particle growth) with increased viscosity.[10]
- The oral solution (1 mL) appeared physically compatible (no phase separation or particle growth) when first added to varying volumes (15–240 mL) of EN formulas (Ensure, Ensure Plus, Osmolite), but a rubbery mass developed over time.[1]
- The solution (2 mL) appeared physically compatible (no phase separation or particle growth) when first added to varying volumes (15–240 mL) of EN formulas (Ensure HN, Ensure Plus HN, Osmolite HN, Vital), but a rubbery mass developed over time.[11]
- Doses of oral liquid added to 240 mL of an EN product (Ensure) appeared physically compatible (no phase separation, clumping, or gelling) with a slight increase in osmolality but no pH change.[12]
- The oral liquid (5 mL) appeared physically compatible when admixed with 10 mL of EN formulas (Enrich, TwoCal HN, Vivonex T.E.N.).[13]
- Bioavailability may be reduced in patients with short bowel syndrome, but it is increased in the presence of P-glycoprotein inhibition.[14,15]

Drug-Nutrition Interactions
- Drug may influence nutrition status directly or indirectly:
  - Weight loss
  - CNS: headache, drowsiness, lethargy, disorientation, confusion, visual disturbances
  - GI: anorexia, nausea, vomiting, abdominal pain
  - Metabolic: hyperkalemia; scalp alopecia, facial/laryngeal edema, finger- or toenail shedding (associated with rare hypersensitivity reaction)
  - Other: muscle weakness
- Influence of malnutrition or obesity on drug disposition:
  - The body weight–normalized volume of distribution is lower in obesity; base dose on an estimated lean body weight.
- Influence of food on oral absorption or bioavailability:
  - Food may delay the rate but not the extent of absorption from tablet formulation.
  - Taken following a meal, oral bioavailability from the elixir may increase by ~40%.
  - High-fiber-containing meals may reduce oral bioavailability.

Recommendations

Gastric	• Disperse tablet in water prior to administration. • Alternative: Dilute liquid with water (at least 1:1) just prior to administration. • Separate from fiber-containing EN formula; otherwise, no need to hold EN beyond the time required to flush-administer-flush.
Postpyloric	• As above. • Monitor for any unexpected change in effect.
Other	• Caution: Manage hypokalemia, hypomagnesemia, and hypercalcemia to avoid drug toxicity.

References

1. Cutie AJ, Altman E, Lenkel L. Compatibility of enteral products with commonly employed drug additives. *JPEN J Parenter Enteral Nutr.* 1983;7:186–191.
2. Obladen M, Mutz A. Orale medikation bei frühgeborenen? *Monatsschr Kinderheilkd.* 1985;133:669–674.
3. Klang M, McLymont V, Ng N. Osmolality, pH, and compatibility of selected oral liquid medications with an enteral nutrition product. *JPEN J Parenter Enteral Nutr.* 2013;37: 689–694.
4. Dickerson RN, Melnik G. Osmolality of oral drug solutions and suspensions. *Am J Hosp Pharm.* 1988;45:832–834.
5. Fernández Polo A, Cabañas Poy MJ, Clemente Bautista S, et al. Osmolality of oral liquid dosage forms to be administered to newborns in a hospital. *Farm Hosp.* 2007;31: 311–314.
6. Kuhlman J, Abshagen U, Rietbrock N. Cleavage of glycosidic bonds of digoxin and derivatives as function of pH and time. *Naunyn Schmiedeberg Arch Pharmacol.* 1973;276: 149–156.
7. Gault MH, Charles JD, Sugden DL, et al. Hydrolysis of digoxin by acid. *J Pharm Pharmacol.* 1977;29:27–32.
8. Sternson LA, Shaffer RD. Kinetics of digoxin stability in aqueous solution. *J Pharm Sci.* 1978;67:327–330.
9. Khalil SA, El-Masury S. Instability of digoxin in acid medium using a nonisotopic method. *J Pharm Sci.* 1978;67:1358–1360.
10. Ortega de la Cruz C, Fernández Gallardo LC, Damas Fernández-Figares M, García Martínez E. Compatibilidad físico-química de medicamentos con nutrición enteral. *Nutr Hosp.* 1993;8:105–108.
11. Altman E, Cutie AJ. Compatibility of enteral products with commonly employed drug additives. *Nutr Supp Serv.* 1984;4:8–17.
12. Holtz L, Milton J, Sturek JK. Compatibility of medications with enteral feedings. *JPEN J Parenter Enteral Nutr.* 1987;11:183–186.
13. Burns PE, McCall L, Wirsching R. Physical compatibility of enteral formulas with various common medications. *J Am Diet Assoc.* 1988;88:1094–1096.
14. Igel S, Drescher S, Mürdter T, et al. Increased absorption of digoxin from the human jejunum due to inhibition of intestinal transporter-mediated efflux. *Clin Pharmacokinet.* 2007;46:777–785.
15. Weiss M, Sermsappasuk P, Siegmund W. Modeling the kinetics of digoxin absorption: enhancement by P-glycoprotein inhibition. *J Clin Pharmacol.* 2012;52:381–387.

Diltiazem Hydrochloride

Product Availability

Solid	• Tablet: 　　○ Immediate-release: 30 mg, 60 mg, 90 mg, 120 mg (salt) 　　　(Cardizem® [Valeant]; others) 　　○ Extended-release: 120 mg, 180 mg, 240 mg, 300 mg, 360 mg, 　　　420 mg (salt) (Cardizem® LA [Valeant]; others) • Capsule (extended-release): 60 mg, 90 mg, 120 mg, 180 mg, 　240 mg, 300 mg, 360 mg, 420 mg (salt) (various)

Physicochemical (drug)

Molecular weight: • 414.52 (salt 450.98)	Permeability: • LogP 2.70 • LogD 2.22 (pH 7.4)	Water solubility: • 0.5 mg/mL
pKa: • 8.1	Classification: • BCS Class 1; BDDCS Class 1	

Pharmaceutical (product)

Solid	• Immediate-release tablets do not disperse in water and may be difficult to crush. • Do not crush, chew, or disassemble extended-release tablets or capsules containing modified-release granules.

Pharmacokinetic (patient)

Absorption	• Proximal small intestine; t_{max} ~2–3 hours after an oral dose (immediate-release) • Bioavailability varies with dosage form and dose (~30%–50%).
Transport	• Substrate for P-glycoprotein efflux • Plasma protein binding ~70%–85%, with albumin accounting for no more than half of the binding • V_d ~3.4 L/kg
Metabolism	• Extensive metabolism via CYP3A and others to several active and inactive metabolites, subsequently conjugated and eliminated in urine and bile mostly as metabolites • Cl ~36 L/h

Enteral Administration and Nutrition Considerations

Compatibility, Stability, Bioavailability Considerations
- Diltiazem HCl in aqueous solution is most stable at a pH of 5–6, with degradation when pH is higher.[1,2]
- The official USP formulation (12 mg/mL solution or suspension) is expected to have a pH of 3.7–4.7, should be stored at controlled room temperature or 2°C–8°C, with a BUD of 60 days.

- Extemporaneously compounded oral suspensions (12 mg/mL) prepared from tablets in OraSweet/OraPlus (1:1), OraSweet SF/OraPlus (1:1), or cherry/simple syrup (1:4), stored in amber polyethylene terephthalate plastic bottles at 5°C or 25°C away from light, remained stable (HPLC analysis) at 60 days.[2]
- An extemporaneously compounded oral suspension (12 mg/mL) prepared from drug powder in SyrSpend SF PH4, stored in bottles at 2°C–8°C or 20°C–25°C, remained stable (HPLC analysis) at both temperatures for 90 days.[3]
- Oral solution preparations (1 mg/mL) in a variety of different sugar solutions (including dextrose, fructose, or sucrose), each at 0.28 mmol/L at 25°C, were expected to remain stable (HPLC analysis) for about 1 month.[4]

Drug-Nutrition Interactions
- Drug may influence nutrition status directly or indirectly:
  - Weight gain
  - CNS: headache, dizziness, asthenia, gait abnormality, tremor
  - GI: anorexia, dysgeusia, nausea, vomiting, abdominal pain, ileus, diarrhea, transient LFT elevations
  - Metabolic: hyperglycemia, hyperuricemia, polyuria, crystalluria, albuminuria
  - Other: muscle cramps, myalgia, arthralgia
- No data on the influence of malnutrition or obesity on drug disposition.
- Influence of food on oral absorption or bioavailability:
  - No influence of food on the immediate-release formulation, although the rate of absorption may be quicker in the fasted state.
  - Grapefruit juice (250 mL) may increase oral bioavailability (by ~20%), but with significant interindividual variability, compared with water (250 mL).[5,6]

Recommendations

Gastric	• If there is no therapeutic alternative, crush and disperse tablet (immediate-release) in water just prior to administration. • Alternative: Consider using a stable extemporaneous suspension, diluted further in water just prior to administration. • No need to hold EN beyond the time required to flush-administer-flush.
Postpyloric	• As above. • Monitor for any unexpected change in effect.

References
1. Kawano K, Matsunaga A, Terade K, et al. Loss of diltiazem hydrochloride in solutions in polyvinyl chloride containers or intravenous administration set—hydrolysis and sorption. *Jap J Hosp Pharm.* 1994;20:537–541.

2. Allen LV, Erickson MA. Stability of baclofen, captopril, diltiazem hydrochloride, dipyridamole, and flecainide acetate in extemporaneously compounded oral liquids. *Am J Health-Syst Pharm.* 1996;53:2179–2184.
3. Polonini HC, Loures S, Lima LC, et al. Stability of atenolol, clonazepam, dexamethasone, diclofenac sodium, diltiazem, enalapril maleate, ketoprofen, lamotrigine, penicillamine-D and thiamine in SyrSpend SF PH4 oral suspensions. *Int J Pharm Compd.* 2016;20:167–174.
4. Suleiman MS, Najib NM, Abdelhameed ME. Stability of diltiazem hydrochloride in aqueous sugar solutions. *J Clin Pharm Ther.* 1988;13:417–422.
5. Sigusch H, Henschel L, Kraul H, et al. Lack of effect of grapefruit juice on diltiazem bioavailability in normal subjects. *Pharmazie.* 1994;49:675–679.
6. Christensen H, Asberg A, Holmboe AB, Berg KJ. Coadministration of grapefruit juice increased systemic exposure of diltiazem in healthy volunteers. *Eur J Clin Pharmacol.* 2002;515–520.

Divalproex Sodium

Product Availability

Solid	• Tablet:
	  ○ Delayed-release: 125 mg, 250 mg, 500 mg (valproic acid) (Depakote® [AbbVie]; others)
	  ○ Extended-release: 250 mg, 500 mg (valproic acid) (Depakote® ER [AbbVie]; others)
	• Capsule (delayed-release): 125 mg (valproic acid) (Depakote® Sprinkle [AbbVie]; others)

Liquid	• Oral solution: 250 mg/5 mL (valproic acid) (Depakene® [AbbVie]; others)

Physicochemical (drug)

Molecular weight:
• 144.21
  ○ sodium salt 166.20
  ○ divalproex sodium 310.41
	Permeability:
	• LogP 2.50
	• LogD n/a
		Water solubility:
		• 2.4 mg/mL (valproic acid)
		• 200 mg/mL (sodium salt)

pKa: • 4.6 (valproic acid) • 4.8 (sodium salt)	Classification: • BCS Class n/a; BDDCS Class n/a	

Pharmaceutical (product)

Solid	• Divalproex is composed of valproic acid and valproate sodium (1:1). • Do not crush tablets or capsule contents; mucosal membrane irritant.

Liquid	• Oral solution:
	  ○ Contains valproate sodium
	  ○ pH n/a
	  ○ Osmolality n/a
	  ○ Viscosity n/a
	  ○ May contain glycerin, sorbitol, and sucrose
	  ○ Maintain at controlled room temperature

Pharmacokinetic (patient)

Absorption	• Proximal small intestine; t_{max} ~1–4 hours after an oral dose, depending on formulation • Bioavailability ~90%–100% (formulation-dependent)
Transport	• Plasma protein binding ~80%–90% • V_d ~11 liters

| Metabolism | • Divalproex sodium is a prodrug, which dissociates in the gut to valproic acid.
• Undergoes hepatic glucuronidation (via UGT) and mitochondrial β-oxidation and minor CYP detoxification
• Cl ~0.6 L/h |

Enteral Administration and Nutrition Considerations

Compatibility, Stability, and Bioavailability Considerations
- The oral solution (2 mL) stored in polypropylene syringes and protected from light at 4°C and 25°C did not remain stable (gas chromatographic analysis) at 90 days (refrigeration) or at 20 days (room temperature), compared with storage in glass, possibly due to drug sorption to the plastic.[1]
- Magnesium valproate solution, suspension, and tablet formulations are considered to be bioequivalent.[2]
- A dose of the liquid admixed with 200 mL of an EN product (Precitene) appeared physically compatible (no phase separation or particle growth).[3]

Drug-Nutrition Interactions
- Drug may influence nutrition status directly or indirectly:
  - Weight gain is more common than weight loss.
  - CNS: headache, somnolence, tremor
  - GI: anorexia, nausea, vomiting, abdominal pain, diarrhea or constipation, increased AST and ALT
  - Metabolic: peripheral edema
  - Other: arthralgia, myalgia
- No data on the influence of malnutrition or obesity on drug disposition.
- Influence of food on oral absorption or bioavailability:
  - Food may slow the rate of absorption but without a significant influence on oral bioavailability.[4]

Recommendations

| Gastric | • If there is no therapeutic alternative, dilute oral solution in water (at least 1:1) prior to administration.
• No need to hold EN beyond the time required to flush-administer-flush. |
| Postpyloric | • As above.
• Monitor for any unexpected change in effect. |

References
1. Sartnurak S, Christensen JM. Stability of valproate sodium syrup in various unit dose containers. *Am J Hosp Pharm*. 1982;39:627–629.
2. Marcelín-Jiménez G, Angeles-Moreno AP, Contreras-Zavala L, et al. A single-dose, three-period, six-sequence crossover study comparing the bioavailability of solution, suspension, and enteric-coated tablets of magnesium valproate in healthy Mexican volunteers under fasting conditions. *Clin Ther*. 2009;31:2002–2011.

3. Ortega de la Cruz C, Fernández Gallardo LC, Damas Fernández-Figares M, García Martínez E. Compatibilidad físico-química de medicamentos con nutrición enteral. *Nutr Hosp.* 1993;8:105–108.

4. Dutta S, Reed RC. Distinct absorption characteristics of oral formulations of valproic acid/divalproex available in the United States. *Epilepsy Res.* 2007;73:275–283.

Donepezil Hydrochloride

Product Availability

Solid	• Tablet: ○ Immediate-release: 5 mg, 10 mg, 23 mg (Aricept® [Eisai]; others) ○ Orally disintegrating: 5 mg, 10 mg (Aricept® ODT [Eisai]; others)
Liquid	• Oral solution: 1 mg/mL (discontinued)

Physicochemical (drug)

Molecular weight: • 379.50 (salt 415.96)	Permeability: • LogP 4.60 (calc) • LogD n/a	Water solubility: • 0.003 mg/mL
pKa: • 8.6	Classification: • BCS Class 1; BDDCS Class 2	

Pharmaceutical (product)

Solid	• Immediate-release tablet products are film-coated. • Do not crush high-dose (23 mg) product to avoid increased absorption rate. • Film-coated and orally disintegrating tablet products are considered to be bioequivalent.
Liquid	• The discontinued oral solution contained sorbitol (70%) and propylene glycol; strawberry-flavored.

Pharmacokinetic (patient)

Absorption	• Small intestine; t_{max} ~3–4 hours after an oral dose • Bioavailability may approach 90%–100%
Transport	• Plasma protein binding ~96%, mostly to albumin, and some to α_1-acid glycoprotein • V_d ~12–16 L/kg
Metabolism	• Extensively metabolized to 4 metabolites (2 of them are active) via CYP2D6 and CYP3A4; they undergo glucuronidation and are excreted in urine. • Cl ~0.13–0.19 L/h/kg

Enteral Administration and Nutrition Considerations

Compatibility, Stability, and Bioavailability Considerations
• Orally disintegrating tablet products may need to include an ingredient to mask taste (although that is not necessary for diluting and administering them via an enteral access device); they otherwise provide similar bioavailability to immediate-release tablet.[1]

- An extemporaneously compounded oral liquid (1 mg/mL) prepared from tablets (5 mg) in deionized water/70% sorbitol (1:1), stored in polyethylene terephthalate plastic bottles at 4°C–8°C or 22°C–26°C, remained stable (HPLC analysis) for 4 weeks.[2]

Drug-Nutrition Interactions

- Drug may influence nutrition status directly or indirectly:
  - Weight loss
  - CNS: insomnia, fatigue
  - GI: anorexia, nausea, vomiting, gastric hypersecretion, diarrhea
  - Other: muscle cramps
- No data on the influence of malnutrition or obesity on drug disposition.
- No known influence of food on oral absorption or bioavailability.

Recommendations

Gastric	• Disperse orally disintegrating tablet in water prior to administration. • Alternative: Crush and/or disperse tablet (5 mg or 10 mg) in water prior to administration. • No need to hold EN beyond the time required to flush-administer-flush.
Postpyloric	• As above. • Monitor for any unexpected change in effect.

References

1. Yan YD, Woo JS, Kang JH, Yong CS, Choi HG. Preparation and evaluation of taste-masked donepezil hydrochloride orally disintegrating tablets. *Biol Pharm Bull.* 2010;33:1364–1370.
2. Yamreudeewong W, Dolence EK, Pahl D. Stability of donepezil in an extemporaneously prepared oral liquid. *J Pharm Pract.* 2006;19:282–285.

Doxazosin Mesylate

Product Availability

Solid	• Tablet:
	    ○ Immediate-release: 1 mg, 2 mg, 4 mg, 8 mg (Cardura® [Pfizer]; others)
	    ○ Extended-release: 4 mg, 8 mg (Cardura® XL [Pfizer])

Physicochemical (drug)

Molecular weight: • 451.48 (mesylate 547.58)	Permeability: • LogP 3.53 (calc) • LogD 0.60 (pH 7.4)	Water solubility: • 6.67 mg/mL
pKa: • n/a	Classification: • BCS Class 1; BDDCS Class 1	

Pharmaceutical (product)

Solid	• Immediate-release tablet disperses in water (20 mL) in 1 minute. • Do not crush, break, or chew extended-release tablets. • Immediate- and extended-release tablets are not bioequivalent; the bioavailability of the latter is only ~50%–60% of the bioavailability of the immediate-release product.

Pharmacokinetic (patient)

Absorption	• Specific site not known; t_{max} ~2–4 hours after an oral dose (immediate-release) • Bioavailability ~65%
Transport	• Plasma protein binding ~98% • V_d ~1–1.9 L/kg
Metabolism	• Extensively metabolized in liver by O-demethylation or hydroxylation via CYP3A4 as well as CYP2D6 and CYP2C9, with most metabolites excreted through bile into feces; enterohepatic recycling is possible • Cl ~1–2 mL/min/kg

Enteral Administration and Nutrition Considerations

Compatibility, Stability, and Bioavailability Considerations
• No data are available.

Drug-Nutrition Interactions
• Drug may influence nutrition status directly or indirectly:
    ○ Weight gain
    ○ CNS: dizziness, headache, lethargy, fatigue, visual abnormalities
    ○ GI: dry mouth, nausea, abdominal pain, diarrhea
    ○ Metabolic: edema, hypokalemia
    ○ Other: arthralgia, myalgia, muscle weakness

- No data on the influence of malnutrition or obesity on drug disposition.
- Influence of food on oral absorption or bioavailability:
  - Food may decrease the rate of absorption, with a slight (but not clinically significant) reduction of oral bioavailability.

Recommendations

Gastric	• Disperse immediate-release tablet in water just prior to administration. • No need to hold EN beyond the time required to flush-administer-flush.
Postpyloric	• As above. • Monitor for any unexpected change in effect.

Doxycycline

Product Availability

Solid	• Tablet, immediate-release: ○ As the *hyclate:* 50 mg, 75 mg, 100 mg, 150 mg (base) (various) ○ As the *monohydrate:* 50 mg, 75 mg, 100 mg, 150 mg (base) (various) • Tablet, delayed-release: ○ As the *hyclate:* 50 mg, 75 mg, 80 mg, 100 mg, 120 mg, 150 mg, 200 mg (base) (Doryx® MPC [Mayne Pharma]) • Tablet, mixed-release: 40 mg (various) • Capsule, immediate-release: ○ As the *hyclate:* 50 mg, 75 mg, 100 mg (base) (Vibramycin® Hyclate [Pfizer]; others) ○ As the *monohydrate:* 50 mg, 75 mg, 100 mg (base) (Monodox® [Aqua Pharms]; others) • Capsule, mixed-release: 40 mg (various)
Liquid	• Powder for oral suspension: ○ As the *monohydrate:* 25 mg/5 mL (base) (Vibramycin® Monohydrate [Pfizer]) • Oral syrup: ○ As the *calcium:* 50 mg/5 mL (base) (Vibramycin® Calcium [Pfizer])

Physicochemical (drug)

Molecular weight:	Permeability:	Water solubility:
• 444.45 ○ monohydrate 462.46 ○ hyclate 1025.88	• LogP –0.02 • Log D –0.06 (pH 7.4)	• 0.63 mg/mL (hyclate is more soluble)
pKa: • 3.02, 7.97, 9.15	**Classification:** • BCS Class 4; BDDCS Class 3	

Pharmaceutical (product)

Solid	• Immediate-release tablets do not disperse in water. • Do not open immediate-release capsule (irritant). • Delayed-release products contain enteric-coated granules. • Mixed-release products contain both immediate-release and delayed-release granules; do not crush.

Liquid	• Suspension (reconstituted):
	o pH n/a
	o Osmolality n/a
	o Viscosity n/a
	o May contain sucrose
	o Store at controlled room temperature
	• Oral syrup:
	o pH n/a
	o Osmolality n/a
	o Viscosity n/a
	o May contain glycerin, propylene glycol, and sorbitol; raspberry-flavored
	o Store at controlled room temperature.

Pharmacokinetic (patient)

Absorption	• In stomach and proximal small bowel; t_{max} within ~1.5–2 hours after an oral dose (immediate-release)
	• Bioavailability >90%
Transport	• Plasma protein binding >90%
	• V_d ~0.75 L/kg
Metabolism	• Some gut lumen inactivation, but otherwise not metabolized
	• Eliminated through bile and urine
	• Cl ~0.53 mL/min/kg

Enteral Administration and Nutrition Considerations

Compatibility, Stability, and Bioavailability Considerations

- An aqueous solution of doxycycline hyclate (10 mg/mL) expected to have a pH of 2–3, while an aqueous dispersion of doxycycline (10 mg/mL) would have a pH of 5–6.5.
- Extemporaneously compounded oral suspensions (33 mg/mL, 167 mg/mL) prepared from doxycycline hyclate tablets in OraSweet/OraPlus (1:1), stored in amber plastic bottles at 2°C–8°C or 22°C–26°C, remained stable (HPLC analysis) for no more than 7 days.[1]
- An extemporaneous oral suspension (5 mg/mL) prepared from doxycycline tablets in either simple syrup/1% methylcellulose (1:10) or OraSweet/OraPlus (1:1), stored in plastic bottles at 4°C or 25°C, remained stable (HPLC analysis) for 14 days.[2]
- Crushed doxycycline tablets are most stable (7 days) in low-fat chocolate milk (refrigerated); when mixed with other common products (eg, water, apple juice, jelly, pudding), crushed tablets are stable for no more than 24 hours.[3]
- Doxycycline has the least affinity for calcium ions, compared with other available tetracyclines.

Drug-Nutrition Interactions
- Drug may influence nutrition status directly or indirectly:
  - GI: stomatitis, glossitis, anorexia, dysphagia, nausea, vomiting, abdominal discomfort, diarrhea (including *Clostridium difficile*–associated)
  - Metabolic: elevated BUN, urinary nitrogen, and urinary ascorbic acid
- No data on the influence of malnutrition or obesity on drug disposition.
- Influence of food on oral bioavailability:
  - A high-fat, high-protein meal (1000 kcal) that included dairy products decreased the rate of absorption and reduced oral bioavailability by ~20%; influence may vary with the product.

Recommendations

Gastric	• Crush and/or disperse immediate-release tablet in water just prior to administration. • Consider separating administration from intermittent bolus feeds; otherwise, no need to hold continuous EN beyond the time required to flush-administer-flush.
Postpyloric	• As above. • Monitor for any unexpected change in effect.
Other	• As with all antimicrobials, consider parenteral alternative for acutely ill patients to ensure therapeutic concentrations.

References

1. Papich MG, Davidson GS, Fortier LA. Doxycycline concentration over time after storage in a compounded veterinary preparation. *J Am Vet Med Assoc.* 2013;242:1674–1678.
2. Nahata MC. Stability of levothyroxine, doxycycline, hydrocortisone, and pravastatin in liquid dosage forms stored at two temperatures. *Int J Pharm Compd.* 2015;19:428–431.
3. Sadrieh N, Brower J, Yu L, et al. Stability, dose uniformity, and palatability of three counterterrorism drugs: human subject and electronic tongue studies. *Pharm Res.* 2005; 22:1747–1756.

Duloxetine Hydrochloride

Product Availability

Solid	• Capsule: 20 mg, 30 mg, 60 mg (base) (Cymbalta® [Lilly]; others)

Physicochemical (drug)

Molecular weight: • 297.42 (salt 333.87)	Permeability: • LogP 4.0 • Log D n/a	Water solubility: • 0.02 mg/mL
pKa: • 9.7	Classification: • BCS Class n/a; BDDCS Class 1	

Pharmaceutical (product)

Solid	• Do not open, chew, or crush capsule. • Capsule contains delayed-release (enteric-coated) granules.

Pharmacokinetic (patient)

Absorption	• Specific site not known; t_{max} ~6 hours after an oral dose (modified-release) • Bioavailability ~30%–80%
Transport	• Plasma protein binding >90% to albumin and α_1-acid glycoprotein • V_d ~1640 liters
Metabolism	• Extensive metabolism by oxidation through CYP1A2 and CYP2D6, with further conjugation to glucuronic acid or sulfate before excretion, mostly via urine • Cl ~10 mL/min/kg

Enteral Administration and Nutrition Considerations

Compatibility, Stability, and Bioavailability Considerations
- The enteric-coated granules require a pH >5.5 to dissolve.
- In subjects who had undergone gastric bypass, oral bioavailability was reduced by ~40% compared with control subjects (all with extensive metabolizer phenotype).[1]

Drug-Nutrition Interactions
- Drug may influence nutrition status directly or indirectly:
  - Decreased appetite
  - CNS: fatigue, somnolence
  - GI: dry mouth, nausea, vomiting, constipation
  - Metabolic: hyponatremia, SIADH
- No data on the influence of malnutrition or obesity on drug disposition.
- Influence of food on oral absorption or bioavailability:
  - Food may delay the rate of absorption with a slight reduction (~10%) in oral bioavailability.

Recommendations

Gastric	• Use a therapeutic alternative.
	• Do not administer by enteral access device.
Postpyloric	• As above.

Reference

1. Roerig JL, Steffen KJ, Zimmerman C, et al. A comparison of duloxetine plasma levels in postbariatric surgery patients versus matched nonsurgical control subjects. *J Clin Psychopharmacol.* 2013;33:479–484.

Dutasteride

Product Availability

Solid	• Capsule: 0.5 mg (Avodart® [GSK]; others)

Physicochemical (drug)

Molecular weight: • 528.54	Permeability: • LogP 6.8 • LogD n/a	Water solubility: • <0.001 mg/mL
pKa: • n/a	Classification: • BCS Class n/a; BDDCS Class 2	

Pharmaceutical (product)

Solid	• Do not chew, crush, or attempt to open capsule (oropharyngeal mucosal irritant). • Women of childbearing potential should not handle (cutaneous absorption and fetal abnormalities).

Pharmacokinetic (patient)

Absorption	• Specific site not known; t_{max} ~2–3 hours after an oral dose • Bioavailability ~40%–94% (60%)
Transport	• Plasma protein binding >96% to albumin and α_1-acid glycoprotein • V_d ~300–500 liters
Metabolism	• Metabolized to at least 3 major and 2 minor metabolites, in part via CYP3A4, then excreted mainly in feces • Cl ~0.2–0.4 mL/min/kg

Enteral Administration and Nutrition Considerations

Compatibility, Stability, and Bioavailability Considerations
- Drug formulations in development using self-microemulsifying formulations may improve both dissolution and oral bioavailability.[1,2]

Drug-Nutrition Interactions
- Drug may influence nutrition status directly or indirectly:
  - CNS: malaise, fatigue, headache
  - Other: musculoskeletal pain
- No data on the influence of malnutrition or obesity on drug disposition.
- Influence of food on oral absorption or bioavailability:
  - Food may decrease the rate of absorption but without influencing oral bioavailability.

Recommendations

Gastric	• Use a therapeutic alternative. • Do not administer by enteral access device.
Postpyloric	• As above.

References

1. Baek I-H, Ha E-S, Yoo J-W, Jung Y, Kim M-S. Design of a gelatin microparticle-containing self-microemulsifying formulation for enhanced oral bioavailability of dutasteride. *Drug Des Dev Ther*. 2015;9:3231–3238.
2. Kim M-S, Ha E-S, Choo G-H, Baek I-H. Preparation and in vivo evaluation of a dutasteride-loaded solid-supersaturatable self-microemulsifying drug delivery system. *Int J Mol Sci*. 2015;16:10821–10833.

Enalapril Maleate

Product Availability

Solid	• Tablet: 2.5 mg, 5 mg, 10 mg, 20 mg (Vasotec® [Valeant]; others)
Liquid	• Oral solution: 1 mg/mL (Epaned® [Silvergate])

Physicochemical (drug)

Molecular weight: • 376.45 (maleate 492.53)	Permeability: • LogP 0.67 (calc) • LogD −2.79 (pH 6.5), −3.69 (pH 7.4) (calc)	Water solubility: • 25 mg/mL (room temperature)
pKa: • 3.0, 5.4	Classification: • BCS Class 1 or 3; BDDCS Class n/a	

Pharmaceutical (product)

Solid	• Tablets do not disperse in water without crushing. • Crush using a closed system (to avoid exposure in pregnancy).
Liquid	• Oral solution: ○ pH n/a ○ Osmolality n/a ○ Viscosity n/a ○ May contain sucralose; mixed berry-flavored ○ Store at refrigeration; may store at controlled room temperature for up to 60 days. ○ Also available as a powder for oral solution; commercially provided diluent may contain glycerin, sorbitol, and saccharin.
Note	• The tablets and oral solution are considered bioequivalent.

Pharmacokinetic (patient)

Absorption	• Specific site not known; t_{max} ~1 hour after an oral dose • Bioavailability ~55%–75%
Transport	• Possible substrate for peptide transporter(s) uptake • Plasma protein binding ~50%–60% • V_d ~1.7 L/kg
Metabolism	• The prodrug is hydrolyzed by carboxylesterase-1 (intestine and liver) to the active metabolite (enalaprilat). • Cl ~150 mL/h

Enteral Administration and Nutrition Considerations

Compatibility, Stability, and Bioavailability Considerations
- Enalapril decomposition is pH-dependent with maximal stability at
pH ~3 with degradation rate increasing at pH >5.[1,2]
- A 1% aqueous solution is expected to have a pH of ~2.6.

- The official USP oral suspension (1 mg/mL) is expected to have a pH of ~2.6–3.6 and a BUD of 60 days whether at controlled room temperature or under refrigeration.
- An extemporaneously compounded solution (0.1 mg/mL, 1 mg/mL) prepared from tablets in sterile water, stored in amber glass bottles at 20°C–24°C, remained stable (HPLC analysis) for 14 days.[3]
- Oral suspensions (1 mg/mL) prepared from crushed tablets in buffer solution and then in a number of vehicles, stored at room temperature or refrigeration, remained stable (HPLC analysis) for at least 30 days.[1,4–7]
- Another extemporaneously compounded suspension (1 mg/mL) prepared from drug powder in SyrSpend SF PH4, stored out of light at 2°C–8°C or 20°C–25°C, remained stable (HPLC analysis) for 90 days.[8]
- Another aqueous preparation (1 mg/mL) using powdered drug in buffered solution and simple syrup, stored in glass and protected from light at 2°C–8°C or 23°C–27°C, remained stable (HPLC analysis) for 50 days or 30 days, respectively.[9]
- A formulation under study that included polyelectrolytes was able to improve stability and bioavailability.[10]

Drug-Nutrition Interactions
- Drug may influence nutrition status directly or indirectly:
  - CNS: dizziness, headache, fatigue
  - GI: dysgeusia, stomatitis, nausea, abdominal pain, diarrhea
  - Metabolic: hyperkalemia, anemia, hypoglycemia
- No data on the influence of malnutrition or obesity on drug disposition.
- Influence of food on oral absorption or bioavailability:
  - A high-fat meal may reduce the rate of absorption and decrease oral bioavailability by ~23%.

Recommendations

Gastric	• Crush and disperse tablet in water just prior to administration. • Alternative: Dilute liquid with water (at least 1:1) just prior to administration. • No need to hold EN beyond the time required to flush-administer-flush.
Postpyloric	• As above. • Monitor for any unexpected change in effect.

References
1. Boulton DW, Woods DJ, Fawcett JP, et al. The stability of an enalapril maleate oral solution prepared from tablets. *Aust J Hosp Pharm.* 1994;24:151–156.
2. Glass BD, Haywood A. Stability considerations in liquid dosage forms extemporaneously prepared from commercially available products. *J Pharm Pharmaceut Sci.* 2006;9:398–426.

3. Schlatter J, Saulnier JL. Stability of enalapril solutions prepared from tablets in sterile water. *Aust J Hosp Pharm.* 1997;27:395–397.

4. Nahata MC, Morosco RS, Hipple TF. Stability of enalapril maleate in three extemporaneously prepared oral liquids. *Am J Health-Syst Pharm.* 1998;55:1155–1157.

5. Allen LV, Erickson MA. Stability of alprazolam, chloroquine phosphate, cisapride, enalapril maleate, and hydralazine hydrochloride in extemporaneously compounded oral liquids. *Am J Health-Syst Pharm.* 1998;55:1915–1920.

6. Sosnowska K, Winnicka K, Czajkowska-Kosnik A. Stability of extemporaneous enalapril maleate suspensions for pediatric use prepared from commercially available tablets. *Acta Pol Pharm.* 2009;66:321–326.

7. Sosnowska K, Winnicka K, Czajkowska-Kosnik A. Comparison of the stability of pediatric enalapril maleate suspensions prepared from various commercially available tablets. *Farmacja Polska.* 2009;65:243–246.

8. Polonini HC, Loures S, Lima LC, et al. Stability of atenolol, clonazepam, dexamethasone, diclofenac sodium, diltiazem, enalapril maleate, ketoprofen, lamotrigine, penicillamine-D and thiamine in SyrSpend SF PH4 oral suspensions. *Int J Pharm Compd.* 2016;20:167–174.

9. Casas M, Álvarez J, Lucero MJ. Physicochemical stability of captopril and enalapril extemporaneous formulations for pediatric patients. *Pharm Dev Technol.* 2013;20:271–278.

10. Ramirez-Rigo MV, Olivera ME, Rubio M, Manzo RH. Enhanced intestinal permeability and oral bioavailability of enalapril maleate upon complexation with the cationic polymethacrylate Eudragit E100. *Eur J Pharm Sci.* 2014;55:1–11.

Escitalopram Oxalate

Product Availability

Solid	• Tablet: 5 mg, 10 mg, 20 mg (base) (Lexapro® [Forest]; others)
Liquid	• Oral solution: 5 mg/5 mL (base) (Lexapro® [Allergan]; others)

Physicochemical (drug)

Molecular weight: • 324.40 (oxalate 414.43)	Permeability: • LogP 3.5 • LogD n/a	Water solubility: • 0.006 mg/mL
pKa: • 9.8	Classification: • BCS Class 1; BDDCS Class 1	

Pharmaceutical (product)

Solid	• Most tablet products are film-coated.
Liquid	• Oral solution: o pH 4.5 o Osmolality 6030 mOsm/kg (calculated based on measurement of 1:5 dilution with sterile water)[1] o Viscosity n/a o May contain sorbitol, glycerin, and propylene glycol; peppermint-flavored o Store at controlled room temperature.
Note	• Tablets and oral solution are considered bioequivalent.

Pharmacokinetic (patient)

Absorption	• Specific site not known; t_{max} ~4 hours after an oral dose • Bioavailability ~80%
Transport	• Plasma protein binding ~56% • V_d ~12 L/kg
Metabolism	• Extensively metabolized (N-demethylation) to several much less active or totally inactive metabolites via CYP2C19 and CYP3A4 • Cl ~600 mL/min

Enteral Administration and Nutrition Considerations

Compatibility, Stability, and Bioavailability Considerations
- Commercial liquid combined (1:1) with Osmolite 1.2, under simulated clinical conditions, would be expected to result in clogging of an 8 Fr or a 20 Fr feeding tube.[1]

Drug-Nutrition Interactions
- Drug may influence nutrition status directly or indirectly:
  o CNS: insomnia, fatigue, blurred vision
  o GI: dry mouth, nausea, abdominal pain, diarrhea

o Metabolic: hyponatremia, hyperglycemia
o Other: arthralgia, myalgia
- No data on the influence of malnutrition or obesity on drug disposition.
- No known influence of food on oral absorption or bioavailability.

Recommendations

Gastric	• Dilute liquid with water (at least 1:1) just prior to administration. • No need to hold EN beyond the time required to flush-administer-flush.
Postpyloric	• As above but may require further dilution given high osmolality. • Monitor for any unexpected change in effect.

Reference

1. Klang M, McLymont V, Ng N. Osmolality, pH, and compatibility of selected oral liquid medications with an enteral nutrition product. *JPEN J Parenter Enteral Nutr.* 2013;37: 689–694.

Esomeprazole Magnesium

Product Availability

Solid	• Tablet:
	  o Extended-release: 20 mg (base) (Nexium® 24HR [AstraZeneca])
	• Capsule:
	  o Delayed-release: 20 mg, 40 mg (base) (Nexium® [AstraZeneca]; others)
	  o Extended-release: 20 mg (base) (Nexium® 24HR [AstraZeneca])

Liquid	• Granules for oral suspension: 2.5 mg, 5 mg, 10 mg, 20 mg, 40 mg per packet (base) (Nexium® [AstraZeneca])

Physicochemical (drug)

Molecular weight:
• 345.42
  o anhydrous 713.12
  o trihydrate 767.17
	Permeability:
	• LogP 2.23
	• LogD n/a
		Water solubility:
		• 0.5 mg/mL

pKa: • 3.97	Classification: • BCS Class n/a; BDDCS Class 1	

Pharmaceutical (product)

Solid	• Do not crush tablets (extended-release) or capsule contents (enteric-coated granules).

Liquid	• Suspension (reconstituted):
	  o Do not crush the granules for suspension (enteric-coated).
	  o The content of each packet for suspension is mixed with 5 mL (2.5 mg, 5 mg) or 15 mL (10 mg, 20 mg, 40 mg) of water; the admixture thickens over 2–3 minutes.
	  o pH n/a
	  o Osmolality n/a
	  o Viscosity n/a
	  o May contain dextrose
	  o Maintain at controlled room temperature and administer within 30 minutes of preparing.

Pharmacokinetic (patient)

Absorption	• Proximal small bowel; t_{max} ~1–2 hours after an oral dose • Bioavailability ~90% (with repeated dosing)
Transport	• Plasma protein binding ~97% • V_d ~16 liters
Metabolism	• Extensive metabolism via CYP2C19 (whose activity the drug may also interfere with) and also CYP3A4 to inactive metabolites, mostly excreted in urine • Cl ~0.5–0.6 L/min

Enteral Administration and Nutrition Considerations

Compatibility, Stability, and Bioavailability Considerations

- Drug stability is pH-dependent with rapid decomposition in acidic environments.
- A noncoated packet formulation dissolved in pH 3.4–5 water to final concentrations of 20 mg/15 mL and 40 mg/15 mL in about 2 minutes; dissolution of the formulation took about 10 minutes in apple juice and orange juice. All of these remained stable (HPLC analysis) for ~60 minutes without altering oral pharmacokinetic profiles in volunteers.[1]
- Granules are smaller than those of lansoprazole or omeprazole, and, when suspended in water (or apple juice) followed by a 10–20 mL flush, are more efficiently delivered (100%) to the end of polyurethane and silicone tubes (16 Fr) compared with the other two proton pump inhibitors (61%–67%).[2]
- In an in vitro study of capsule granules suspended in 50 mL of water, in a 60 mL oral syringe, delivery through an 8 Fr polyurethane nasogastric tube with 20 mL water flush pre/post drug administration was successful when administered immediately; however, when a 15-minute incubation period occurred, there were significant differences between products and between water sources (deionized, tap) attributed to alterations in enteric coating.[3]
- Suspending the granules (40 mg capsule) in 50 mL of water in a 60 mL syringe, replacing the plunger, shaking 15 seconds, and then administering the suspension via 16 Fr nasogastric tubes over 30 seconds, followed by another 30 mL water flush, delivered most of the drug to the distal tip with bioavailability similar to oral dosing in a crossover study with 47 healthy subjects.[4]
- After suspending the granules in water or water-diluted OraPlus diluent (30%, 50%, 70%) in a syringe and shaking the suspension, administration through a 14 Fr nasogastric tube or 20 Fr gastrostomy tube was successful, but it was less efficient through an 8 Fr nasogastric tube.[5]
- Mixing OraPlus with water to suspend the granules was more effective than water alone when administered through an 8 Fr nasogastric tube.[5]
- Another in vitro analysis in which the contents of 40 mg capsules were dispersed in tap water (50 mL, or 25 mL × 2) prior to administration through 8 Fr polyurethane nasogastric tubes, 14 Fr nasogastric tubes, or 20 Fr silicone gastrostomy tubes revealed near complete (≥98%) granule delivery when using the 50 mL volume all at once.[6]
- When a 16 Fr silicone nasogastric tube was also used for a fiber-containing enteral formula (Fresubin Original Fibre) but flushed with 10 mL of water before/after administration of the microgranule tablet dispersed in 50 mL sterile water, all of the drug was delivered to the distal end of the feeding tube.[7]

- In an in vitro study to test the effect of repeated administration on the patency of feeding tubes, a 10 mg product for oral suspension in 15 mL of sterile water was administered twice daily by 30 mL syringe through three different sizes of feeding tubes (6 Fr, 8.5 Fr, 10 Fr), across 7 days under simulated clinical conditions by the administration of 22-hour-per-day enteral feed by pump, with 5 mL water flush before/after. The only change in flow rate or obstruction occurred in the 6 Fr tube by the sixth day.[8]

Drug-Nutrition Interactions
- Drug may influence nutrition status directly or indirectly:
  - CNS: lethargy, fatigue
  - GI: dry mouth, nausea, abdominal pain, diarrhea (including *Clostridium difficile*–associated)
  - Metabolic: hypomagnesemia
  - Other: increased risk of osteoporosis-related fractures (e.g., hip, spine, wrist), muscle weakness and cramps
- No data on the influence of malnutrition or obesity on drug disposition.
- Influence of food on oral absorption or bioavailability:
  - Food intake decreases oral bioavailability by 43%–53% but without clinical significance on gastric pH reduction.

Recommendations

Gastric	• Prepare suspension as directed by manufacturer, dilute further with water just prior to administration through a tube (≥10 Fr). • No need to hold EN beyond the time required to flush-administer-flush.
Postpyloric	• As above. • Monitor for any unexpected change in effect.

References

1. Bladh N, Blychert E, Johansson K, et al. A new esomeprazole packet (sachet) formulation for suspension: in vitro characteristics and comparative pharmacokinetics versus intact capsules/tablets in healthy volunteers. *Clin Ther*. 2007;29:640–649.
2. Messaouik D, Sauto-Miranda V, Bagel-Boithias S, et al. Comparative study and optimization of the administration mode of three proton pump inhibitors by nasogastric tube. *Int J Pharm*. 2005;299:65–72.
3. Hoover A, Sun D, Wen H, et al. In vitro evaluation of nasogastric tube delivery performance of esomeprazole magnesium delayed-release capsules. *J Pharm Sci*. 2017; 106:1859–1864.
4. Sostek MB, Chen Y, Skammer W, et al. Esomeprazole administered through a nasogastric tube provides bioavailability similar to oral dosing. *Aliment Pharmacol Ther*. 2003;18:581–586.
5. Shah SA, Sander S, Coleman CI, et al. Delivery of esomeprazole magnesium through nasogastric and gastrostomy tubes using an oral liquid vehicle as a suspending agent in vitro. *Am J Health-Syst Pharm*. 2006;63:1882–1887.

6. White CM, Kalus JS, Quercia R, et al. Delivery of esomeprazole magnesium enteric-coated pellets through small caliber and standard nasogastric tubes and gastrostomy tubes in vitro. *Am J Health-Syst Pharm.* 2003;59:2085–2088.

7. Messaouik D, Sauto-Miranda V, Balayssac D, et al. Is the administration of esomeprazole through a nasogastric tube modified by concomitant delivery of a nutrition mixture? *Eur J Hosp Pharm Sci.* 2006;12:100–104.

8. Stewart P, Dayneka N, Grenier S, et al. In vitro study of esomeprazole sachet suspension administered via enteral feeding tubes. *CJHP.* 2009;62:48–49.

Estradiol

Product Availability

Solid	• Tablet:
	   ○ Estradiol acetate: 0.45 mg, 0.9 mg, 1.8 mg (Femtrace® [Warner Chilcott])
	   ○ Ethinyl estradiol: 2 µg, 5 µg in combination with a progestin (various)
	   ○ Estradiol: 0.5 mg, 1 mg, 2 mg alone or in combination with a progestin (various)

Physicochemical (drug)

Molecular weight: • 272.39	Permeability: • LogP 4.01 • LogD 4.52 (pH 7) (calc)	Water solubility: • 0.09 mg/mL
pKa: • ~10–11	Classification: • BCS Class 1; BDDCS Class 1	

Pharmaceutical (product)

Solid	• Tablets do not easily disperse in water. • Use a closed system to crush tablet to minimize caregiver exposure.

Pharmacokinetic (patient)

Absorption	• Proximal-to-mid small bowel; t_{max} varies but ~2–3 hours after an oral dose • Bioavailability is variable: ~25%–65%
Transport	• Substrate for P-glycoprotein and BCRP efflux • Plasma protein binding ~97% to albumin • V_d ~14 L/kg
Metabolism	• Undergoes hydroxylation via CYP3A4, is further methylated, and undergoes glucuronic acid and sulfate conjugation; following biliary excretion may undergo deconjugation with enterohepatic recirculation • Cl ~600 mL/h/kg

Enteral Administration and Nutrition Considerations

Compatibility, Stability, and Bioavailability Considerations

- The administration of a 20 µg dose either in tablet form or in a hydroalcoholic solution resulted in similar oral bioavailability in a group of healthy women.[1]
- A formulation using nanoparticle technology increased dissolution and oral bioavailability in an animal model.[2]

Drug-Nutrition Interactions
- Drug may influence nutrition status directly or indirectly:
  - Reduced concentrations of serum α-tocopherol and coenzyme Q_{10}
  - CNS: headache, visual disturbances
  - GI: nausea, vomiting, abdominal pain
  - Metabolic: fluid retention, hypertriglyceridemia, hypocalcemia or rare hypercalcemia
  - Other: arthralgia
- The influence of malnutrition or obesity on drug disposition:
  - Pharmacokinetic variability may be greater in obesity.[3]
- Influence of food on oral absorption or bioavailability:
  - Grapefruit juice may increase oral bioavailability.[4]

Recommendations

Gastric	• If there is no therapeutic alternative (e.g., transdermal formulation), crush tablet (closed) and dilute with water prior to administration. • No need to hold EN beyond the time required to flush-administer-flush.
Postpyloric	• As above. • Monitor for any unexpected change in effect.

References
1. Hunt T, Geetha R, Warga E. The bioavailability of desogestrel/ethinyl estradiol tablets relative to the oral solution. *Clin Drug Invest.* 1998;15:507–514.
2. Mittal G, Ravi Kumar MNV. Impact of polymeric nanoparticles on oral pharmacokinetics: a dose-dependent case study with estradiol. *J Pharm Sci.* 2009;98:3730–3734.
3. Goldzieher JW, Stanczyk FZ. Oral contraceptives and individual variability of circulating levels of ethinyl estradiol and progestins. *Contraception.* 2008;78:4–9.
4. Weber A, Jager R, Borner A, et al. Can grapefruit juice influence ethinyl estradiol bioavailability? *Contraception.* 1996;53:41–47.

Eszopiclone

Product Availability

Solid	• Tablet: 1 mg, 2 mg, 3 mg (Lunesta® [Sunovion]; others)

Physicochemical (drug)

Molecular weight: • 388.82	Permeability: • LogP 0.8 • LogD n/a	Water solubility: • 0.8 mg/mL
pKa: • 5.35	Classification: • BCS Class n/a; BDDCS Class 1	

Pharmaceutical (product)

Solid	• Degree of tablet film-coating may vary by manufacturer.

Pharmacokinetic (patient)

Absorption	• Proximal small bowel; t_{max} ~1 hour after an oral dose • Bioavailability ~80%
Transport	• Plasma protein binding ~52%–59% • V_d ~90 liters
Metabolism	• Extensively metabolized by oxidation and methylation (via CYP3A4, CYP2E1) to both active and inactive metabolites; most of the drug is eliminated in urine • Cl n/a

Enteral Administration and Nutrition Considerations

Compatibility, Stability, Bioavailability Considerations
• Soluble in aqueous buffer at pH 3.2.

Drug-Nutrition Interactions
• Drug may influence nutrition status directly or indirectly:
   o CNS: confusion, psychomotor and cognitive impairment
   o GI: unpleasant taste, dry mouth, nausea, dyspepsia, vomiting, rare hepatitis
   o Metabolic: rare hypokalemia
• No data on the influence of malnutrition or obesity on drug disposition.
• Influence of food on oral absorption or bioavailability:
   o Food, especially a high-fat meal, can reduce the rate of oral absorption but without an influence on oral bioavailability.

Recommendations

Gastric	• Crush and/or disperse tablet in water prior to administration. • No need to hold EN beyond the time required to flush-administer-flush.
Postpyloric	• As above. • Monitor for any unexpected change in effect.

Ezetimibe

Product Availability

Solid	• Tablet: 10 mg (Zetia® [Merck]; others)

Physicochemical (drug)

Molecular weight: • 409.44	Permeability: • LogP 4.5 • LogD n/a	Water solubility: • 0.004 mg/mL
pKa: • 9.72	Classification: • BCS Class 2; BDDCS Class 2	

Pharmaceutical (product)

Solid	• Tablets may disperse in water with time.

Pharmacokinetic (patient)

Absorption	• Proximal small bowel; t_{max} ~1–2 hours after an oral dose (based on metabolite) • Bioavailability ~93%
Transport	• Substrate for P-glycoprotein efflux; substrate for OATP1B1 uptake • Plasma protein binding >90% (both drug and metabolite) • V_d ~1.5 L/kg
Metabolism	• Rapid metabolism to the active phenolic glucuronide metabolite (via UGT1A1, UGT1A3, UGT2B15), but then slowly eliminated; possibly related to enterohepatic recirculation, including accumulation of glucuronide at the intestinal wall • Cl ~6.6 mL/min/kg

Enteral Administration and Nutrition Considerations

Compatibility, Stability, and Bioavailability Considerations

- An amorphous nanosuspension formulation made with distilled water, ethanol, and Tween 80 was studied for improving the drug's solubility and bioavailability.[1]
- A nanocrystal formulation under development used a nonionic surfactant (TPGS) with P-glycoprotein inhibitory activity to improve dissolution and absorption.[2]
- A self-nanoemulsifying delivery system under development improved aqueous solubility and dissolution.[3]
- Including hydroxypropylcellulose in a formulation improved drug dissolution and bioavailability.[4]
- A set of amorphous solid dispersions were studied to characterize phase transformation during dissolution in biorelevant media including Ensure Plus.[5]

Enteral Administration and Nutrition Considerations

Compatibility, Stability, and Bioavailability Considerations
- Degradation of the drug is pH-dependent, being extremely unstable in aqueous solution of pH 2.0 at 25°C, exhibiting more than 60% loss within 24 hours.[1]
- An extemporaneously compounded oral liquid (8 mg/mL) prepared from tablets (40 mg) in distilled water and cherry syrup, stored in amber glass bottles at 4°C or 24°C, remained stable (HPLC analysis) for 20 days or 15 days, respectively.[2]
- An extemporaneously compounded oral suspension (8 mg/mL) prepared from tablets (40 mg) in sterile water and then OraSweet/OraPlus (1:1), stored in amber polyethylene terephthalate bottles at 23°C–25°C, remained stable (HPLC analysis) for 95 days.[3]
- A microemulsion test formulation resulted in a 1.8-fold increased oral bioavailability in an animal model, which is in keeping with improved in vitro intestinal permeation studies.[4]
- A nanoparticle formulation is expected to improve oral bioavailability.[5]

Drug-Nutrition Interactions
- Drug may influence nutrition status directly or indirectly:
  - CNS: headache
  - GI: constipation or diarrhea, LFT elevations
  - Metabolic: elevated BUN or serum creatinine, proteinuria
- No data on the influence of malnutrition or obesity on drug disposition
- No known influence of food on oral absorption or bioavailability

Recommendations

Gastric	• Crush and/or disperse tablet in water prior to administration. • Alternative: Dilute suspension with water (at least 1:1) just prior to administration. • No need to hold EN beyond the time required to flush-administer-flush.
Postpyloric	• As above. • Monitor for any unexpected change in effect.

References
1. Wu Y, Fassihi R. Stability of metronidazole, tetracycline hydrochloride, and famotidine alone and in combination. *Int J Pharmaceut*. 2005;290:1–13.
2. Quercia RA, Jay GT, Fan C, et al. Stability of famotidine in an extemporaneously prepared oral liquid. *Am J Hosp Pharm*. 1993;50:691–693.
3. Dentinger PJ, Swenson CF, Anaizi NH. Stability of famotidine in an extemporaneously compounded oral liquid. *Am J Health-Syst Pharm*. 2000;57:1340–1342.

4. Jha SK, Karki R, Puttegowda VD, Harinarayana D. In vitro intestinal permeability studies and pharmacokinetic evaluation of famotidine microemulsion for oral delivery. *Int Schol Res Not.* 2014;452051.

5. Mokhtar M, Gosselin P, Lacasse F, Hildgen P. Design of PEG-grafted-PLA nanoparticles as oral permeability enhancer for P-gp substrate drug model famotidine. *J Microencapsul.* 2017;34:91–103.

Felodipine
Product Availability

Solid	• Tablet: Extended-release: 2.5 mg, 5 mg, 10 mg (various)

Physicochemical (drug)

Molecular weight: • 384.26	Permeability: • LogP 3.86 • LogD n/a	Water solubility: • 0.02 mg/mL
pKa: • 5.4	Classification: • BCS Class n/a; BDDCS Class 2	

Pharmaceutical (product)

Solid	• Do not crush tablet (modified-release).

Pharmacokinetic (patient)

Absorption	• Specific site not known; t_{max} ~2.5–5 hours after an oral dose • Bioavailability ~20%
Transport	• Plasma protein binding ~99% • V_d ~10 L/kg
Metabolism	• Extensive first-pass metabolism via CYP3A4 • Cl ~0.8 L/min

Enteral Administration and Nutrition Considerations

Compatibility, Stability, and Bioavailability Considerations
• No data are available.

Drug-Nutrition Interactions
• Drug may influence nutrition status directly or indirectly:
  o CNS: headache, tremor
  o GI: nausea, heartburn, abdominal cramps
  o Metabolic: peripheral edema
  o Other: weakness, muscle cramps
• No data on the influence of malnutrition or obesity on drug disposition.
• Influence of food on oral absorption or bioavailability:
  o A high-fat or high-carbohydrate meal can increase the peak concentrations from the extended-release tablet by ~60%, despite no significant influence on oral bioavailability.
  o Grapefruit juice can increase oral bioavailability by up to 2-fold.

Recommendations

Gastric	• Do not administer by enteral access device. • Consider a therapeutic alternative (eg, amlodipine).
Postpyloric	• As above.

Fenofibrate

Product Availability

Solid	• Tablet: Immediate-release: 40 mg, 48 mg, 50 mg, 54 mg, 120 mg, 145 mg, 160 mg (TriCor® [AbbVie]; others)
	• Capsule:
	  o Fenofibrate: 50 mg, 150 mg (Lipofen® [Cipher])
	  o Micronized: 30 mg, 67 mg, 90 mg, 134 mg, 200 mg (choline fenofibrate) (various)
	  o Delayed-release: 45 mg, 135 mg (choline fenofibrate; fenofibric acid) (Trilipix® [AbbVie]; others)

Physicochemical (drug)

Molecular weight: • 360.84	Permeability: • LogP 5.3 • LogD 4.80 (pH 7.4)	Water solubility: • 0.0008 mg/mL
pKa: • 2.9	Classification: • BCS Class 2; BDDCS Class 2	

Pharmaceutical (product)

Solid	• Do not open, chew, or crush modified-release capsules. • Formulations are not necessarily bioequivalent.

Pharmacokinetic (patient)

Absorption	• Specific site not known; t_{max} ~6–8 hours after an oral dose • Bioavailability ~60%–69% (fenofibrate), ~81%–88% (fenofibric acid)
Transport	• Plasma protein binding ~99% • V_d ~0.89 L/kg
Metabolism	• Fenofibrate is a prodrug hydrolyzed by esterases to the active fenofibric acid, subsequently conjugated with glucuronic acid, excreted mostly in urine • Cl ~1.1–1.2 L/h

Enteral Administration and Nutrition Considerations

Compatibility, Stability, and Bioavailability Considerations

- Bioavailability of choline fenofibrate and fenofibric acid is better than fenofibrate.[1,2]
- Fenofibric acid coformulated with magnesium carbonate improved dissolution and bioavailability.[3]
- Several formulations under study may improve drug dissolution and oral bioavailability.[4-6]
- Lipid-containing dispersions under study may improve oral absorption without food dependence of micronized drug product.[7-10]

Drug-Nutrition Interactions
- Drug may influence nutrition status directly or indirectly:
  - CNS: headache
  - GI: nausea, abdominal pain, diarrhea/constipation, LFT abnormalities, cholelithiasis, cholecystitis, pancreatitis
  - Other: myopathy, rhabdomyolysis
- No data on the influence of malnutrition or obesity on drug disposition.
- Influence of food on oral absorption or bioavailability:
  - Most micronized capsule formulations require administration with fat-containing food to meet expectant bioavailability.
  - No known influence of food on oral bioavailability of other formulations.

Recommendations

Gastric	• Crush and/or disperse tablet in water prior to administration. • No need to hold EN beyond the time required to flush-administer-flush.
Postpyloric	• As above. • Monitor for any unexpected change in effect.

References

1. Zhu T, Ansquer J-C, Kelly MT, Sleep DJ, Pradhan RS. Comparison of the gastrointestinal absorption and bioavailability of fenofibrate and fenofibric acid in humans. *J Clin Pharmacol.* 2010;50:914–921.
2. Wei X, Li P, Liu M, et al. Absolute oral bioavailability of fenofibric acid and choline fenofibrate in rats determined by ultra-performance liquid chromatography tandem mass spectrometry. *Biomed Chromatogr.* 2016;31:e3832.
3. Kim KS, Kim JH, Jin SG, et al. Effect of magnesium carbonate on the solubility, dissolution and oral bioavailability of fenofibric acid powder as an alkalinising solubilizer. *Arch Pharm Res.* 2016;39:531–538.
4. Kim GG, Poudel BK, Marasini N, et al. Enhancement of oral bioavailability of fenofibrate by solid self-microemulsifying drug delivery systems. *Drug Dev Ind Pharm.* 2013;39:1431–1438.
5. Yousaf AM, Kim DW, Oh Y-K, et al. Enhanced oral bioavailability of fenofibrate using polymeric nanoparticulated systems: physicochemical characterization and in vivo investigation. *Int J Nanomedicine.* 2015;10:1819–1830.
6. Mohsin K, Alamri R, Ahmad A, et al. Development of self-nanoemulsifying drug delivery systems for the enhancement of solubility and oral bioavailability of fenofibrate, a poorly water-soluble drug. *Int J Nanomedicine.* 2016;11:2829–2838.
7. Mohsin K. Design of lipid-based formulations for oral administration of poorly water-soluble drug fenofibrate: effects of digestion. *AAPS Pharm Sci Tech.* 2012;13:637–646.
8. Zhang X, Chen G, Zhang T, Ma Z, Wu B. Effects of PEGylated lipid nanoparticles on the oral absorption of one BCS II drug: a mechanistic investigation. *Int J Nanomedicine.* 2014;9:5503–5514.
9. Weng T, Qi J, Wang K, et al. The role of lipid based nano delivery systems on oral bioavailability enhancement of fenofibrate, a BCS II drug: comparison with fast-release formulations. *J Nanobiotechnology.* 2014;12:39.
10. O'Shea JP, Faisal W, Ruane-O'Hora T, et al. Lipidic dispersion to reduce food dependent oral bioavailability of fenofibrate: in vitro, in vivo and in silico assessments. *Eur J Pharm Biopharm.* 2015;96:207–216.

Fexofenadine Hydrochloride

Product Availability

Solid	• Tablet: 30 mg, 60 mg, 180 mg (various)
Liquid	• Oral suspension: 30 mg/5 mL (Allegra® [Sanofi Aventis]; others)

Physicochemical (drug)

Molecular weight: • 501.67 (salt 538.13)	Permeability: • LogP 1.96 (calc) • LogD 2.68 (pH 7.4)	Water solubility: • 1.98–2.2 mg/mL (25°C)
pKa: • 4.25, 9.53	Classification: • BCS Class 1 or 3; BDDCS Class 3	

Pharmaceutical (product)

Solid	• Tablet products are often film-coated and may not disperse easily in water.
Liquid	• Oral suspension: ○ pH n/a ○ Osmolality n/a ○ Viscosity n/a ○ May contain polypropylene glycol, sucrose, and xylitol; raspberry-cream-flavored ○ Store at controlled room temperature. ○ Shake product well before measuring dose.
Note	• Tablet and suspension are considered bioequivalent.

Pharmacokinetic (patient)

Absorption	• Specific site not known; t_{max} ~1–3 hours after an oral dose • Bioavailability ~30%
Transport	• Substrate for P-glycoprotein efflux • Substrate for organic anion-transporting polypeptides (OATPs) uptake transporters, including OATP1A2 and OATP2B1 (intestine) and OATP1B1 and OATP1B3 (hepatic) • Plasma protein binding ~60%–70% • V_d ~5.4–5.8 L/kg (in children)
Metabolism	• Only ~5% is metabolized by liver, with drug primarily excreted unchanged in the feces. • Fexofenadine is the active metabolite of terfenadine (no longer commercially available). • Cl ~9.4–14.4 mL/min/kg

Enteral Administration and Nutrition Considerations

Compatibility, Stability, and Bioavailability Considerations
- A microemulsion formulation under study enhanced oral drug bioavailability compared with the commercial liquid formulation.[1]
- A variety of formulations being tested identified a dispersion using Cremophor that increased oral bioavailability by 62% in healthy volunteers.[2]

Drug-Nutrition Interactions
- Drug may influence nutrition status directly or indirectly:
  - CNS: headache, drowsiness, fatigue
  - GI: nausea, dyspepsia
  - Metabolic: angioedema
- No data on the influence of malnutrition or obesity on drug disposition.
- Influence of food on oral absorption or bioavailability:
  - High-fat meal decreases oral bioavailability by ~21% (tablet) or 30% (suspension).
  - Aluminum- and magnesium-containing products may reduce oral bioavailability by ~41% if taken within 15 minutes.
  - Fruit juices (grapefruit, orange, apple) administered at 300–1200 mL with or within 4 hours of drug administration, decreased oral bioavailability (25%–72%) relative to water; that effect may be mitigated by temporal separation.[3,4]
  - Piperine, an alkaloid found in black pepper, administered at a dose of 20 mg/d, as might be found in supplement products, increased oral bioavailability by more than 50% in healthy volunteers, likely through P-glycoprotein inhibition.[5]

Recommendations

Gastric	• If there is no therapeutic alternative (eg, cetirizine), dilute oral liquid in water (at least 1:1) just prior to administration. • No need to hold EN beyond the time required to flush-administer-flush.
Postpyloric	• As above. • Monitor for any unexpected change in effect.

References

1. Gundogdu E, Gonzalez Alvarez I, Karasulu E. Improvement of effect of water-in-oil microemulsion as an oral delivery system for fexofenadine: in vitro and in vivo studies. *Int J Nanomedicine.* 2011;6:1631–1640.
2. Yehia SA, El-Ridi MS, Tadros MI, El-Sherif NG. Enhancement of the oral bioavailability of fexofenadine hydrochloride via Cremophor® EL-based liquisolid tablets. *Adv Pharm Bull.* 2015;5:569–581.
3. Greenblatt DJ. Analysis of drug interactions involving fruit beverages and organic anion-transporting polypeptides. *J Clin Pharmacol.* 2009;49:1403–1407.

4. Bailey DG. Fruit juice inhibition of uptake transport: a new type of food-drug interaction. *Br J Clin Pharmacol.* 2010;70:645–655.
5. Bedada SK, Boga PK. The influence of piperine on the pharmacokinetics of fexofenadine, a P-glycoprotein substrate, in healthy volunteers. *Eur J Clin Pharmacol.* 2017;73: 343–349.

Finasteride

Product Availability

Solid	• Tablet: 1 mg, 5 mg (various)

Physicochemical (drug)

Molecular weight: • 372.56	Permeability: • LogP 3.03 • LogD 3.03 (pH 7.4)	Water solubility: • 0.043 mg/mL
pKa: • n/a	Classification: • BCS Class 1; BDDCS Class 1	

Pharmaceutical (product)

Solid	• Tablet products are often film-coated. • Crush/disperse only using a closed system. • Women of childbearing potential should not handle (risk of fetal abnormalities).

Pharmacokinetic (patient)

Absorption	• Specific site not known; t_{max} ~1–2 hours after an oral dose • Bioavailability ~65%
Transport	• Plasma protein binding ~90% • V_d ~1.1 L/kg
Metabolism	• Extensive metabolism, mostly via CYP3A4 to minimally active metabolites excreted in urine and feces • Cl ~165 mL/min

Enteral Administration and Nutrition Considerations

Compatibility, Stability, and Bioavailability Considerations
- An orally disintegrating tablet under study was found to be bioequivalent to the standard tablet in a group of healthy volunteers.[1]
- A microemulsifying system formulation being considered for development improved bioavailability in human volunteers.[2]

Drug-Nutrition Interactions
- Drug may influence nutrition status directly or indirectly:
  - CNS: dizziness, asthenia
  - GI: nausea, abdominal pain, diarrhea
- No data on the influence of malnutrition or obesity on drug disposition.
- No known influence of food on oral absorption or bioavailability.

Recommendations

Gastric	• If there is no therapeutic alternative, use a closed system to crush and disperse in water prior to administration. • No need to hold EN beyond the time required to flush-administer-flush.
Postpyloric	• As above. • Monitor for any unexpected change in effect.

References

1. Chen L, Jiang X, Huang L, et al. Bioequivalence of a single 10-mg dose of finasteride 5-mg oral disintegrating tablets and standard tablets in healthy adult male Han Chinese volunteers: a randomized sequence, open-label, two-way crossover study. *Clin Ther*. 2009; 31:2242–2248.
2. Fagir W, Hathout RM, Sammour OA, El-Shafeey AH. Self-microemulsifying systems of finasteride with enhanced oral bioavailability: multivariate statistical evaluation, characterization, spray-drying and in vivo studies in human volunteers. *Nanomedicine*. 2015;10:3373–3389.

Fluconazole

Product Availability

Solid	• Tablet: 50 mg, 100 mg, 150 mg, 200 mg (Diflucan® [Pfizer]; others)
Liquid	• Powder for oral suspension: 50 mg/5 mL, 200 mg/5 mL (Diflucan® [Pfizer]; others)

Physicochemical (drug)

Molecular weight: • 306.28	Permeability: • LogP 0.50 • LogD 0.95 (pH 7.4)	Water solubility: • 8–10 mg/mL
pKa: • 1.76	Classification: • BCS Class 1; BDDCS Class 3	

Pharmaceutical (product)

Solid	• Tablet may disperse in water
Liquid	• Oral suspension (reconstituted): o pH 4.2–4.29[1,2] o Osmolality 2185 mOsm/kg (calculated based on measurement of 1:5 dilution with sterile water)[2] o Viscosity n/a o May contain sucrose; orange-flavored o Does not need refrigeration after preparation, and remains stable for 14 days (5°C–30°C)
Note	• Tablet and suspension are considered bioequivalent.

Pharmacokinetic (patient)

Absorption	• Specific site not known; t_{max} ~1–2 hours after an oral dose • Bioavailability >90%
Transport	• Plasma protein binding ~11%–12% • V_d 0.6–1 L/kg
Metabolism	• Eliminated renally, mostly unchanged • Cl ~0.23 mL/min/kg

Enteral Administration and Nutrition Considerations

Compatibility, Stability, and Bioavailability Considerations
- The reconstituted suspension (200 mg/5 mL) with sterile water for irrigation remained stable (HPLC analysis) in amber polyethylene oral syringes at 22°C–25°C for 70 days.[1]
- The commercial suspension combined (1:1) with Osmolite 1.2, under simulated clinical conditions, would result in clogging of both an 8 Fr and a 20 Fr feeding tube.[2]

- An extemporaneously compounded oral liquid (1 mg/mL) prepared from tablets in deionized water and stored in glass bottles at 4°C or 23°C remained stable (HPLC analysis) for 15 days.[3]
- Administration into jejunum results in similar bioavailability.[4]
- Bioavailability was highly variable (32%–100%) in patients with abdominal trauma regardless of whether the abdomen was open or closed.[5]
- Bariatric surgery is not expected to significantly alter oral bioavailability.[6]

Drug-Nutrition Interactions
- Drug may influence nutrition status directly or indirectly:
  o CNS: headache, fatigue tremor
  o GI: dry mouth, anorexia, nausea, vomiting, abdominal pain, diarrhea, LFT elevations and rare hepatic failure
  o Metabolic: edema, hypokalemia
  o Other: arthralgia, myalgia
- Influence of malnutrition or obesity on drug disposition:
  o Reduced weight-normalized volume of distribution and increased clearance suggest that drug dosing in obesity should be based on an estimated lean body weight.[7–9]
- Influence of food on oral absorption or bioavailability:
  o No known influence of food, including a high-fat meal, on oral drug bioavailability.
  o No known influence of EN on enteral (via gastric or postpyloric route) drug bioavailability.[10]

Recommendations

Gastric	• Disperse tablet in water prior to administration. • Alternative: Consider diluting suspension with water (at least 1:1) prior to administration, especially through a long small-bore feeding tube. • No need to hold EN beyond the time required to flush-administer-flush.
Postpyloric	• Dilute the suspension prior to administration. • Monitor for any unexpected change in effect.
Other	• As with all antimicrobials, consider parenteral alternative for acutely ill patients to ensure therapeutic concentrations.

References

1. Dentinger PJ, Swenson CF. Stability of reconstituted fluconazole oral suspension in plastic bottles and oral syringes. *Ann Pharmacother.* 2009;43:485–489.
2. Klang M, McLymont V, Ng N. Osmolality, pH, and compatibility of selected oral liquid medications with an enteral nutrition product. *JPEN J Parenter Enteral Nutr.* 2013;37: 689–694.
3. Yamreudeewong W, Lopez-Anaya A, Rappaport H. Stability of fluconazole in an extemporaneously prepared oral liquid. *Am J Hosp Pharm.* 1993;50:2366–2367.

4. Joe LA, Jacobs RA, Guglielmo BJ. Systemic absorption of oral fluconazole after gastrointestinal resection. *J Antimicrob Chemother.* 1994;33:1070.
5. Barquist ES, Gomez-Fein E, Block EFJ, et al. Bioavailability of oral fluconazole in critically ill abdominal trauma patients with and without abdominal wall closure: a randomized crossover clinical trial. *J Trauma.* 2007;63:159–163.
6. Darwich AS, Pade D, Ammori BJ, et al. A mechanistic pharmacokinetic model to assess modified oral drug bioavailability post bariatric surgery in morbidly obese patients: interplay between CYP3A gut wall metabolism, permeability and dissolution. *J Pharm Pharmacol.* 2012;64:1008–1024.
7. Cohen LG, DiBiasio A, Lisco SJ, et al. Fluconazole serum concentrations and pharmacokinetics in an obese patient. *Pharmacotherapy.* 1997;17:1023–1026.
8. Pittrow L, Penk A. Special pharmacokinetics of fluconazole in septic, obese and burn patients. *Mycoses.* 1999;42(Suppl 2):87–90.
9. Lopez ND, Phillips KM. Fluconazole pharmacokinetics in a morbidly obese, critically ill patient receiving continuous venovenous hemofiltration. *Pharmacotherapy.* 2014; 34:e162–e168.
10. Nicolau DP, Crowe H, Nightingale CH, Quintiliani R. Bioavailability of fluconazole administered via a feeding tube in intensive care unit patients. *J Antimicrob Chemother.* 1995;36:395–401.

Fluoxetine Hydrochloride

Product Availability

Solid	• Tablet: 10 mg, 15 mg, 20 mg, 60 mg (base) (Sarafem® [Apil]; others) • Capsule: 10 mg, 20 mg, 40 mg (base) (Prozac® [Lilly]; others) • Capsule: 90 mg (base) (Prozac® Weekly [Lilly])
Liquid	• Oral solution: 20 mg/5 mL (base) (various)

Physicochemical (drug)

Molecular weight: • 309.33 (salt 345.79)	Permeability: • LogP 4.05 • LogD 1.95 (pH 7.4)	Water solubility: • 14–15.2 mg/mL
pKa: • 9.8	Classification: • BCS Class 1; BDDCS Class 1	

Pharmaceutical (product)

Solid	• Do not crush tablets; disperse in large volume (50–100 mL) of water. • Once-weekly capsule contains enteric-coated granules that should not be crushed.

Liquid	• Oral solution:
	   o pH n/a
	   o Osmolality n/a
	   o Viscosity n/a
	   o May contain alcohol, glycerin, and sucrose
	   o Store at controlled room temperature (20°C–25°C) and protect from light.

Pharmacokinetic (patient)

Absorption	• Specific site not known; t_{max} ~6–8 hours after an oral dose • Bioavailability ~60%–80%
Transport	• Plasma protein binding ~95%, including albumin and α_1-acid glycoprotein • V_d 20–45 L/kg
Metabolism	• Metabolized to an active metabolite (norfluoxetine) via CYP2C19 and CYP2D6 followed by conjugation with glucuronic acid to metabolites, which are eliminated renally • Cl ~350 mL/min

Enteral Administration and Nutrition Considerations

Compatibility, Stability, and Bioavailability Considerations

- The commercial solution (4 mg/mL) diluted to a concentration of 1 mg/mL and 2 mg/mL with deionized water remained stable in amber glass bottles for 8 weeks at 5°C and 30°C.[1]
- The dilution of commercial solution with purified water, simple syrup, or cran-grape juice was reported to be visually compatible.[2]

Drug-Nutrition Interactions

- Drug may influence nutrition status directly or indirectly:
  - Weight loss is associated with decreased appetite and food consumption.
  - CNS: headache, insomnia, anxiety, tremor, dyskinesia (eg, buccolingual and buccoglossal), blurred vision
  - GI: dry mouth, anorexia, nausea, dyspepsia, diarrhea
  - Metabolic: hyponatremia, often secondary to SIADH
- No data on the influence of malnutrition or obesity on drug disposition.
- Influence of food on oral absorption or bioavailability:
  - Food can delay the oral absorption by 3–4 hours but without an influence on the extent of absorption.

Recommendations

Gastric	• Dilute oral solution with water (at least 1:1) prior to administration. • No need to hold EN beyond the time required to flush-administer-flush.
Postpyloric	• As above. • Monitor for any unexpected change in effect.

References

1. Peterson JA, Risley DS, Anderson PN, et al. Stability of fluoxetine hydrochloride in fluoxetine solution diluted with common pharmaceutical diluents. *Am J Hosp Pharm*. 1994;51:1342–1345.
2. Geller JL, Gaulin BD, Barreira PJ. A practitioner's guide to use of psychotropic medication in liquid form. *Hosp Comm Psychiatry*. 1992;43:969–971.

Folic Acid

Product Availability

Solid	• Tablet: 1 mg (various)

Physicochemical (drug)

Molecular weight: • 441.41	Permeability: • LogP –0.52 • LogD n/a	Water solubility: • 0.0016 mg/mL
pKa: • 2.16, 3.79, 4.47, 7.90	Classification: • BCS Class 4; BDDCS Class 2	

Pharmaceutical (product)

Solid	• Tablets may disperse in water within 5 minutes.

Pharmacokinetic (patient)

Absorption	• Small bowel, duodenum, and proximal jejunum; t_{max} ~30–60 minutes after an oral dose • Bioavailability ~85% (folic acid with food) or nearly 100% (folic acid without food); this is greater than bioavailability of food folates
Transport	• Substrate for proton-coupled folate transporter, more so than for reduced folate carrier (at enterocyte) • Plasma protein binding ~50%–64% • V_d ~32 liters
Metabolism	• Folic acid (aka pteroylglutamic acid) needs to be reduced to di- and then tetra-hydrofolate, and methyl-tetra-hydrofolate for transport, but some unmetabolized folic acid may appear unchanged in the circulation; most is eliminated renally with some appearing in feces. • Cl n/a

Enteral Administration and Nutrition Considerations

Compatibility, Stability, and Bioavailability Considerations

- Folic acid solutions are both light- and heat-sensitive, with more rapid photodegradation in acidic media.[1]
- Maximal stability of folic acid aqueous solution occurs at pH 7.6.[2]
- In aqueous solution with pH ≥5.6, folic acid solubility approaches 1 mg/mL, but it may precipitate out of solution when pH is <4.5–5.[3]
- An extemporaneously compounded oral solution (1 mg/mL) prepared from folic acid powder in distilled water (pH adjusted to 8–8.5), stored in dark glass bottles at refrigerator or room temperature, remained stable for at least 30 days.[4]
- Novel folate formulations under study enhanced oral bioavailability in an animal model.[5]

Drug-Nutrition Interactions
- Drug may influence nutrition status directly or indirectly:
  o May mask vitamin B_{12} deficits
  o CNS: confusion
  o GI: anorexia, nausea, abdominal distension (at large doses)
- No data on the influence of malnutrition or obesity on drug disposition.
- No known influence of food on absorption or oral bioavailability.

Recommendations

Gastric	• Disperse tablets in water just prior to administration. • No need to hold EN beyond the time required to flush-administer-flush.
Postpyloric	• As above. • Jejunal administration may be less effective than duodenal. • Monitor for any unexpected change in effect.

References

1. Akhtar MJ, Ataullah Khan M, Ahmad I. Identification of photoproducts of folic acid and its degradation pathways in aqueous solution. *J Pharm Biomed Anal.* 2003;31:579–588.
2. Akhtar MJ, Ataullah Khan M, Ahmad I. Photodegradation of folic acid in aqueous solution. *J Pharm Biomed Anal.* 1999;25:269–275.
3. Barker A, Hebron BS, Beck PR, et al. Folic acid and total parenteral nutrition. *JPEN J Parenter Enteral Nutr.* 1984;8:3–7.
4. Woods D. Extemporaneous formulation in pharmacy practice: folic acid oral solution. *NZ Pharm.* 1993;13:34.
5. Miraglia N, Agostinetto M, Bianchi D, Valoti E. Enhanced oral bioavailability of a novel folate salt: comparison with folic acid and a calcium folate salt in a pharmacokinetic study in rats. *Minerva Ginecol.* 2016;68:99–105.

Furosemide (frusemide)

Product Availability

Solid	• Tablet: 20 mg, 40 mg, 80 mg (Lasix® [Sanofi Aventis]; others)
Liquid	• Oral solution: 40 mg/5 mL, 10 mg/mL (various)

Physicochemical (drug)

Molecular weight:
• 330.75
	Permeability:
	• LogP 2.03
	• Log D –1.54 (pH 7.4);
	  –1.26 (pH 6.5) and
	  –2.16 (pH 7.4) (calc)
		Water solubility:
		• 0.07 mg/mL

pKa: • 3.90	Classification: • BCS Class 4; BDDCS Class 4	

Pharmaceutical (product)

Solid	• Tablets may disperse in water (20 mL) within 5 minutes.

Liquid	• Oral solution:
	• pH 9.77 (40 mg/5 mL)
	• Osmolality:
	  ○ 1737 mOsm/kg (2 mg/mL product), 350 mOsm/kg when diluted 4:1 with water[1]
	  ○ 2050 mOsm/kg (10 mg/mL product)[2]
	  ○ 3375 mOsm/kg[3]
	  ○ 3938 mOsm/kg (10 mg/mL product)[4]
	  ○ 8975 mOsm/kg (calculated based on measurement of 1:5 dilution of 40 mg/5 mL product with sterile water)[5]
	• Viscosity n/a
	• Often contains sorbitol
	• Store solution at 15°C–30°C and protect from light.

Pharmacokinetic (patient)

Absorption	• Jejunum; t_{max} ~1 hour after an oral dose • Bioavailability is variable, ~60%; variability is related to solubility that is correlated with both pH and buffer capacity in the gut.[6]
Transport	• Substrate for MRP2 efflux and OAT3 uptake • Plasma protein binding ~95% • V_d ~0.13 L/kg
Metabolism	• Minimal metabolism with rapid renal elimination • Cl ~1.7 mL/min/kg

Enteral Administration and Nutrition Considerations

Compatibility, Stability, and Bioavailability Considerations
- Refrigeration increases the risk for crystalline precipitate.
- Hydrolysis of furosemide occurs in solution of pH <3.5 but is negligible at pH ≥8.[7]
- The photodegradation of furosemide in solution is least at pH ~7.[8]
- Aqueous vehicles containing sugar worsen the stability of furosemide.[9]
- Repackaging furosemide oral solution (10 mg/mL) as 20 mg (2 mL) doses in 5 mL syringes (oral, amber, polypropylene) stored at 4°C and 25°C sustained ≤5% drug loss (HPLC analysis) when stored for up to 180 days.[10]
- Oral powder (from crushed tablets) diluted in lactose powder and stored in polyethylene coated glassine papers at room temperature for 28 days resulted in no loss of drug (HPLC analysis).[11]
- An extemporaneously compounded oral suspension (5 mg/mL) prepared from drug powder in a complex diluent including carboxymethylcellulose and propylene glycol, stored in amber glass at 2°C–8°C or 23°C–27°C, remained stable (HPLC analysis) for up to 7 days[12]
- An extemporaneously compounded oral suspension (10 mg/mL) prepared from drug powder in SyrSpend SF ALKA and stored in amber plastic container at 2°C–8°C remained stable (HPLC analysis) at 14 days.[13]
- Furosemide oral solution (10 mg/mL) was visually compatible with three EN formulations (Vital, Osmolite, Osmolite HN) when mixed in equal volumes, but no further analysis was available.[14]
- At higher concentrations (40 mg/mL and 80 mg/mL), furosemide solutions were visually compatible (no phase separation, clumping, or gelling) over 12 hours in Ensure, Ensure Plus, or Osmolite, while osmolality of the mixtures increased (≤10%) relative to EN alone.[3]
- A dose of 40 mg (10 mg/mL solution) was visually compatible (no phase separation or particle formation) in 10 mL of Enrich, TwoCal HN, or Vivonex TEN.[15]
- The commercial solution combined (1:1) with Osmolite 1.2, under simulated clinical conditions, would result in no clogging of either an 8 Fr or a 20 Fr feeding tube.[5]
- In a crossover study in healthy subjects, administration of the tablet sublingually to allow dispersion over 5 minutes resulted in improved bioavailability compared with swallowing the tablet intact.[16]
- Although a change in bioavailability was not reported, the rate of drug absorption was faster following gastric bypass, with no differences in natriuresis compared with control patients.[17]
- Drug was adequately absorbed in a patient with multiple small bowel enterocutaneous fistulas.[18]
- Bioavailability is similar when administered by jejunostomy.[19]
- Nanoparticle formulation under study improved oral bioavailability in an animal model.[20]

Drug-Nutrition Interactions

- Drug may influence nutrition status directly or indirectly:
  - Weight loss associated with diuresis
  - CNS: dizziness, lightheadedness, blurred vision
  - GI: oral (and gastric) irritation, anorexia, nausea, vomiting, abdominal cramps, diarrhea
  - Metabolic: volume depletion, hypokalemia, hypomagnesemia, hypocalcemia, contraction alkalosis, hyperglycemia and glycosuria, hyperlipidemia (LDL-cholesterol, triglycerides), hyperammonemia
  - Other: muscle spasm
- No data on the influence of malnutrition or obesity on drug disposition.
- Influence of food on oral absorption or bioavailability:
  - A standard breakfast reduced the rate of absorption and oral bioavailability by ~30%.[21]

Recommendations

Gastric	• Disperse tablets in water prior to administration.
	• Alternative: Dilute oral solution just prior to administration.
	• No need to hold EN beyond the time required to flush-administer-flush.
Postpyloric	• Disperse tablets in water prior to administration.
	• Monitor for any unexpected change in effect.

References

1. Fernández Polo A, Cabañas Poy MJ, Clemente Bautista S, et al. Osmolality of oral liquid dosage forms to be administered to newborns in a hospital. *Farm Hosp.* 2007;31: 311–314.
2. Dickerson RN, Melnik G. Osmolality of oral drug solutions and suspensions. *Am J Hosp Pharm.* 1988;45:832–834.
3. Holtz L, Milton J, Sturek JK. Compatibility of medications with enteral feedings. *JPEN J Parenter Enteral Nutr.* 1987;11:183–186.
4. Niemiec PW, Vanderveen TW, Morrison JI, et al. Gastrointestinal disorders caused by medication and electrolyte solution osmolality during enteral nutrition. *JPEN J Parenter Enteral Nutr.* 1983;7:387–389.
5. Klang M, McLymont V, Ng N. Osmolality, pH, and compatibility of selected oral liquid medications with an enteral nutrition product. *JPEN J Parenter Enteral Nutr.* 2013;37: 689–694.
6. Rabbie SC, Flanagan T, Martin PD, Basit AW. Inter-subject variability in intestinal drug solubility. *Int J Pharm.* 2015;485:229–234.
7. Cruz JE, Maness DD, Yakatan GJ. Kinetics and mechanism of hydrolysis of furosemide. *Int J Pharm.* 1979;2:275–281.
8. Asker AF, Ferdous AJ. Photodegradation of furosemide solutions. *PDA J Pharm Sci Technol.* 1996;50:158–162.
9. Ghanekar AG, Gupta VD, Gibbs CW. Stability of furosemide in aqueous systems. *J Pharm Sci.* 1978;67:808–811.
10. Christensen JM, Lee RY, Parrott KA. Stability of three oral drug products repackaged in unit dose containers. *Am J Hosp Pharm.* 1983;40:612–615.

11. Yang YHK, Lin TR, Huang YF, et al. Stability of furosemide, nadolol and propranolol hydrochloride in extemporaneously compounded powder packets from tablets. *Chin Pharm J.* 2000;52:51–58.
12. Mendes C, Costa AP, Oliveira PR, et al. Physicochemical and microbiological stability studies of extemporaneous anti-hypertensive pediatric suspensions for hospital use. *Pharm Dev Technol.* 2013;18:813–820.
13. Geiger CM, Sorenson B, Whaley P. Stability assessment of 10 active pharmaceutical ingredients compounded in SyrSpend SF. *Int J Pharm Compd.* 2015;19:420–427.
14. Fagerman KE, Ballou AE. Drug compatibilities with enteral feeding solutions coadministered by tube. *Nutr Supp Serv.* 1988;8:31–32.
15. Burns PE, McCall L, Wirsching R. Physical compatibility of enteral formulas with various common medications. *J Am Diet Assoc.* 1988;88:1094–1096.
16. Haegeli L, Brunner-La Rocca HP, Wenk M, et al. Sublingual administration of furosemide: new application of an old drug. *Br J Clin Pharmacol.* 2007;64:804–809.
17. Tandra S, Chalasani N, Jones DR, et al. Pharmacokinetic and pharmacodynamics alterations in the Roux-en-Y gastric bypass recipients. *Ann Surg.* 2013;258:262–269.
18. Viswesh VV. Unpredictable absorption of oral opioid medications in a quadriplegic patient with chronic enterocutaneous fistulas. *J Pain Palliat Care Pharmacother.* 2012;26: 254–256.
19. Adams D. Administration of drugs through a jejunostomy tube. *Br J Intens Care.* 1994; 4:10–17.
20. El-Sayed Radwan S, Samir Sokar M, Ali Abdelmonsif D, Hassan El-Kamel A. Mucopenetrating nanoparticles for enhancement of oral bioavailability of furosemide: in vitro and in vivo evaluation/sub-acute toxicity study. *Int J Pharm.* 2017;526:366–379.
21. McCrindle JL, Li KAM, Wa TC, Barron W, Prescott LF. Effect of food on the absorption of frusemide and bumetanide in man. *Br J Clin Pharmacol.* 1996;42:743–746.

Gabapentin

Product Availability

Solid	• Tablet:
	  ○ Immediate-release: 100 mg, 300 mg, 400 mg, 600 mg, 800 mg (Neurontin® [Pfizer]; others)
	  ○ Delayed-release: 300 mg, 600 mg (Gralise® [Depomed])
	  ○ Extended-release: 300 mg, 600 mg (enacarbil) (Horizant® [Arbor Pharms])
	• Capsule (immediate-release): 100 mg, 300 mg, 400 mg, 800 mg (Neurontin® [Pfizer]; others)

Liquid	• Oral solution: 250 mg/5 mL (Neurontin® [Pfizer]; others)

Physicochemical (drug)

Molecular weight: • 171.24	Permeability: • LogP –1.10 • LogD –1.31 (pH 7.4)	Water solubility: • >100 mg/mL (pH 7.4)
pKa: • 3.7, 10.7	Classification: • BCS Class 3; BDDCS Class 3	

Pharmaceutical (product)

Solid	• Many tablet products are film-coated. • Do not crush modified-release or film-coated tablet. • Capsule contents may disperse in water. • Solid formulations are not interchangeable.

Liquid	• Oral solution:
	  ○ pH 5.62–6.31
	  ○ Osmolality 8275 mOsm/kg (calculated based on measurement of 1:5 dilution of the product with sterile water)[1]
	  ○ Viscosity n/a
	  ○ May contain glycerin and xylitol; strawberry-anise flavored
	  ○ Store at 2°C–8°C (refrigerator).

Pharmacokinetic (patient)

Absorption	• Small bowel; t_{max} ~2–3 hours after an oral dose (immediate-release) • Bioavailability varies with the dose: ~60% at 300 mg, ~27% at 1600 mg
Transport	• Substrate for P-glycoprotein efflux • Substrate for L-type amino acid transport system (LAT1) for uptake at proximal small bowel (capacity limited) • Substrate for organic cation transporter (OCTN1) uptake • Plasma protein binding <3% • V_d ~0.8 L/kg

Metabolism	• Minimal metabolism with subsequent renal excretion
	• Cl ~11 L/h

Enteral Administration and Nutrition Considerations

Compatibility, Stability, and Bioavailability Considerations
- Gabapentin degradation is lowest at pH 5.5–6.5.[2]
- Three different preparation methods for tablets were compared: (a) open crushing with mortar and pestle followed by suspension in water; (b) closed crushing in a commercial tablet crusher and then open suspension in water; and (c) closed crushing and confined suspension in water in a different commercial device. Although the methods were similar in the efficiency of preparation, the fully closed method prevented particle aerosolization.[3]
- An extemporaneously compounded oral suspension prepared from capsules using either simple syrup/1% methylcellulose (1:1) or OraPlus/OraSweet (1:1), stored in amber plastic bottles at 4°C or 25°C, remained stable (HPLC analysis) for 91 days (refrigerated) or 56 days (room temperature).[4]
- An extemporaneously compounded oral suspension (50 mg/mL) prepared from drug powder in SyrSpend SF, stored in light-resistant containers at 2°C–8°C or at 18°C–26°C, remained stable (HPLC analysis) for 120 days (refrigerated) or 90 days (room temperature).[5]
- The commercial solution combined (1:1) with Osmolite 1.2, under simulated clinical conditions, would result in no clogging of either an 8 Fr or a 20 Fr feeding tube.[1]

Drug-Nutrition Interactions
- Drug may influence nutrition status directly or indirectly:
  - Weight gain
  - CNS: ataxia, fatigue, somnolence, headache, depression, visual disturbances (eg, diplopia, amblyopia)
  - GI: dry mouth, nausea, vomiting, diarrhea
  - Metabolic: peripheral edema, hyponatremia, hyperglycemia
  - Other: back and extremity pain
- No data on the influence of malnutrition or obesity on drug disposition.
- Influence of food on oral bioavailability:
  - No known influence of food on the oral bioavailability of immediate-release formulations.
  - Low-fat (200–300 kcal, 6% fat), moderate-fat (500–600 kcal, 30% fat), and high-fat (1000 kcal, 50% fat) meals increased the rate of absorption and oral bioavailability of the modified-release formulation by 23%, 31%, and 43%, respectively, relative to the fasted condition.[6]
  - Coadministration of magnesium reduced bioavailability of gabapentin by 43%.[7]

    o Mixing capsule contents with protein-containing food increased oral bioavailability (~26%) compared with non-protein-containing food.[8]

Recommendations

Gastric	• Disperse capsule contents in water prior to administration. • Alternative: Dilute oral solution with water (at least 1:1) prior to administration. • No need to hold EN beyond the time required to flush-administer-flush.
Postpyloric	• Disperse capsule contents in water prior to administration. • Monitor for any unexpected change in effect.

References

1. Klang M, McLymont V, Ng N. Osmolality, pH, and compatibility of selected oral liquid medications with an enteral nutrition product. *JPEN J Parenter Enteral Nutr.* 2013;37: 689–694.
2. Zour E, Lodhi SA, Nesbitt RU, et al. Stability studies of gabapentin in aqueous solutions. *Pharm Res.* 1992;9:595–600.
3. Salmon D, Pont E, Chevallard H, et al. Pharmaceutical and safety considerations of tablet crushing in patients undergoing enteral intubation. *Int J Pharm.* 2013;443:146–153.
4. Nahata MC. Development of two stable oral suspensions for gabapentin. *Pediatr Neurol.* 1999;20:195–197.
5. Sorenson B, Voudrie MA, Gehrig D. Stability of gabapentin in SyrSpend SF. *Int J Pharm Compd.* 2012;16:347–349.
6. Lal R, Sukbntherng J, Luo W, et al. The effect of food with varying fat content on the clinical pharmacokinetics of gabapentin after oral administration of gabapentin enacarbil. *Int J Clin Pharmacol Ther.* 2010;48:120–128.
7. Yagi T, Naito T, Mino Y, Umemura K, Kawakami J. Impact of concomitant antacid administration on gabapentin plasma exposure and oral bioavailability in healthy adult subjects. *Drug Metab Pharmacokinet.* 2012;27:248–254.
8. Gidal BE, Maly MM, Kowalsi JW, et al. Gabapentin absorption: effect of mixing with foods of varying macronutrient composition. *Ann Pharmacother.* 1998;32:405–409.

Gemfibrozil

Product Availability

| Solid | • Tablet: 600 mg (Lopid® [Pfizer]; others) |

Physicochemical (drug)

Molecular weight: • 250.34	Permeability: • LogP 3.94 • LogD 1.33 (pH 7.4)	Water solubility: • 0.02 mg/mL
pKa: • 4.42	Classification: • BCS Class n/a; BDDCS Class 2	

Pharmaceutical (product)

| Solid | • Tablets are film-coated and may not disperse in water. |

Pharmacokinetic (patient)

Absorption	• Specific site not known; t_{max} ~1–2 hours after an oral dose • Bioavailability ~97%
Transport	• Plasma protein binding ~95% • V_d ~0.14 L/kg
Metabolism	• Metabolized to 4 metabolites via hydroxylation and oxidation followed by conjugation and then excreted mainly through the urine; likely undergoes some enterohepatic recirculation • Cl ~1.7 mL/min/kg

Enteral Administration and Nutrition Considerations

Compatibility, Stability, and Bioavailability Considerations
- No data are available.

Drug-Nutrition Interactions
- Drug may influence nutrition status directly or indirectly:
  o Weight loss
  o CNS: headache, drowsiness, blurred vision
  o GI: altered taste, dry mouth, nausea, vomiting, epigastric pain, diarrhea, rare cholestatic jaundice
  o Metabolic: anemia, impaired glucose tolerance, decreased lipolysis (adipose tissue) and hepatic uptake of free fatty acids, while increasing plasma lipoprotein lipase activity
- No data on the influence of malnutrition or obesity on drug disposition.
- Influence of food on oral absorption or bioavailability:
  o Food may reduce both rate and extent of absorption compared with administration 30 minutes prior to a meal.

Recommendations

Gastric	• Crush and/or disperse tablet in water prior to administration. • No need to hold EN beyond the time required to flush-administer-flush.
Postpyloric	• As above. • Monitor for any unexpected change in effect.

Glipizide

Product Availability

Solid	• Tablet: o Immediate-release: 5 mg, 10 mg (Glucotrol® [Pfizer]; others) o Extended-release: 2.5 mg, 5 mg, 10 mg (Glucotrol-XL® [Pfizer]; others)

Physicochemical (drug)

Molecular weight: • 445.54	Permeability: • LogP 1.91 • LogD –0.40 (pH 7.4)	Water solubility: • 0.355 mg/mL (room temperature, pH 7.5)
pKa: • 5.9	Classification: • BCS Class 2; BDDCS Class 2	

Pharmaceutical (product)

Solid	• Immediate-release tablet may disperse in water (20 mL) in about 1 minute. • Do not divide, chew, or crush the sustained-release tablet (tablet shell is indigestible).

Pharmacokinetic (patient)

Absorption	• Specific site not known; t_{max} ~1–3 hours after an oral dose (immediate-release) • Bioavailability ~80%–100%
Transport	• Plasma protein binding ~92%–99% via a nonionic mechanism • V_d ~10–12 liters
Metabolism	• Near complete metabolism, especially via hydroxylation to at least 4 metabolites, which are excreted renally • Cl ~21–38 mL/kg/h

Enteral Administration and Nutrition Considerations

Compatibility, Stability, and Bioavailability Considerations
• Solubility and dissolution were enhanced by a nanocomposite formulation.[1]

Drug-Nutrition Interactions
• Drug may influence nutrition status directly or indirectly:
  o Weight gain (likely secondary to increased appetite and stimulated lipogenesis)
  o CNS: asthenia, headache, depression, confusion
  o GI: anorexia, pyrosis, nausea, vomiting, diarrhea

- ○ Metabolic: hypoglycemia, hyponatremia (including that related to SIADH)
- ○ Other: arthralgia, myalgia, leg cramps
- No data on the influence of malnutrition or obesity on drug disposition.
- Influence of food on oral absorption or bioavailability:
  - ○ May be best administered on an empty stomach (separated 30 minutes from food).

Recommendations

Gastric	• Crush and/or disperse immediate-release tablet in water just prior to administration. • No need to hold EN beyond the time required to flush-administer-flush.
Postpyloric	• As above. • Monitor for any unexpected change in effect.

Reference

1. Kushare SS, Gattani SG. Microwave-generated bionanocomposites for solubility and dissolution enhancement of poorly water-soluble drug glipizide: in-vitro and in-vivo studies. *J Pharm Pharmacol.* 2013;65:79–93.

Glyburide (Glibenclamide)

Product Availability

Solid	• Tablet:
	    ○ Conventional: 1.25 mg, 2.5 mg, 5 mg (DiaBeta® [Sanofi-Aventis]; others)
	    ○ Micronized: 1.5 mg, 3 mg, 6 mg (Glynase® [Pharmacia & Upjohn]; others)

Physicochemical (drug)

Molecular weight: • 494.01	Permeability: • LogP 4.24 (calc) • LogD 1.41 (pH 7.4)	Water solubility: • 0.004 mg/mL
pKa: • 5.3	Classification: • BCS Class 2; BDDCS Class 2	

Pharmaceutical (product)

Solid	• Immediate-release tablet may disperse in water (20 mL) within 5 minutes. • Micronized tablet formulations are not considered bioequivalent with the conventional tablets.

Pharmacokinetic (patient)

Absorption	• Specific site not known; t_{max} ~2–4 hours after an oral dose • Bioavailability ~65%–90% (micronized), 90%–100% (conventional)
Transport	• Substrate for OATP uptake • Plasma protein binding approaches ~99% • V_d ~0.125 L/kg
Metabolism	• Completely metabolized (via CYP2C9), with elimination via both hepatic and renal routes • Cl ~1.3 mL/min/kg

Enteral Administration and Nutrition Considerations

Compatibility, Stability, and Bioavailability Considerations

- The drug's aqueous solubility improves with higher pH due to salt formation (4 µg/mL at pH 4; 600 µg/mL at pH 9).
- The further reduction in drug particle size through a nanosizing process resulted in enhanced dissolution and increased bioavailability in an animal model.[1]
- Lipid nanoparticle formulations under study may remain stable and improve bioavailability, but they would in effect be an extended-release form of the drug.[2]
- A self-nanoemulsifying delivery system allowed quicker drug dissolution and improved bioavailability in an animal model.[3]

- Another self-emulsification delivery system, when dispersed in distilled water (1%), remained stable (HPLC analysis) at 25°C/60% relative humidity for 2 weeks; drug decomposition was associated with three of the four delivery system components.[4]

Drug-Nutrition Interactions
- Drug may influence nutrition status directly or indirectly:
  - Weight gain (likely secondary to increased appetite and stimulated lipogenesis)
  - GI: nausea, epigastric fullness, cholestatic jaundice
  - Metabolic: hypoglycemia, hyponatremia (including that related to SIADH)
- Influence of malnutrition or obesity on drug disposition:
  - Weight-normalized volume of distribution (L/kg) is lower in obese patients, who may also be more sensitive to the drug's action.[5,6]
- Influence of food on oral absorption or bioavailability:
  - Although orange juice and grapefruit juice impair drug transport into the cell in vitro, a clinical study indicated no difference in oral bioavailability when grapefruit juice was consumed with or within 4 hours before/after drug administration compared to water.[7]

Recommendations

Gastric	• Crush and/or disperse tablet in water just prior to administration. • No need to hold EN beyond the time required to flush-administer-flush.
Postpyloric	• As above. • Monitor for any unexpected change in effect.

References

1. Wang Y, Yang W, Fu Q, et al. The role of particle size of glyburide crystals in improving its oral absorption. *Drug Deliv Transl Res.* 2017;7:428–438.
2. Goncalves LMD, Maestrelli F, Di Cesare Mannelli L, et al. Development of solid lipid nanoparticles as carriers for improving oral bioavailability of glibenclamide. *Eur J Pharm Biopharm.* 2016;102:41–50.
3. Liu H, Shang K, Liu W, et al. Improved oral bioavailability of glyburide by a self-nanoemulsifying drug delivery system. *J Microencapsul.* 2014;31:277–283.
4. Bachhav Y, Patravale V. SMEDDs of glyburide: formulation, in vitro evaluation, and stability studies. *AAPS PharmSciTech.* 2009;10:482–487.
5. Jaber LA, Antal EJ, Slaughter RL, et al. The pharmacokinetics and pharmacodynamics of 12 weeks of glyburide therapy in obese diabetics. *Eur J Clin Pharmacol.* 1993;45: 459–463.
6. Jaber LA, Ducharme MP, Halapy H. The effects of obesity on the pharmacokinetics and pharmacodynamics of glipizide in patients with non-insulin-dependent diabetes mellitus. *Ther Drug Monitor.* 1996;18:6–13.
7. Lilja JJ, Niemi M, Fredrikson H, Neuvonen PJ. Effects of clarithromycin and grapefruit juice on the pharmacokinetics of glibenclamide. *Br J Clin Pharmacol.* 2007;63:732–740.

Guaifenesin

Product Availability

Solid	• Tablet:
	  ○ Immediate-release: 200 mg (various)
	  ○ Extended-release: 600 mg, 1.2 g (Mucinex® [Reckitt Benckiser]; others)

Liquid	• Oral solution: 100 mg/5 mL, 200 mg/5 mL (various)

Physicochemical (drug)

Molecular weight: • 198.2	Permeability: • LogP 1.39 • LogD 0.84 (pH 5.5)	Water solubility: • 50 mg/mL (25°C)
pKa: • 13.5	Classification: • BCS Class n/a; BDDCS Class n/a	

Pharmaceutical (product)

Solid	• Do not crush tablet because products are often modified-release (alone or in combination products).

Liquid	• Oral solution (syrup):
	  ○ pH 2.6 (200 mg/5 mL)
	  ○ pH 2.78 (100 mg/5 mL)
	  ○ Osmolality 278 mOsm/kg (100 mg/5 mL)[1]
	  ○ Viscosity n/a
	  ○ May contain glycerin, high-fructose corn syrup, propylene glycol, and saccharin
	  ○ Store at controlled room temperature.

Pharmacokinetic (patient)

Absorption	• Specific site not known; t_{max} ~30 minutes after an oral dose • Bioavailability n/a
Transport	• Plasma protein binding n/a • V_d ~2.4–2.8 L/kg
Metabolism	• Cl ~100–130 L/h

Enteral Administration and Nutrition Considerations

Compatibility, Stability, and Bioavailability Considerations

- A 1% aqueous solution has a pH between 5 and 7.
- An oral solution (10 mL) is physically incompatible (increased viscosity; flocculent precipitate) when added to varying volumes (15–240 mL) of EN products (Ensure, EnsurePlus, Osmolite, Ensure HN, Ensure Plus HN, Osmolite HN).[2,3]

- An oral solution (5 mL) is physically incompatible (forming a thick gelatinous mass, or particulates and phase separation) when added to 10 mL of EN products (Enrich, TwoCal HN).[4]
- No visible incompatibilities were noted when an oral solution (10 mL) was mixed with Vital (15–240 mL) or when 5 mL was mixed with 10 mL of Vivonex TEN.[3,4]
- Commercially available oral solution (100 mg/5 mL) combined (1:1) with Osmolite 1.2, under simulated clinical conditions, would result in clogging of both an 8 Fr and a 20 Fr feeding tube.[1]

Drug-Nutrition Interactions
- Drug may influence nutrition status directly or indirectly:
  o GI: vomiting
- No data on the influence of malnutrition or obesity on drug disposition.
- No known influence of food on oral absorption or bioavailability.

Recommendations

Gastric	• Dilute oral solution in water (at least 1:1) prior to administration. • Consider holding EN beyond the time required to flush-administer-flush.
Postpyloric	• As above. • Monitor for any unexpected change in effect.

References

1. Klang M, McLymont V, Ng N. Osmolality, pH, and compatibility of selected oral liquid medications with an enteral nutrition product. *JPEN J Parenter Enteral Nutr.* 2013;37:689–694.
2. Cutie AJ, Altman E, Lenkel L. Compatibility of enteral products with commonly employed drug additives. *JPEN J Parenter Enteral Nutr.* 1983;7:186–191.
3. Altman E, Cutie AJ. Compatibility of enteral products with commonly employed drug additives. *Nutr Supp Serv.* 1984;4:8–17.
4. Burns PE, McCall L, Wirsching R. Physical compatibility of enteral formulas with various common medications. *J Am Diet Assoc.* 1988;88:1094–1096.

Hydralazine Hydrochloride

Product Availability

| Solid | • Tablet: 10 mg, 25 mg, 50 mg, 100 mg (various) |

Physicochemical (drug)

Molecular weight: • 160.18	Permeability: • LogP 1.00 • LogD 0.56 (pH 7.4)	Water solubility: • 40–44 mg/mL (25°C)
pKa: • 7.3	Classification: • BCS Class 1 or 3; BDDCS Class 1	

Pharmaceutical (product)

| Solid | • Tablets do not disperse in water. |

Pharmacokinetic (patient)

Absorption	• Specific site not known; t_{max} ~0.5–1.5 hours after an oral dose • Bioavailability ~10%–26%
Transport	• Plasma protein binding ~85%–87% • V_d ~2.2 L/kg
Metabolism	• Extensive metabolism (gut mucosa and liver) by acetylation and hydroxylation, followed by conjugation with glucuronic acid before renal elimination • Cl depends on acetylation metabolic phenotype

Enteral Administration and Nutrition Considerations

Compatibility, Stability, and Bioavailability Considerations
- The optimal aqueous solubility occurs at pH 3.2–4.4.[1]
- A 2% aqueous oral solution has a pH 3.5–4.2.
- In an aqueous solution, the drug is incompatible (discoloration with yellow precipitate) with edetate sodium or sodium bisulfite.[2]
- The official USP oral solution using purified water has a final pH between 3 and 5 and is to be stored at 2°C–8°C.
- Lactose in the commercial tablets may accelerate hydralazine degradation when used in an oral liquid.[3]
- As a 1% aqueous solution, the drug was unstable (HPLC analysis) within 24 hours if sucrose, dextrose, fructose, lactose, or maltose were included in the solution stored in amber bottles at 24°C.[1]
- A prepared oral solution should be refrigerated and is more likely to decompose at pH >7.[4]
- A 10 mg/mL aqueous oral solution was more stable (up to 3 months) than a 1 mg/mL solution (2 weeks) stored in amber bottles (glass or polyethylene terephthalate) at 25°C.[4]

- Extemporaneously compounded oral solutions (1 mg/mL, 10 mg/mL) prepared from drug powder with sorbitol, parabens, propylene glycol, aspartame, and purified water, stored in amber polyethylene terephthalate plastic bottles or amber glass bottles at 5°C or 25°C (60% relative humidity), remained stable (HPLC analysis) for 14 days (1 mg/mL) or 92 days (10 mg/mL) at room temperature, and for up to 92 days at refrigeration.[4]
- Extemporaneously compounded oral liquids prepared from tablets (50 mg) in distilled water, then in a mixture of maltitol, edetate, saccharine, parabens, and propylene glycol and adjusted to pH 3.7, stored in amber glass bottles at 5°C, remained stable (HPLC analysis) at 2 weeks.[2]
- Extemporaneously compounded oral suspensions (4 mg/mL) prepared from tablets (100 mg) in cherry syrup/simple syrup (1:4), OraSweet/OraPlus (1:1), or OraSweet SF/OraPlus (1:1), stored in amber polyethylene terephthalate plastic bottles at 5°C or 25°C, were unstable (HPLC analysis) within 1 day at room temperature, and by 1–2 days at refrigeration.[3]

Drug-Nutrition Interactions
- Drug may influence nutrition status directly or indirectly:
  o CNS: headache
  o GI: anorexia, nausea, vomiting, adynamic ileus
  o Other: arthralgia, edema and myalgia (as part of a systemic lupus-like syndrome), peripheral neuritis (paresthesia)
- No data on the influence of malnutrition or obesity on drug disposition.
- Influence of food on oral absorption or bioavailability:
  o Both a standard breakfast (470 mL, 17.5 g protein, 17.4 g fat, 68.2 g carbohydrate) and an EN bolus (470 mL, 17.5 g protein, 17.5 g fat, 68.2 g carbohydrate), administered over 20 minutes by mouth, reduce oral bioavailability by at least 50% compared with the fasted state. When the drug was administered during nasogastric infusion of the same volume of EN over 6 hours, there was no observed effect on bioavailability. The volunteers involved in the crossover study included both slow and fast acetylation phenotypes.[5]

Recommendations

Gastric	• Crush and disperse tablet in water just prior to administration. • No need to hold EN beyond the time required to flush-administer-flush.
Postpyloric	• As above. • Monitor for any unexpected change in effect.

References

1. Gupta VD, Stewart KR, Bethea C. Stability of hydralazine hydrochloride in aqueous vehicles. *J Clin Hosp Pharm.* 1986;11:215–223.
2. Alexander KS, Pudipeddi M, Parker GA. Stability of hydralazine hydrochloride syrup compounded from tablets. *Am J Hosp Pharm.* 1993;50:683–686.
3. Allen LV, Erickson MA. Stability of alprazolam, chloroquine phosphate, cisapride, enalapril maleate, and hydralazine hydrochloride in extemporaneously compounded oral liquids. *Am J Health-Syst Pharm.* 55:1915–1920.
4. Okeke CC, Medwick T, Nairn G, et al. Stability of hydralazine hydrochloride in both flavored and nonflavored extemporaneous preparations. *Int J Pharm Compd.* 2003;7: 313–319.
5. Semple HA, Koo W, Tam YK, Ngo L-Y, Coutts RT. Interactions between hydralazine and oral nutrients in humans. *Ther Drug Monit.* 1991;13:304–308.

Hydrochlorothiazide

Product Availability

Solid	• Tablet: 12.5 mg, 25 mg, 50 mg (various) • Capsule: 12.5 mg (Microzide® [Watson]; others)

Physicochemical (drug)

Molecular weight:
• 297.74
	Permeability:
	• LogP –0.07
	• Log D –0.07 (pH 7.4),
	  –0.98 (pH 7.4, calc),
	  –1.78 (pH 6.5, calc)
		Water solubility:
		• 0.6 mg/mL

pKa: • 7.9, 9.2	Classification: • BCS Class 3 or 4; BDDCS Class 3	

Pharmaceutical (product)

Solid	• Tablet may disperse in water (20 mL) within about 5 minutes.

Pharmacokinetic (patient)

Absorption	• Specific site not known; t_{max} ~1–3 hours after an oral dose • Bioavailability ~65%–75%
Transport	• Plasma protein binding ~40%–68% • V_d ~0.83 L/kg
Metabolism	• Does not undergo metabolism but is eliminated renally • Cl ~4.9 mL/min/kg

Enteral Administration and Nutrition Considerations

Compatibility, Stability, and Bioavailability Considerations

- The drug is subject to hydrolysis at pH extremes, complete and irreversible at pH >8.2; however, at pH 1.5–8.2, the equilibrium process is considered to favor the drug.[1-3]
- An extemporaneously compounded oral suspension (2 mg/mL) prepared from crushed tablets or drug powder using distilled water, citric acid, and Methocel E50, stored in containers at room temperature and protected from light, remained stable (HPLC analysis) for 10 weeks.[4]
- The above preparation had a pH of ~3, with low viscosity and low osmolality (20 mOsm/kg), with pure drug powder considered better than using crushed tablets.[4]
- A pharmacy-prepared hydrochlorothiazide oral suspension (10 mg/mL) had an osmolality of 1837 mOsm/kg, which decreased to 370 mOsm/kg when diluted 4:1 with water.[5]
- An extemporaneously compounded oral suspension (2 mg/mL) prepared from drug powder in glycerol 20% or methylcellulose 1% with citric acid buffer (pH 3–3.5), stored at 5°C or 25°C and protected from light, remained stable (HPLC analysis) for 3 weeks.[6]

- An extemporaneously compounded oral suspension (5 mg/mL) prepared from drug powder in a vehicle that included carboxymethylcellulose, propylene glycol, saccharin, parabens, ethanol, and sterile water with citric acid for pH 3.3, stored in amber glass at 2°C–8°C or 23°C–27°C, remained stable (HPLC analysis) for 7 days.[3]
- A self-nanoemulsifying delivery system allowed for quicker drug dissolution and improved bioavailability in an animal model.[7]

Drug-Nutrition Interactions
- Drug may influence nutrition status directly or indirectly:
  - May increase urinary zinc excretion
  - CNS: dizziness, headache
  - GI: anorexia, nausea, vomiting, abdominal cramping, diarrhea
  - Metabolic: hypokalemia, hypomagnesemia, contraction (hypochloremic) alkalosis, hypercalcemia, hyperglycemia, glycosuria
  - Other: muscle weakness
- No data on the influence of malnutrition or obesity on drug disposition.
- Influence of food on oral absorption or bioavailability:
  - Food may reduce the rate and extent (10%–20%) of oral absorption from the capsule formulation.
  - Data based on an in situ intestinal perfusion study showed increased bioavailability with concurrent use of Zhenju.[8]

Recommendations

Gastric	• Disperse tablet in water prior to administration. • No need to hold EN beyond the time required to flush-administer-flush.
Postpyloric	• As above. • Monitor for any unexpected change in effect.

References

1. Deventer K, Baele G, Van Eenoo P, et al. Stability of selected chlorinated thiazide diuretics. *J Pharm Biomed Anal*. 2009;49:519–524.
2. Tagliari MP, Stulzer HK, Assreuy J, et al. Evaluation of physicochemical characteristics of suspensions containing hydrochlorothiazide developed for pediatric use. *Lat Am J Pharm*. 2009;28:734–740.
3. Mendes C, Costa AP, Oliveira PR, et al. Physicochemical and microbiological stability studies of extemporaneous antihypertensive pediatric suspensions for hospital use. *Pharm Dev Technol*. 2013;18:813–820.
4. Totterman AM, Luukkonen P, Riukka L, et al. Formulation of enteral hydrochlorothiazide suspension for premature infants. *Eur J Hosp Pharm*. 1994;4:65–69.
5. Fernández Polo A, Cabañas Poy MJ, Clemente Bautista S, et al. Osmolality of oral liquid dosage forms to be administered to newborns in a hospital. *Farm Hosp*. 2007;31: 311–314.
6. Santoveña A, Hernández-Paiz Z, Fariña JB. Design of a pediatric oral formulation with a low proportion of hydrochlorothiazide. *Int J Pharm*. 2012;423:360–364.

7. Yadav PS, Yadav E, Verma A, Amin S. Development, characterization, and pharmacodynamics evaluation of hydrochlorothiazide loaded self-nanoemulsifying drug delivery systems. *Sci World J.* 2014:274823.

8. Qin J, Wang L, Bai Y, et al. Enhanced absorption and bioavailability of hydrochlorothiazide by Chinese medicines in the Zhenju antihypertensive compound. *J Pharm Pharmacol.* 2014;66:855–864.

Hydrocodone Bitartrate

Product Availability

Solid	• Tablet: 20 mg, 30 mg, 40 mg, 60 mg, 80 mg, 100 mg, 120 mg (Hysingla®-ER [Purdue Pharma]; others) • Capsule: 10 mg, 15 mg, 20 mg, 30 mg, 40 mg, 50 mg (Zohydro® ER [Pernix]; others)

Physicochemical (drug)

Molecular weight: • 299.37	Permeability: • LogP 1.27 • LogD 3.38 (pH 7.4)	Water solubility: • 62.5 mg/mL
pKa: • 8.2	Classification: • BCS Class n/a; BDDCS Class 1	

Pharmaceutical (product)

Solid	• Do not crush, break, or chew solid products. • Tablet formulations are extended-release and often film-coated. • Capsule formulations contain extended-release granules. • Immediate-release combination products (solid and liquid) contain acetaminophen at varying concentrations.

Pharmacokinetic (patient)

Absorption	• Specific site not known; t_{max} ~1–2 hours (immediate-release) or ~5 hours (modified-release) after an oral dose • Bioavailability n/a
Transport	• Plasma protein binding ~36% • V_d ~3.4–4.7 L/kg

Metabolism	• Metabolized to norhydrocodone via CYP3A4 and to hydromorphone via CYP2D6; may also undergo metabolism through CYP2B6 and CYP2C19; most metabolites excreted renally
	 • Cl (varies by CYP2D6 metabolic phenotype):
	   o Extensive metabolizer ~11 mL/min/kg
	   o Poor metabolizer ~6.5 mL/min/kg

Enteral Administration and Nutrition Considerations

Compatibility, Stability, and Bioavailability Considerations
• No data are available.

Drug-Nutrition Interactions
• Drug may influence nutrition status directly or indirectly:
  o CNS: dizziness, fatigue, headache
  o GI: dry mouth, anorexia, nausea, vomiting, abdominal cramping, constipation

- o Metabolic: peripheral edema
- o Other: back pain, muscle spasms
- No data on the influence of malnutrition or obesity on drug disposition.
- Influence of food on oral absorption or bioavailability:
  - o A high-fat or standard meal may increase the rate of oral absorption but not overall bioavailability of an extended-release product; this effect may be less pronounced with chronic use.[1,2]

Recommendations

Gastric	• Do not administer by enteral access device; consider a therapeutic alternative.
Postpyloric	• As above.

References

1. Farr SJ, Robinson CY, Rubino CM. Effects of food and alcohol on the pharmacokinetics of an oral, extended-release formulation of hydrocodone in healthy volunteers. *Clin Pharmacol Adv Appl.* 2015;7:1–9.
2. Bond M, Rabinovich-Guilatt L, Selim S, et al. Effect of food on the pharmacokinetics of single- and multiple-dose hydrocodone extended release in healthy subjects. *Clin Drug Investig.* 2017;37:1153–1163.

Hydroxyzine Hydrochloride or Pamoate

Product Availability

Solid	• Tablet (hydrochloride): 10 mg, 25 mg, 50 mg, 100 mg (salt) (various) • Capsule (pamoate): 25 mg, 50 mg, 100 mg (as HCl salt equivalent) (Vistaril® [Pfizer]; others)
Liquid	• Solution (hydrochloride): 10 mg/5 mL (salt) (various) • Suspension (pamoate): 25 mg/5 mL (HCl salt) (Vistaril® [Pfizer]; others)

Physicochemical (drug)

Molecular weight: • 374.91	Permeability: • LogP 3.50 • LogD 2.37 (pH 7.4)	Water solubility: • Hydrochloride 700 mg/mL • Pamoate <0.1 mg/mL
pKa: • 2.6, 7.0	Classification: • BCS Class 2; BDDCS Class 1	

Pharmaceutical (product)

Solid	• Difficult to crush, most tablets are film-coated and do not disperse in water. • Capsule contents may disperse in water.
Liquid	• Solution: o pH 3.16[1] o Osmolality 3540 mOsm/kg (calculated based on measurement of 1:5 dilution with sterile water);[1] 4450 mOsm/kg.[2] o Viscosity n/a o May contain ethanol, corn syrup, propylene glycol, and sucrose; peppermint-flavored o Store at controlled room temperature. • Suspension: o pH 4.5–7 o Osmolality n/a o Viscosity n/a o May contain propylene glycol and sorbitol; lemon-flavored o Shake very well prior to measuring out a dose.
Note	• Hydroxyzine pamoate 170 mg ≈ 100 mg hydroxyzine hydrochloride

Pharmacokinetic (patient)

Absorption	• Specific site not known; t_{max} ~2 hours after an oral dose • Bioavailability ~72%
Transport	• Plasma protein binding ~93% • V_d ~16 L/kg
Metabolism	• Complete hepatic metabolism is followed by biliary excretion. • An active metabolite includes cetirizine. • Cl ~9.8 mL/min/kg

Enteral Administration and Nutrition Considerations

Compatibility, Stability, and Bioavailability Considerations

- The commercial solution combined (1:1) with Osmolite 1.2, under simulated clinical conditions, would result in clogging of an 8 Fr feeding tube, but not a 20 Fr feeding tube.[1]

Drug-Nutrition Interactions

- Drug may influence nutrition status directly or indirectly:
  - CNS: sedation, tremor
  - GI: dry mouth
- No data on the influence of malnutrition or obesity on drug disposition.
- No known influence of food on oral absorption or bioavailability.

Recommendations

Gastric	• Dilute a liquid form of the medication with water just prior to administration. • No need to hold EN beyond the time required to flush-administer-flush.
Postpyloric	• May require significant dilution with water to allow tolerance; consider a therapeutic alternative. • Monitor for any unexpected change in effect.

References

1. Klang M, McLymont V, Ng N. Osmolality, pH, and compatibility of selected oral liquid medications with an enteral nutrition product. *JPEN J Parenter Enteral Nutr.* 2013;37: 689–694.
2. Dickerson RN, Melnik G. Osmolality of oral drug solutions and suspensions. *Am J Hosp Pharm.* 1988;45:832–834.

Ibandronate Sodium

Product Availability

Solid	• Tablet: 2.5 mg, 150 mg (base) (Boniva® [Hoffman La Roche]; others)

Physicochemical (drug)

Molecular weight:	Permeability:	Water solubility:
• 319.23	• LogP –2.10	• >100 mg/mL
	• LogD n/a	
pKa:	**Classification:**	
• 9.9	• BCS Class n/a; BDDCS Class 3	

Pharmaceutical (product)

Solid	• Do not crush; oropharyngeal mucosal irritation.
	• Tablets are film-coated and do not disperse in water.

Pharmacokinetic (patient)

Absorption	• Specific site not known; t_{max} ~1 hour after an oral dose
	• Bioavailability ≤1%
Transport	• Plasma protein binding ~90%
	• V_d ~90 liters (at least)
Metabolism	• No known metabolism
	• At least 50% of the absorbed drug is excreted unchanged in the urine, while much of the remainder is taken up by bone tissue.
	• Cl ~84–160 mL/h

Enteral Administration and Nutrition Considerations

Compatibility, Stability, Bioavailability Considerations
 • A preparation that incorporated a deoxycholic acid derivative improved intestinal permeability and bioavailability (4-fold) when administered intrajejunally in an animal model.[1]

Drug-Nutrition Interactions
 • Drug may influence nutrition status directly or indirectly:
   o CNS: headache
   o GI: dysphagia, odynophagia associated with oropharyngeal and esophageal ulceration (local effect of drug), possible gastric/duodenal ulcers, abdominal pain, diarrhea
   o Metabolic: hypocalcemia, hypercholesterolemia
   o Other: bone, joint, and/or muscle pain
 • No data on the influence of malnutrition or obesity on drug disposition.

- Influence of food on oral absorption or bioavailability:
  ○ A standard breakfast reduces bioavailability by ~90%.
  ○ Administration within 2 hours of food or the standard test meal reduces drug bioavailability by ~75%.
  ○ Multivalent cation-containing (aluminum, calcium, magnesium, iron) products or foods reduce oral absorption.

Recommendations

Gastric	• Do not administer by enteral access device.
Postpyloric	• As above.
Other	• Maintain calcium and vitamin D status.

Reference

1. Park JW, Hwang SR, Jeon O-C, Moon HT, Byun Y. Enhanced oral absorption of ibandronate via complex formation with bile acid derivative. *J Pharm Sci*. 2013;102: 341–346.

Ibuprofen

Product Availability

Solid	• Tablet: 200 mg, 400 mg, 600 mg, 800 mg (Motrin® [McNeil]; others) • Tablet (chewable): 50 mg, 100 mg (Advil® Children's [Pfizer]; Motrin® Children's [Johnson & Johnson Consumer]) • Capsule: 200 mg (various)
Liquid	• Oral suspension: 40 mg/mL, 100 mg/5 mL (free acid and potassium salt) (various)

Physicochemical (drug)

Molecular weight: • 206.29	Permeability: • LogP 3.97 • LogD 0.81 (pH 7.4)	Water solubility: • 0.038 mg/mL
pKa: • 4.43	Classification: • BCS Class 2; BDDCS Class 2	

Pharmaceutical (product)

Solid	• Tablets may be film-coated and do not disperse in water. • Do not crush (taste is unacceptable).

Liquid	• Oral suspension:
	  ○ pH 3.6–4.6 (eg, 100 mg/5 mL suspension pH 3.9)
	  ○ Osmolality 2350 mOsm/kg (calculated based on measurement of 1:5 dilution of 100 mg/5 mL product with sterile water).[1]
	  ○ Viscosity is significant (>300 mPa·s)
	  ○ May contain glycerin, propylene glycol, sorbitol, and/or sucrose
	  ○ Store at controlled room temperature.

Pharmacokinetic (patient)

Absorption	• Specific site not known; t_{max} ~1–2 hours after an oral dose • Bioavailability ~80%
Transport	• Plasma protein binding ~90%–99% • V_d 0.16 L/kg
Metabolism	• Oxidized to 2 inactive metabolites (via CYP2C9), some of which undergoes glucuronidation and account for over 50% of renal excretion • Cl ~60 mL/min

Enteral Administration and Nutrition Considerations

Compatibility, Stability, and Bioavailability Considerations

- The dissolution of drug in suspension preparations is dependent on pH (slowest at pH 1).[2]
- Drug solubility increases in propylene glycol and in ethanol; sorbitol and glycerol had a more modest influence on solubility.[3]
- An extemporaneously compounded oral suspension (20 mg/mL) prepared from ibuprofen powder, stored in amber glass bottles at 28°C–32°C and protected from light, resulted in a viscous (320–353 mPa·s) preparation, with a pH ~3.8, with good stability (HPLC analysis) for 24 months.[4]
- An oral suspension preparation of ibuprofen lysinate exhibits a quicker rate of absorption and enhanced bioavailability relative to the reference suspension in healthy volunteers.[5]
- A commercial suspension combined (1:1) with Osmolite 1.2, under simulated clinical conditions, would result in clogging of both an 8 Fr and a 20 Fr feeding tube.[1]
- A formulation under study that incorporates ibuprofen in an organic-alkali metal framework has similar absorption to the standard potassium salt but with longer durability in the circulation.[6]
- Microemulsion formulations under study resulted in higher (~40%) oral bioavailability.[7]
- Compared with pure powder, a solid dispersion formulation improved solubility and bioavailability in an animal model.[8]
- Based on findings with an orodispersible tablet formulation, oral bioavailability in the postoperative phase (following lumbar back surgery) was significantly lower (~50%) than that determined preoperatively despite no change in t_{max}.[9]

Drug-Nutrition Interactions

- Drug may influence nutrition status directly or indirectly:
  - CNS: dizziness, headache, nervousness, fatigue, confusion, amblyopia
  - GI: stomatitis, anorexia, nausea, vomiting, dyspepsia, epigastric pain, ulceration, bleeding, bloating, constipation or diarrhea, LFT elevations including rare jaundice or hepatitis
  - Metabolic: peripheral edema, azotemia, hyperkalemia (associated with renal impairment)
- Influence of malnutrition or obesity on drug disposition:
  - Weight-normalized volume of distribution (L/kg) was slightly lower and clearance (mL/min) was increased in the obese.[10]
- Influence of food on oral absorption or bioavailability:
  - Food may reduce the rate of oral absorption without an influence on the bioavailability.

Recommendations

Gastric	• If there is no therapeutic alternative, dilute oral suspension with water (at least 1:1) just prior to administration. • No need to hold EN beyond the time required to flush-administer-flush.
Postpyloric	• As above. • Monitor for any unexpected change in effect.
Other	• Maintain hydration during therapy.

References

1. Klang M, McLymont V, Ng N. Osmolality, pH, and compatibility of selected oral liquid medications with an enteral nutrition product. *JPEN J Parenter Enteral Nutr.* 2013;37: 689–694.
2. Rivera-Leyva JC, García-Flores M, Valladares-Méndez A, Orozco-Castellanos LM, Martínez-Alfaro M. Comparative studies on the dissolution profiles of oral ibuprofen suspension and commercial tablets using biopharmaceutical classification system criteria. *Indian J Pharm Sci.* 2012;74:312–318.
3. Devi PN, Rao YM. Solubilization of ibuprofen by using cosolvents, surfactants and formulation of an elixir and injectable preparation. *East Pharm.* 1995;38:137–140.
4. Martin-Viana NDLP, Lacarrere IGM, Apan JMG, et al. Development of formulation for oral suspension ibuprofen 100 mg/5 mL for pediatric use. *Rev Cubana Farm.* 2009; 43(2):1–11.
5. Ferrero-Cafiero JM, Gich I, Puntes M, et al. Ibuprofen lysinate, quicker and less variable: relative bioavailability compared to ibuprofen base in a pediatric suspension dosage form. *Int J Clin Pharmacol Ther.* 2015;53:972–979.
6. Hartlieb KJ, Ferris DP, Holcroft JM, et al. Encapsulation of ibuprofen in CD-MOF and related bioavailability studies. *Mol Pharm.* 2017;14:1831–1839.
7. You X, Xing Q, Tuo J, et al. Optimizing surfactant content to improve oral bioavailability of ibuprofen in microemulsions: just enough or more than enough? *Int J Pharm.* 2014; 471:276–284.
8. Park Y-J, Kwon R, Quan QZ, et al. Development of novel ibuprofen-loaded solid dispersion with improved bioavailability using aqueous solution. *Arch Pharm Res.* 2009; 32:767–772.
9. Piirainen A, Kokki M, Lidsle HM, et al. Absorption of ibuprofen orodispersible tablets in early postoperative phase—a pharmacokinetic study. *Curr Med Res Opin.* 2017;1394832.
10. Abernathy DR. Greenblatt DJ. Ibuprofen disposition in obese individuals. *Arth Rheum.* 1985;28:1117–1121.

Irbesartan

Product Availability

Solid	• Tablet: 75 mg, 150 mg, 300 mg (Avapro® [Sanofi Aventis]; others)

Physicochemical (drug)

Molecular weight: • 428.54	Permeability: • LogP 6.04 (calc) • LogD 1.00 (pH 7.4)	Water solubility: • 0.08 mg/mL
pKa: • 4.08, 4.29	Classification: • BCS Class 2; BDDCS Class 2	

Pharmaceutical (product)

Solid	• Tablet products may be film-coated and do not disperse well in water. • Avoid exposure during pregnancy.

Pharmacokinetic (patient)

Absorption	• Specific site not known; t_{max} ~1–1.5 hours after an oral dose • Bioavailability ~60%–80%
Transport	• Plasma protein binding ~90% to albumin and α_1-acid glycoprotein • V_d ~53–93 liters
Metabolism	• Metabolized predominantly by CYP2C9 as well as by glucuronic acid conjugation, with most excretion into feces • Cl ~157–176 mL/min

Enteral Administration and Nutrition Considerations

Compatibility, Stability, and Bioavailability Considerations
- A self-nanoemulsifying formulation under development and study improved drug dissolution and increased oral bioavailability by 1.8-fold compared with commercial tablets in an animal model.[1,2]

Drug-Nutrition Interactions
- Drug may influence nutrition status directly or indirectly:
  - CNS: fatigue, dizziness
  - GI: dyspepsia, diarrhea
  - Metabolic: azotemia, oliguria
- No data on the influence of malnutrition or obesity on drug disposition.
- No known influence of food on oral bioavailability.

Recommendations

Gastric	• Crush and disperse tablet in water just prior to administration. • No need to hold EN beyond the time required to flush-administer-flush.
Postpyloric	• As above. • Monitor for any unexpected change in effect.

References

1. Patel J, Patel A, Raval M, Sheth N. Formulation and development of a self-nanoemulsifying drug delivery system of irbesartan. *J Adv Pharm Technol Res.* 2011;2:9–16.
2. Patel J, Dhingani A, Garala K, Raval M, Sheth N. Quality by design approach for oral bioavailability enhancement of irbesartan by self-nanoemulsifying tablets. *Drug Deliv.* 2014;21:412–435.

Ivermectin

Product Availability

| Solid | • Tablet: 3 mg (Stromectol® [Merck]; others) |

Physicochemical (drug)

Molecular weight: • 875.11	Permeability: • LogP 5.39 (calc) • LogD 6.82 (pH 7.4)	Water solubility: • 0.004 mg/mL
pKa: • 13.2	Classification: • BCS Class 2; BDDCS Class 1	

Pharmaceutical (product)

| Solid | • Tablets may not easily disperse in water without crushing first. |

Pharmacokinetic (patient)

Absorption	• Specific site not known; t_{max} ~4 hours after an oral dose • Bioavailability n/a
Transport	• Substrate for P-glycoprotein efflux • Plasma protein binding ~93%, mainly to albumin and less to α_1-acid glycoprotein • V_d ~3.5 L/kg (healthy); ~9.9 L/kg (infected)
Metabolism	• Hepatic metabolism (primarily by CYP3A4) with biliary excretion of unchanged drug and metabolites • Cl ~2.1 mL/min/kg

Enteral Administration and Nutrition Considerations

Compatibility, Stability, and Bioavailability Considerations
• No data are available.

Drug-Nutrition Interactions
• Drug may influence nutrition status directly or indirectly:
  o CNS: dizziness, asthenia, headache, tremor
  o GI: anorexia, nausea, vomiting, abdominal pain, diarrhea or constipation, elevated concentrations of AST, ALT, and bilirubin
  o Metabolic: peripheral edema
  o Other: arthralgia, myalgia
• No data on the influence of malnutrition or obesity on drug disposition.
• Influence of food on absorption or oral bioavailability:
  o High-fat meal (~50 g fat) increases oral bioavailability by ~2.5-fold.
  o An in vitro model was developed and proved successful to predict positive food effect studies of BCS Class 2 agents including ivermectin.[1]

Recommendations

Gastric	• Crush and disperse tablet in water just prior to administration. • Hold EN for 1 hour before and 1 hour after each drug dose.
Postpyloric	• As above. • Monitor for any unexpected change in effect.

Reference

1. Raman S, Polli JE. Prediction of positive food effect: bioavailability enhancement of BCS class II drugs. *Int J Pharm.* 2016;506:110–115.

Ketoconazole

Product Availability

Solid	• Tablet: 200 mg (various)

Physicochemical (drug)

Molecular weight: • 531.44	Permeability: • LogP 4.35 • LogD 4.05 (pH 7.4)	Water solubility: • 0.007 mg/mL
pKa: • 2.9, 6.5	Classification: • BCS Class 2; BDDCS Class 2	

Pharmaceutical (product)

Solid	• Tablets may disperse in water (20 mL) within 5 minutes. • Commercial suspension (100 mg/5 mL) is no longer available.

Pharmacokinetic (patient)

Absorption	• Specific site not known; t_{max} ~1–2 hours after an oral dose • Requires acidic gastric environment for absorption • Bioavailability ~50%
Transport	• Plasma protein binding ~84%–99%, mostly to albumin • V_d ~0.4–0.5 L/kg
Metabolism	• Partially metabolized to several inactive metabolites, mostly via CYP3A4, with biliary excretion into feces • Cl ~0.16 L/h/kg

Enteral Administration and Nutrition Considerations

Compatibility, Stability, and Bioavailability Considerations

- Drug stability is pH-dependent and optimal at pH 5–9, with instability evident at pH <5.[1]
- At aqueous dispersions between 0.25% and 2%, the drug was stable at pH 7 as long as the antioxidant (BHT) concentration was ≤0.1%.[1]
- The official USP formulation for oral suspension (20 mg/mL) prepared from drug powder or from tablets can be stored at room temperature with a BUD of 14 days.
- Extemporaneously compounded oral solutions (2.5 mg/mL, 5 mg/mL) prepared in ethanol and water, stored at refrigerator or room temperature and protected from or exposed to light, remained stable (HPLC analysis) for 29 days.[2]
- Extemporaneously compounded oral suspensions (20 mg/mL) prepared from tablets with OraSweet/OraPlus (1:1) or OraSweet SF/OraPlus (1:1) or cherry syrup/simple syrup (1:4), stored in clear polyethylene terephthalate plastic bottles at 5°C or 25°C and protected from light, remained stable (HPLC analysis) for 60 days.[3]

- An extemporaneously compounded oral suspension (20 mg/mL) prepared from drug powder in SyrSpend SF PH4, stored in low-actinic bottles at 2°C–8°C or 20°C–25°C, remained stable (HPLC analysis) for 90 days.[4]
- Incorporating organic acids (eg, citric acid) into the preparation of an oral formulation enhanced dissolution and increased oral bioavailability 1.7-fold in an animal model.[5,6]
- A formulation under development may diminish the poor bioavailability that accompanies nonacidic gastric conditions.[7]

Drug-Nutrition Interactions
- Drug may influence nutrition status directly or indirectly:
  - Increased appetite, inhibited synthesis of 1,25-dihydroxy-vitamin D
  - CNS: headache, dizziness, fatigue
  - GI: dry mouth; dysgeusia; anorexia; nausea; vomiting; abdominal pain; diarrhea or constipation; elevated concentrations of AST, ALT, and alkaline phosphatase; rare hepatotoxicity
  - Metabolic: peripheral edema; decreased serum concentrations of cortisol, testosterone and estradiol; hyperlipidemia
  - Other: arthralgia, myalgia
- No data on the influence of malnutrition or obesity on drug disposition.
- Influence of food on absorption or oral bioavailability:
  - Food may improve oral absorption and bioavailability, but effects can vary by individual.

Recommendations

Gastric	• If there is no therapeutic alternative, disperse tablet in water just prior to administration. • Consider holding EN for 1 hour before and 1 hour after each drug dose.
Postpyloric	• As above. • Monitor for any unexpected change in effect.
Other	• As with all antimicrobials, consider parenteral alternative for acutely ill patients to ensure therapeutic concentrations.

References

1. Skiba M, Skiba-Lahiani M, Marchais H, et al. Stability assessment of ketoconazole in aqueous formulations. *Int J Pharm.* 2000;198:1–6.
2. Kumer KP, Oonomah AD, Bradshaw WG, et al. Stability of ketoconazole in ethanolic solutions. *Drug Dev Ind Pharm.* 1991;17:577–580.
3. Allen LV, Erickson MA. Stability of ketoconazole, metolazone, metronidazole, procainamide hydrochloride, and spironolactone in extemporaneously compounded oral liquids. *Am J Health-Syst Pharm.* 1996;53:2073–2078.
4. Polonini HC, Loures S, de Araujo EP, et al. Stability of allopurinol, amitriptyline hydrochloride, carbamazepine, domperidone, isoniazid, ketoconazole, lisinopril, naproxen, paracetamol (acetaminophen), and sertraline hydrochloride in SyrSpend SF PH4 oral suspensions. *Int J Pharm Compd.* 2016;20:426–434.

5. Adachi M, Hinatsu Y, Kusamori K, et al. Improved dissolution and absorption of ketoconazole in the presence of organic acids as pH-modifiers. *Eur J Pharm Sci.* 2015;76: 225–230.

6. Adachi M, Hinatsu Y, Kusamori K, et al. Effects of manufacturing methods on dissolution and absorption of ketoconazole in the presence of organic acid as a pH modifier. *AAPS PharmSciTech.* 2017;18:1203–1212.

7. Xin C, Li-Hong W, Jing Y, et al. Ketoconazole ion-exchange fiber complex: a novel method to reduce the individual difference of bioavailability in oral administration caused by gastric anacidity. *Pharm Dev Technol.* 2013;18:1346–1354.

Lamotrigine

Product Availability

Solid	• Tablet:
	   ○ Immediate-release: 25 mg, 100 mg, 150 mg, 200 mg (Lamictal® [GSK]; others)
	   ○ Orally disintegrating: 25 mg, 50 mg, 100 mg, 200 mg (Lamictal® ODT [GSK]; others)
	   ○ Chewable, dispersible: 2 mg, 5 mg, 25 mg (Lamictal® CD [GSK]; others)
	   ○ Extended-release: 25 mg, 50 mg, 100 mg, 200 mg, 250 mg, 300 mg (Lamictal® XR [GSK]; others)

Physicochemical (drug)

Molecular weight: • 256.10	Permeability: • LogP 2.53 (calc) • LogD –0.19 (pH 7.4)	Water solubility: • 0.17 mg/mL (25°C)
pKa: • 5.7	Classification: • BCS Class 2; BDDCS Class 2	

Pharmaceutical (product)

Solid	• Immediate-release tablet is intended to be administered whole. • Do not crush the extended-release tablet. • Only the dispersible tablet may be dispersed in liquid. • The orally dispersible tablet is considered bioequivalent to the immediate-release tablet. • The extended-release tablet is considered bioequivalent to the immediate-release tablet.

Pharmacokinetic (patient)

Absorption	• Specific site not known; t_{max} ~2 hours after an oral dose (immediate-release) • Bioavailability ~98% • Nasogastric tube administration has not been evaluated.
Transport	• Plasma protein binding ~55% • V_d 0.9–1.3 L/kg
Metabolism	• Metabolized by glucuronic acid conjugation to inactive metabolites that can be excreted renally • Cl ~0.58 mL/min/kg

Enteral Administration and Nutrition Considerations

Compatibility, Stability, and Bioavailability Considerations

- Lamotrigine hydrolysis is rapid at alkaline pH but slower at acidic pH.[1]
- The official USP formulation for oral suspension (1 mg/mL) is expected to have a pH of 4–5 and is given a BUD of 90 days.

- An extemporaneously compounded oral liquid (20 mg/mL) has a pH of 4.97.
- An extemporaneously compounded oral suspension (1 mg/mL) prepared from tablets (100 mg) using OraSweet or OraSweet SF with OraPlus as a vehicle and stored in amber polyethylene terephthalate bottles at 4°C and 25°C remained stable (HPLC analysis) for 91 days; however, no data on osmolality or viscosity were reported.[2]
- Another extemporaneously compounded oral suspension (1 mg/mL) prepared from drug powder in SyrSpend SF PH4, stored out of light at 2°C–8°C or 20°C–25°C, remained stable (HPLC analysis) for 90 days.[3]
- A formulation in development revealed similar dissolution profiles to marketed products.[4]

Drug-Nutrition Interactions
- Drug may influence nutrition status directly or indirectly:
  - Weight loss is more likely than weight gain.
  - May reduce serum folate concentrations.
  - CNS: dizziness, headache, confusion, ataxia, tremor, diplopia
  - GI: dry mouth, altered taste, stomatitis, dysphagia, nausea, vomiting, abdominal pain, constipation or diarrhea, LFT abnormalities
  - Metabolic: edema, hyperglycemia, anemia
  - Other: arthralgia, myalgia
- No data on the influence of malnutrition or obesity on drug disposition.
- No known influence of food on oral absorption or bioavailability.

Recommendations

Gastric	• Disperse appropriate tablet in water just prior to administration. • No need to hold EN beyond the time required to flush-administer-flush.
Postpyloric	• As above. • Monitor for any unexpected change in effect.

References

1. Shrivastava PK, Shrivastava SK. Stress studies and the estimation of lamotrigine in pharmaceutical formulation by validated RP-HPLC method. *Indian J Pharm Educ Res.* 2009;43:156–161.
2. Nahata MC, Morosco RS, Hipple TF. Stability of lamotrigine in two extemporaneously prepared oral suspensions at 4 and 25°C. *Am J Health-Syst Pharm.* 1999;56:240–242.
3. Polonini HC, Loures S, Lima LC, et al. Stability of atenolol, clonazepam, dexamethasone, diclofenac sodium, diltiazem, enalapril maleate, ketoprofen, lamotrigine, penicillamine-D and thiamine in SyrSpend SF PH4 oral suspensions. *Int J Pharm Compd.* 206;20:167–174.
4. Koteswari P, Sunium S, Srinivasababu P, Babu GK, Nithya PD. Formulation development and evaluation of fast disintegrating tablets of lamotrigine using liquid-solid technique. *Int J Pharm Invest.* 2014;4:207–214.

Lansoprazole

Product Availability

Solid	• Tablet (orally disintegrating): 15 mg, 30 mg (Prevacid® SoluTab® [Takeda]; others) • Capsule: 15 mg, 30 mg (Prevacid® [Takeda]; others)

Physicochemical (drug)

Molecular weight: • 369.37	Permeability: • LogP 1.90 • LogD 2.36 (pH 7.4)	Water solubility: • 0.001 mg/mL
pKa: • 4.01	Classification: • BCS Class 1; BDDCS Class 2	

Pharmaceutical (product)

Solid	• Do not crush tablet or capsule contents as they contain enteric-coated granules. • The tablet will, however, completely disperse in 10 mL of water. • Packets for oral suspension (no longer available) contained xanthan gum among the ingredients, which formed a viscous suspension that would clog small-bore feeding tubes.

Pharmacokinetic (patient)

Absorption	• Specific site not known; t_{max} ~2 hours after an oral dose • Bioavailability ≥80% (better in CYP2C19 poor metabolizer phenotype)
Transport	• Substrate for P-glycoprotein efflux • Plasma protein binding ~97% • V_d ~15.7 liters
Metabolism	• Metabolized extensively by hydroxylation (via CYP2C19) and sulfoxidation (via CYP3A4/5) and excreted in urine and feces • Cl ~11.1 mL/min

Enteral Administration and Nutrition Considerations

Compatibility, Stability, and Bioavailability Considerations
- Aqueous degradation half-life is estimated to be 30 minutes at pH 5.
- Aqueous solutions decompose at a greater rate at lower pH, and the orally dispersible tablet is moisture sensitive.[1]
- The official USP formulation for oral suspension (25 mg/mL) prepared from capsule contents with sodium bicarbonate and OraBlend is expected to have a pH of 8–8.5 and provide a BUD of 90 days.
- Enteric-coated granules (15 or 30 mg) can be prepared as a suspension within 20 minutes in 8.4% sodium bicarbonate (2.5 mL, 5 mL, 10 mL, 20 mL) and sterile water in a 30 mL syringe.[2]

- Another extemporaneously compounded oral suspension (3 mg/mL), prepared from capsule contents (30 mg) in 8.4% sodium bicarbonate (10 mL) and stored in 10 mL amber oral syringes remained stable (HPLC analysis) for up to 8 hours at room temperature, and for 14 days at 4°C; viscosity was not reported.[3]
- An extemporaneously compounded oral suspension (3 mg/mL) prepared from capsule contents in 8.4% sodium bicarbonate, stored in amber plastic syringes and protected from light at 3°C–4°C or 20°C–22°C, remained stable (HPLC analysis) for only 72 hours (room temperature) or 8 days (refrigerated).[4]
- An extemporaneously compounded oral suspension (3 mg/mL) prepared from 30 mg capsule contents in 8.4% sodium bicarbonate, and further diluted with OraSweet/OraPlus (1:1) with pH adjusted to 8.8, remained stable (HPLC analysis) when stored in amber glass bottles at 4°C and 25°C for 91 days.[5]
- An oral suspension (3 mg/mL) using disintegrating tablets (30 mg) in OraBlend (10 mL), which remained stable for up to 3 days at room temperature and for 7 days refrigerated, occluded a 5 Fr nasogastric tube but not an 8 Fr or 10 Fr tube.[6]
- Dispersing capsule contents in 10 mL of 8.4% sodium bicarbonate and administered by nasogastric tube (8 Fr) is clinically effective.[7]
- The extemporaneously compounded suspension (3 mg/mL) administered via nasogastric tube (8 Fr) to 36 healthy subjects controlled 24-hour gastric pH despite lower bioavailability than from administration of intact oral capsules.[8]
- Gastric acid suppression was similar when lansoprazole (30 mg) was administered through a gastrostomy (size not reported) as dry non-encapsulated granules in orange juice (45 mL) or when suspended in 8.4% sodium bicarbonate (10 mL) before administration.[9,10]
- When the capsule contents were suspended in apple juice (15–40 mL) prior to administration, only ~30% of granules were delivered to the end of a 14 Fr nasogastric tube; in contrast, about two-thirds of drug granules were delivered all the way through a 16 Fr tube; in that case, 42% of samples clogged the feeding tube, although the delivered suspension resulted in similar bioavailability to an orally administered capsule.[11–13]
- The administration for 3 days of the orally disintegrating tablet (30 mg) mixed in water (10 mL) through a nasogastric tube (Fr size, material, and length not reported) to 10 critically ill patients resulted in an average bioavailability of 76% relative to 30 mg intravenously delivered to 9 critically ill patients over the same time period, but the enterally administered regimen maintained gastric pH >4 for a longer period of time than the intravenous one; patients did not receive gastric EN.[14]
- When drug capsule contents were mixed one at a time with a number of different oral liquids (e.g., apple juice, orange juice, ginger ale [all with pH <7], water) and administered through a nasogastric tube (18 Fr,

Argyle Salem sump), only the 8.4% sodium bicarbonate preparation delivered all the drug through the tube and that preparation was the only one not to occlude the tube.[15]
- Alternative enteric-coating substances for drug granules have been studied.[16]

Drug-Nutrition Interactions
- Drug may influence nutrition status directly or indirectly:
  - CNS: lethargy, fatigue
  - GI: dry mouth, nausea, prolonged gastric emptying, abdominal pain, diarrhea (including *Clostridium difficile*–associated)
  - Metabolic: hypomagnesemia
  - Other: increased risk of osteoporosis-related fracture; muscle weakness and cramps
- No data on the influence of malnutrition or obesity on drug disposition.
- Influence of food on oral absorption or bioavailability:
  - Food can significantly reduce oral bioavailability (by ~50%) when administered ~30 minutes after the meal.

Recommendations

Gastric	• Disperse tablet (or capsule contents) in 10 mL of 8.4% sodium bicarbonate prior to administration. • Consider holding EN for 1 hour before and after each dose.
Postpyloric	• As above. • Monitor for any unexpected change in effect.

References
1. Church C, Smith J. How stable are medicines moved from original packs into compliance aids? *Pharm J.* 2006;276:75–81.
2. McAndrews KL, Eastham JH. Omeprazole and lansoprazole suspensions for nasogastric administration. *Am J Health-Syst Pharm.* 1999;56:81.
3. DiGiacinto JL, Olsen KM, Bergman KL, et al. Stability of suspension formulations of lansoprazole and omeprazole stored in amber-colored plastic oral syringes. *Ann Pharmacother.* 2000;34:600–605.
4. Morrison JT, Lugo RA, Thigpen JC, et al. Stability of extemporaneously prepared lansoprazole suspension at two temperatures. *J Pediatr Pharmacol Ther.* 2013;18:122–127.
5. Ensom MHH, Decarie D, Sheppard I. Stability of lansoprazole in extemporaneously compounded suspensions for nasogastric or oral administration. *Can J Hosp Pharm.* 2007;60:184–191.
6. Melkoumov A, Soukrati A, Elkin I, et al. Quality evaluation of extemporaneous delayed-release liquid formulations of lansoprazole. *Am J Health-Syst Pharm.* 2011;68:2069–2074.
7. Taubel JJ, Sharma VK, Chiu YL, et al. A comparison of simplified lansoprazole suspension administered nasogastrically and pantoprazole administered intravenously: effects on 24-h intragastric pH. *Aliment Pharmacol Ther.* 2001;15:1807–1817.
8. Doan TT, Wang Q, Griffen JS, et al. Comparative pharmacokinetics and pharmacodynamics of lansoprazole oral capsules and suspension in healthy subjects. *Am J Health-Syst Pharm.* 2001;58:1512–1519.

9. Sharma VK, Ugheoke EA, Vasudeva R, et al. The pharmacodynamics of lansoprazole administration via gastrostomy as intact non-encapsulated granules. *Aliment Pharmacol Ther.* 1998;12:1171–1174.

10. Sharma VK, Vasudeva R, Howden CW. Simplified lansoprazole suspension—a liquid formulation of lansoprazole—effectively suppresses intragastric acidity when administered through a gastrostomy. *Am J Gastroenterol.* 1999;94:1813–1817.

11. Chun AHC, Shi HH, Achai R, et al. Lansoprazole: administration of the contents of a capsule dosage formulation through a nasogastric tube. *Clin Ther.* 1996;18:833–842.

12. Dunn A, White CM, Reddy P, et al. Delivery of omeprazole and lansoprazole granules through a nasogastric tube in vitro. *Am J Health-Syst Pharm.* 1999;56:2327–2330.

13. Messaouik D, Sauto-Miranda V, Bagel-Boithias S, et al. Comparative study and optimization of the administration mode of three proton pump inhibitors by nasogastric tube. *Int J Pharm.* 2005;299:65–72.

14. Olsen KM, Devlin JW. Comparison of the enteral and intravenous lansoprazole pharmacodynamics responses in critically ill patients. *Aliment Pharmacol Ther.* 2008;28: 326–333.

15. Olabisi A, Chen J, Garala M. Evaluation of different lansoprazole formulations for nasogastric or orogastric administration. *Hosp Pharm.* 2007;42:537–542.

16. Fang Y, Wang G, Zhang R, et al. Eudragit L/HPMCAS blend enteric-coated lansoprazole pellets: enhanced drug stability and oral bioavailability. *AAPS PharmSciTech.* 2014;15:513–521.

Levetiracetam

Product Availability

Solid	• Tablet:
	   ○ Immediate-release: 250 mg, 500 mg, 750 mg, 1000 mg (Keppra® [UCB Pharma]; others)
	   ○ Orally disintegrating: 250 mg, 500 mg, 750 mg, 1000 mg (Spritam® [Aprecia Pharms])
	   ○ Extended-release: 500 mg, 750 mg (Keppra® XR [UCB Pharma]; others)

Liquid	• Oral solution: 100 mg/mL (Keppra® Oral Solution [UCB Pharma]; others)

Physicochemical (drug)

Molecular weight: • 170.21	Permeability: • LogP –0.34 to –0.67 (calc) • LogD n/a	Water solubility: • 104 mg/mL
pKa: • 15.7	Classification: • BCS Class 1; BDDCS Class 3	

Pharmaceutical (product)

Solid	• Immediate-release tablet products may be film-coated; do not crush (unacceptable taste). • Orally disintegrating tablet may disperse easily in small volume of water. • Do not crush extended-release tablet.

Liquid	• Oral solution:
	   ○ pH 6.03
	   ○ Osmolality 5075 mOsm/kg (calculated based on measurement of 1:5 dilution of 100 mg/mL product with sterile water)[1]
	   ○ Viscosity not significant
	   ○ May contain glycerin, maltitol, and potassium acesulfame; grape-flavored
	   ○ Store solution at controlled room temperature.

Pharmacokinetic (patient)

Absorption	• Specific site not known; t_{max} ~60–80 minutes after an oral dose (fasted) • Bioavailability ~95%–100% • Conventional tablet, orally disintegrating tablet, and solution are considered bioequivalent.
Transport	• Plasma protein binding <10% • V_d ~0.5–0.7 L/kg

Metabolism	• Not extensively metabolized; ~24% hydrolyzed to inactive metabolite • Cl ~0.96 mL/min/kg

Enteral Administration and Nutrition Considerations

Compatibility, Stability, and Bioavailability Considerations

- An extemporaneously compounded oral suspension (50 mg/mL) prepared from tablets in OraSweet/OraPlus (1:1) and stored in amber plastic bottles at 4°C or 25°C remained stable (HPLC analysis) for 91 days.[2]
- The commercial solution combined (1:1) with Osmolite 1.2, under simulated clinical conditions, would result in no clogging of either an 8 Fr or a 20 Fr feeding tube.[1]
- The tablet (500 mg) taken with water (120 mL) or crushed and mixed with 120 mL EN (Sustacal) and administered by mouth resulted in similar oral bioavailability in a crossover study of 10 healthy volunteers.[3]
- Delivery of pure drug directly into the proximal small bowel or distal small bowel resulted in bioavailability comparable to oral administration of immediate-release tablet in a crossover study of healthy subjects.[4]

Drug-Nutrition Interactions

- Drug may influence nutrition status directly or indirectly:
  - CNS: somnolence, fatigue, coordination difficulties (eg, ataxia), behavioral abnormalities (eg, apathy, depression)
  - GI: anorexia
  - Metabolic: decreased hemoglobin and RBC count
- No data on the influence of malnutrition or obesity on drug disposition.
- Influence of food on oral absorption or bioavailability:
  - Food may decrease rate of absorption but without an influence on oral bioavailability.
  - A high-fat meal (57.5 g fat, 71 g carbohydrate, 34 g protein) decreased the rate of absorption from the orally disintegrating tablet but had no influence on oral bioavailability.[5]

Recommendations

Gastric	• Dilute oral solution with water prior to administration. • No need to hold EN beyond the time required to flush-administer-flush.
Postpyloric	• As above. • Monitor for any unexpected change in effect.

References

1. Klang M, McLymont V, Ng N. Osmolality, pH, and compatibility of selected oral liquid medications with an enteral nutrition product. *JPEN J Parenter Enteral Nutr.* 2013;37: 689–694.

2. Ensom MHH, Décarie D, Rudolph S. Stability of levetiracetam in extemporaneously compounded suspensions. *Can J Hosp Pharm*. 2011;64:207–211.
3. Fay MA, Sheth RD, Gidal BE. Oral absorption kinetics of levetiracetam: the effect of mixing with food or enteral nutrition formula. *Clin Ther*. 2005;27:594–598.
4. Stockis A, Sargentini-Maier ML, Otoul C, et al. Assessment of levetiracetam bioavailability from targeted sites in the human intestine using remotely activated capsules and gamma scintigraphy: open-label, single-dose, randomized, four-way crossover study in healthy male volunteers. *Clin Ther*. 2010;32:1813–1821.
5. Boudriau S, Hanzel C, Massicotte J, et al. Randomized comparative bioavailability of a novel three-dimensional printed fast-melt formulation of levetiracetam following the administration of a single 1000-mg dose to healthy human volunteers under fasting and fed conditions. *Drugs R D*. 2016;16:229–238.

Levofloxacin

Product Availability

Solid	• Tablet: 250 mg, 500 mg, 750 mg (anhydrous base) (Levaquin® [Janssen]; others)
Liquid	• Oral solution: 125 mg/5 mL (Levaquin® [Janssen]; others)

Physicochemical (drug)

Molecular weight: • 361.38	Permeability: • LogP 2.1 • LogD −0.40 (pH 7.4)	Water solubility: • 50 mg/mL (pH 6.9)
pKa: • 6.24	Classification: • BCS Class 1; BDDCS Class 3	

Pharmaceutical (product)

Solid	• Tablets may be film-coated.
Liquid	• Oral solution: ○ pH 5.13 (pH 5–6) ○ Osmolality 2115 mOsm/kg (calculated based on measurement of 1:5 dilution of a 125 mg/5 mL product with sterile water)[1] ○ Viscosity n/a ○ May contain sucrose, glycerin, sucralose, and propylene glycol ○ Solution may be stored at controlled room temperature.
Note	• Tablets and solution are considered bioequivalent.

Pharmacokinetic (patient)

Absorption	• Specific site not known; t_{max} ~1–2 hours after an oral dose • Bioavailability ~99%
Transport	• Substrate for P-glycoprotein efflux, substrate for OATP1A2 uptake • Plasma protein binding ~24%–38%, mostly to albumin • V_d ~74–112 liters
Metabolism	• Minimally metabolized to N-oxide and desmethyl metabolites; otherwise, most of the drug is excreted unchanged, primarily in urine • Cl ~144–226 mL/min

Enteral Administration and Nutrition Considerations

Compatibility, Stability, and Bioavailability Considerations
• Aqueous solubility is pH-dependent: constant between pH 0.6 and 5.8, higher at pH 5.8–6.7, and dropping off at higher pH.

- An extemporaneously compounded oral suspension (50 mg/mL) prepared from crushed tablets (500 mg) with OraPlus/strawberry syrup, NF (1:1) and stored in amber plastic bottles stored at room temperature (23°C–25°C) or refrigerated (3°C–5°C) remained stable (HPLC analysis) for 57 days.[2]
- The commercial solution combined (1:1) with Osmolite 1.2, under simulated clinical conditions, would result in clogging of both an 8 Fr and a 20 Fr feeding tube.[1]
- The admixture of crushed tablet (500 mg) with an EN product (Ensure, 240 mL) was incompatible, decreasing drug availability (61%); this did not occur when drug was admixed in water or water containing calcium and/or magnesium, and regardless of temperature (5°C–37°C).[3]
- Administration into the jejunum of crushed tablets results in adequate (perhaps higher) bioavailability.[4]
- A novel formulation incorporating surfactant being considered has exhibited enhanced bioavailability in an animal model.[5]

Drug-Nutrition Interactions
- Drug may influence nutrition status directly or indirectly:
  - CNS: agitation, anxiety, insomnia, confusion, depression, blurry vision
  - GI: anorexia, bad taste, oral pain, vomiting, abdominal discomfort, diarrhea (including *Clostridium difficile*–associated), LFT elevations and rare hepatotoxicity
  - Metabolic: hyperamylasemia, hypoglycemia, crystalluria
  - Other: peripheral neuropathy (sensory or sensorimotor), tendonitis, arthralgia, weakness
- Influence of malnutrition or obesity on drug disposition:
  - Drug volume of distribution and clearance are not significantly different in obesity, suggesting that dosing should not be based on total body weight.[6,7]
- Influence of food on oral absorption or bioavailability:
  - No known influence of food on oral absorption of tablets, but food may reduce absorption from oral solution.
  - Divalent and trivalent cation-containing products may interfere with oral drug absorption (Al^{+3} > Cu^{+2} > Zn^{+2} > Mg^{+2} > Ca^{+2}). Separating cations (ie, 200 mg elemental calcium as carbonate) by 2 hours from drug (750 mg) administration prevents the interaction at steady state in healthy volunteers but not in adults with cystic fibrosis.[8]
  - Although not expected to be clinically significant, orange juice (~350 mL) may reduce oral bioavailability when administered with or within 4 hours of drug administration, especially if the juice is calcium-fortified.[9]

Recommendations

Gastric	• Dilute oral solution with water (at least 1:1) prior to administration. • Consider holding EN for 1 hour before and 2 hours after each drug dose.
Postpyloric	• As above. • Monitor for any unexpected change in effect.
Other	• As with all antimicrobials, consider parenteral alternative for acutely ill patients to ensure therapeutic concentrations.

References

1. Klang M, McLymont V, Ng N. Osmolality, pH, and compatibility of selected oral liquid medications with an enteral nutrition product. *JPEN J Parenter Enteral Nutr.* 2013;37: 689–694.
2. VandenBussche HL, Johnson CE, Fontana EM, et al. Stability of levofloxacin in an extemporaneously compounded oral liquid. *Am J Health-Syst Pharm.* 1999;56: 2316–2318.
3. Wright DH, Pietz SL, Konstantinides FN, Rotschafer JC. Decreased in vitro fluoroquinolone concentrations after admixture with an enteral feeding formulation. *JPEN J Parenter Enteral Nutr.* 2000;24:42–48.
4. Reid J, Marciniuk D, Peloquin CA, Hoeppner V. Pharmacokinetics of antituberculosis medications delivered via percutaneous gastrojejunostomy tube. *Chest.* 2002;121:281–284.
5. Imran M, Shah MR, Ullah F, et al. Sugar-based novel niosomal nanocarrier system for enhanced oral bioavailability of levofloxacin. *Drug Deliv.* 2016;23:3653–3664.
6. Luque S, Grau S, Valle M, et al. Levofloxacin weight-adjusted dosing and pharmacokinetic disposition in a morbidly obese patient. *J Antimicrob Chemother.* 2011;66:1653–1654.
7. Cook AM, Martin C, Adams VR, et al. Pharmacokinetics of intravenous levofloxacin administered at 750 mg in obese adults. *Antimicrob Agents Chemother.* 2011;55: 3240–3243.
8. Pai MP, Allen SE, Amsden GW. Altered steady state pharmacokinetics of levofloxacin in adult cystic fibrosis patients receiving calcium carbonate. *J Cyst Fibrosis.* 2006;5:153–157.
9. Bailey DG. Fruit juice inhibition of uptake transport: a new type of food-drug interaction. *Br J Clin Pharmacol.* 2010;70:645–655.

Levothyroxine Sodium

Product Availability

Solid	• Tablet: 25 µg, 50 µg, 75 µg, 88 µg, 100 µg, 112 µg, 125 µg, 137 µg, 150 µg, 175 µg, 200 µg, 300 µg (various)

Physicochemical (drug)

Molecular weight:	Permeability:	Water solubility:
• 776.88 (salt 798.86)	• LogP 4.0 • LogD 0.65 (pH 7.4)	• 0.15 mg/mL
pKa: • 0.27, 7.43, 9.43	**Classification:** • BCS Class 3; BDDCS Class 2	

Pharmaceutical (product)

Solid	• Closed crushing to avoid exposure. • Avoid exposure to temperatures >15°C.

Pharmacokinetic (patient)

Absorption	• Specific site not known; jejunum > duodenum; t_{max} ~2 hours after an oral dose (fasted) • Bioavailability varies (~40%–80%) • Various commercial products are not generally considered bioequivalent or interchangeable.
Transport	• Substrate for several uptake transporters, including OATP1A2 • Plasma protein binding ~99%, including albumin, thyroxine-binding prealbumin, and thyroxine-binding globulin • V_d ~14.7 liters
Metabolism	• Metabolized through hepatic conjugation and may undergo enterohepatic recirculation • Cl n/a

Enteral Administration and Nutrition Considerations

Compatibility, Stability, and Bioavailability Considerations
- The drug is unstable in the presence of heat, light, air, and humidity.
- Saturated aqueous solutions have a pH >8.
- Aqueous solubility is pH-dependent, with best solubility at pH <2 and >8.[1]
- Aqueous solutions exposed to UV light are at risk for deiodination of the drug.[1]
- For immediate use, crushed tablets can be suspended in 5–10 mL water
- An aqueous preparation (25 µg/mL) prepared from tablets or bulk powder (yellow suspension or clear solution, respectively), stored in amber polyethylene bottles, resulted in significant degradation (HPLC analysis) at 4°C, 25°C, and 40°C, with or without preservatives.[2]

- The best stability (8 days) was with nonpreserved suspension prepared from tablets stored at 4°C or 25°C.[2]
- An extemporaneously compounded oral suspension (25 µg/mL) prepared from tablets in either simple syrup/1% methylcellulose (1:10) or OraSweet/OraPlus (1:1), stored in plastic bottles at 4°C or 25°C, remained stable (HPLC analysis) for 7 days (room temperature) or 14 days (refrigerated).[3]
- A complex oral levothyroxine syrup (40 µg/mL) is expected to be stable (HPLC analysis) for 2 weeks at 25°C; viscosity and osmolality were not reported.[4]
- Tablets crushed to a powder were better absorbed than the intact tablet in several patients; effect is most likely an improvement in dissolution and may be product-specific.[5]
- Oral liquid formulations may have a better bioavailability with less likelihood of interaction with calcium and iron salts.[6]
- An oral levothyroxine solution was shown to be bioequivalent to a commercial tablet formulation in an open, randomized, single-dose crossover study in healthy volunteers.[7]
- When an oral liquid formulation was mixed in breakfast beverages (orange juice, milk, tea, coffee), the drug remained stable (LC-MS/MS analysis) for ~20 minutes.[8]
- EN formula containing iron, fiber, or soybean should be avoided as a carrier for drug administration.
- Based on an in vitro study, percutaneous endoscopic gastrostomy tubes (14 Fr silicone) pretreated with EN (Jevity) were associated with a 45% relative increase in drug adsorption compared with tubes not used for EN, although the clinical significance of this finding is not clear.[9]
- Oral bioavailability of the drug is not altered following Roux-en-Y gastric bypass.[10]

Drug-Nutrition Interactions

- Drug may influence nutrition status directly or indirectly:
  - CNS: insomnia
  - GI: dysphagia
  - Metabolic: hyperthyroidism
- No data on the influence of malnutrition or obesity on drug disposition.
- Influence of food on oral absorption or bioavailability:
  - In general, food decreases drug absorption; drug is best administered on an empty stomach.
  - Dietary fiber, as well as calcium- and iron-salts decrease oral absorption.[11]
  - Divalent and trivalent cation–containing products may reduce oral bioavailability and are best separated by at least 2–4 hours.
  - Soybeans, but not soy isoflavone supplements, may decrease oral drug absorption.[12]

- ○ EN may reduce absorption; if the formula contains iron, fiber, or soybean, it should be avoided.[13]
- ○ Grapefruit juice (~600 mL) may reduce oral bioavailability (~10%) when administered with or within 4 hours of drug administration.[14]

Recommendations

Gastric	• Crush and/or disperse tablet in water just prior to administration. • Hold EN 1 hour before and after drug administration if EN is expected to last >5 days.
Postpyloric	• As above. • Monitor for any unexpected change in effect.

References

1. Won CM. Kinetics of degradation of levothyroxine in aqueous solution and in solid state. *Pharm Res.* 1992;9:131–137.
2. Boulton DW, Fawcett JP, Woods DJ. Stability of an extemporaneously compounded levothyroxine sodium oral liquid. *Am J Health-Syst Pharm.* 1996;53:1157–1161.
3. Nahata MC. Stability of levothyroxine, doxycycline, hydrocortisone, and pravastatin in liquid dosage forms stored at two temperatures. *Int J Pharm Compd.* 2015;19:428–431.
4. Alexander KS, Kothapalli MR, Dollimor D. Stability of an extemporaneously formulated levothyroxine sodium syrup compounded from commercial tablets. *Int J Pharm Compd.* 1997;1:60–64.
5. Yamamoto T. Tablet formulation of levothyroxine is absorbed less well than powdered levothyroxine. *Thyroid.* 2003;13:1177–1181.
6. Guglielmi V, Bellia A, Bianchini E, et al. Drug interactions in users of tablet vs. oral liquid levothyroxine formulations: a real-world evidence study in primary care. *Endocrine.* 2018;59:585–592.
7. Yannovits N, Zintzaras E, Pouli A, et al. A bioequivalence study of levothyroxine tablets versus an oral levothyroxine solution in healthy volunteers. *Eur J Drug Metab Pharmacokinet.* 2006;31:73–78.
8. Bernareggi A, Grata E, Pinorini MT, Conti A. Oral liquid formulation of levothyroxine is stable in breakfast beverages and may improve thyroid patient compliance. *Pharmaceutics.* 2013;5:621–633.
9. Manessis A, Lascher S, Bukberg P, et al. Quantifying amount of adsorption of levothyroxine by percutaneous endoscopic gastrostomy tubes. *JPEN J Parenter Enteral Nutr.* 2008;32:197–200.
10. Rubio IG, Galrao AL, Santo MA, et al. Levothyroxine absorption in morbidly obese patients before and after Roux-en-Y gastric bypass (RYGB) surgery. *Obes Surg.* 2012;22: 253–258.
11. Ianiro G, Mangiola F, DiRienzo TA, et al. Levothyroxine absorption in health and disease, and new therapeutic perspectives. *Eur Rev Med Pharmacol Sci.* 2014;18:451–456.
12. Persiani S, Sala F, Manzotti C, et al. Evaluation of levothyroxine bioavailability after oral administration of a fixed combination of soy isoflavones in post-menopausal female volunteers. *Drug Res.* 2016;66:136–140.
13. Smyrniotis V, Vaos N, Arkadopoulos N, et al. Severe hypothyroidism in patients dependent on prolonged thyroxine infusion through a jejunostomy. *Clin Nutr.* 2000; 19:65–67.
14. Bailey DG. Fruit juice inhibition of uptake transport: a new type of food-drug interaction. *Br J Clin Pharmacol.* 2010;70:645–655.

Linaclotide

Product Availability

Solid	• Capsule: 72 µg, 145 µg, 290 µg (Linzess® [Allergan])

Physicochemical (drug)

Molecular weight: • 1526.8	Permeability: • LogP n/a • LogD n/a	Water solubility: • 0.7 mg/mL
pKa: • n/a	Classification: • BCS Class n/a; BDDCS Class n/a	

Pharmaceutical (product)

Solid	• Do not break open or chew capsule.

Pharmacokinetic (patient)

Absorption	• Minimally absorbed • Locally acting at the gut epithelium to activate guanylate cyclase
Transport	• Not applicable
Metabolism	• Active metabolite formed by carboxypeptidase-A within the GI tract lumen

Enteral Administration and Nutrition Considerations

Compatibility, Stability, Bioavailability Considerations
- Linaclotide, a 14-amino acid peptide, was shown to remain stable in simulated acidic gastric fluid.[1]

Drug-Nutrition Interactions
- Drug may influence nutrition status directly or indirectly:
  - CNS: headache
  - GI: abdominal pain, distension, diarrhea
- No data on the influence of malnutrition or obesity on drug disposition.
- Influence of food on oral absorption or bioavailability:
  - A high-fat meal will increase risk for loose stools.
  - Best administered on an empty stomach.

Recommendations

Gastric	• Do not administer by enteral access device.
Postpyloric	• As above.

Reference

1. Busby RW, Kessler MM, Bartolini WP, et al. Pharmacologic properties, metabolism, and disposition of linaclotide, a novel therapeutic peptide approved for the treatment of irritable bowel syndrome with constipation and chronic idiopathic constipation. *J Pharmacol Exp Ther*. 2013;344:196–206.

Lisdexamfetamine Dimesylate

Product Availability

Solid	• Tablet: Chewable: 10 mg, 20 mg, 30 mg, 40 mg, 50 mg, 60 mg (salt) (Vyvanse® [Shire]) • Capsule: Immediate-release: 10 mg, 20 mg, 30 mg, 40 mg, 50 mg, 60 mg, 70 mg (salt) (Vyvanse® [Shire]; others)

Physicochemical (drug)

Molecular weight: • 263.34 (salt 455.60)	Permeability: • LogP 1.06 • LogD n/a	Water solubility: • 792 mg/mL (salt)
pKa: • 10.2	Classification: • BCS Class n/a; BDDCS Class n/a	

Pharmaceutical (product)

Solid	• Tablets can be crushed and dispersed in water. • Capsule contents can be dispersed in water.

Pharmacokinetic (patient)

Absorption	• Specific site not known; t_{max} ~3–4 hours after an oral dose • Bioavailability n/a
Transport	• Plasma protein binding n/a • V_d ~190 liters
Metabolism	• This prodrug of dextroamphetamine is converted on first pass (gut and liver) with subsequent renal elimination. • Cl ~15–18 L/h

Enteral Administration and Nutrition Considerations

Compatibility, Stability, and Bioavailability Considerations
- In a crossover study of healthy adults, active drug (D-amphetamine) bioavailability of capsule contents mixed with orange juice and consumed orally for several days was similar to bioavailability of intact capsules.[1]

Drug-Nutrition Interactions
- Drug may influence nutrition status directly or indirectly:
  - Weight loss
  - CNS: abuse potential, behavior disorders, insomnia
  - GI: decreased appetite, dry mouth, nausea, upper abdominal pain, vomiting
  - Metabolic: growth suppression
- No data on the influence of malnutrition or obesity on drug disposition.

- Influence of food on oral absorption or bioavailability:
  - Food may decrease the rate of absorption but without influence on oral bioavailability of the intact capsule or capsule contents dispersed in water.[2]
  - A high-fat meal slightly reduces bioavailability of the chewable tablet.

Recommendations

Gastric	• Dissolve capsule contents in water just prior to administration. • Alternative: Disperse chewable tablet in water just prior to administration. • No need to hold EN beyond the time required to flush-administer-flush.
Postpyloric	• As above. • Monitor for any unexpected change in effect.

References

1. Ermer J, Corcoran M, Lasseter K Martin PT. Relative bioavailabilities of lisdexamfetamine dimesylate and D-amphetamine in healthy adults in an open-label, randomized, crossover study after mixing lisdexamfetamine dimesylate with food or drink. *Ther Drug Monit.* 2016;38:769–776.
2. Krishnan S, Zhang Y. Relative bioavailability of lisdexamfetamine 70-mg capsules in fasted and fed healthy adult volunteers and in solution: a single-dose, crossover pharmacokinetic study. *J Clin Pharmacol.* 2008;48:293–302.

Lisinopril

Product Availability

Solid	• Tablet: 2.5 mg, 5 mg, 10 mg, 20 mg, 30 mg, 40 mg (Prinivil® [Merck]; Zestril® [Alvogen Malta]; others)
Liquid	• Oral solution: 1 mg/mL (Qbrelis® [Silvergate Pharms])

Physicochemical (drug)

Molecular weight: • 405.50	Permeability: • LogP –1.22 • Log D –3.40 (pH 7.4); –6.64 (pH 6.5 calc)	Water solubility: • 97 mg/mL
pKa: • 3.6, 4.3, 7.1, 10.2	Classification: • BCS Class 3; BDDCS Class 3	

Pharmaceutical (product)

Solid	• Tablets disperse in water (10–20 mL) in about 1 minute.
Liquid	• Oral solution: o pH 4.3–5.1 o Osmolality n/a o Viscosity n/a o May contain xylitol o Store at 20°C–25°C.

Pharmacokinetic (patient)

Absorption	• Specific site not known; variable absorption with t_{max} ~7 hours after an oral dose • Bioavailability variable ~25% (6%–60%)
Transport	• Possible substrate for peptide transporter(s) • Minimal plasma protein binding but highly bound with angiotensin-converting enzyme • V_d ~2.4 L/kg
Metabolism	• Excreted unchanged in the urine • Cl ~4.2 mL/min/kg

Enteral Administration and Nutrition Considerations

Compatibility, Stability, and Bioavailability Considerations
- The official USP oral suspension (1 mg/mL) prepared from tablets in OraSweet/OraPlus (1:1) is expected to have a pH of 4.3–5.3 with a BUD of 90 days.
- An extemporaneously compounded oral syrup (2 mg/mL) prepared from powder in distilled water and syrup, stored in amber plastic bottles at 5°C or 23°C, remained stable (HPLC analysis) for a 30-day study period.[1]

- An oral syrup (2 mg/mL) prepared from crushed tablets and stored in amber bottles at 5°C or 23°C remained stable for 30 days.[2]
- An oral liquid (1 mg/mL) prepared from tablets (20 mg) in purified water, sodium citrate/citric acid, and OraSweet SF, stored in amber polyethylene terephthalate bottles at 25°C (35% relative humidity), remained stable (HPLC analysis) regardless of light exposure for 6 weeks.[3]
- Two oral liquid recipes (1 mg/mL) prepared from tablets (10 mg), varying in suspending vehicle (OraSweet/OraPlus [1:1] or 1% methylcellulose/simple syrup [1:13]) and stored in amber plastic bottles at 4°C or 25°C, remained stable (HPLC analysis) for 91 days (refrigerated) or 56 days (room temperature).[4]
- An extemporaneously compounded oral suspension (1 mg/mL) prepared from drug powder in SyrSpend SF PH4 and stored in a low-actinic bottle at 2°C–8°C or 20°C–25°C remained stable (HPLC analysis) for 90 days.[5]

Drug-Nutrition Interactions
- Drug may influence nutrition status directly or indirectly:
  - CNS: headache, dizziness, fatigue
  - GI: nausea, vomiting, diarrhea
  - Metabolic: hyperkalemia
- No data on the influence of malnutrition or obesity on drug disposition.
- No known influence of food on oral absorption or bioavailability.

Recommendations

Gastric	• Disperse tablet in water prior to administration.
	• Alternative: Dilute oral solution in water prior to administration.
	• No need to hold EN beyond the time required to flush-administer-flush.
Postpyloric	• As above.
	• Monitor for any unexpected change in effect.

References

1. Webster AA, English BA, Rose DJ. The stability of lisinopril as an extemporaneous syrup. *Int J Pharm Compd.* 1997;1:352–353.
2. Rose DJ, Webster AA, English BA, et al. Stability of lisinopril syrup (2 mg/mL) extemporaneously compounded from tablets. *Int J Pharm Compd.* 2000;4:398–399.
3. Thompson KC, Zhao Z, Mazakis JM, et al. Characterization of an extemporaneous liquid formulation of lisinopril. *Am J Health-Syst Pharm.* 2003;60:69–74.
4. Nahata MC, Morosco RS. Stability of lisinopril in two liquid dosage forms. *Ann Pharmacother.* 2004;38:396–399.
5. Polonini HC, Loures S, de Araujo EP, et al. Stability of allopurinol, amitriptyline hydrochloride, carbamazepine, domperidone, isoniazid, ketoconazole, lisinopril, naproxen, paracetamol (acetaminophen), and sertraline hydrochloride in SyrSpend SF PH4 oral suspensions. *Int J Pharm Compd.* 2016;20:426–434.

Lomitapide Mesylate

Product Availability

Solid	• Capsule: 5 mg, 10 mg, 20 mg, 30 mg, 40 mg, 60 mg (base) (Juxtapid® [Aegerion])

Physicochemical (drug)

Molecular weight:	Permeability:	Water solubility:
• 693.7 (mesylate 789.8)	• LogP 9.07 • LogD n/a	• 3.5 mg/mL (at pH 4)
pKa: • 9.02, 10.35	Classification: • BCS Class n/a; BDDCS Class n/a	

Pharmaceutical (product)

Solid	• Capsules should not be opened, crushed, chewed, or dissolved (pregnancy category X).

Pharmacokinetic (patient)

Absorption	• Specific site not known; t_{max} ~6 hours after an oral dose • Bioavailability ~7%
Transport	• Not a P-glycoprotein substrate • Plasma protein binding ~99.8% • V_d ~985–1292 liters
Metabolism	• Hepatic metabolism to at least two metabolites, via CYP3A4 more than by CYP1A2, CYPB6, CYP2C8, or CYP2C19, before renal and biliary excretion • Cl n/a

Enteral Administration and Nutrition Considerations

Compatibility, Stability, and Bioavailability Considerations
• Aqueous solutions at pH 2–5 may be slightly soluble.

Drug-Nutrition Interactions
• Drug may influence nutrition status directly or indirectly:
  o Malabsorption of fat-soluble vitamins and fatty acids
  o Weight loss
  o CNS: headache, fatigue
  o GI: nausea, vomiting, dyspepsia, abdominal discomfort, distension or pain, diarrhea (including urgency/tenesmus) more than constipation, hepatic steatosis, hepatotoxicity (AST, ALT elevations >3 times upper normal)
  o Other: back pain
• No data on the influence of malnutrition or obesity on drug disposition.

- Influence of food on oral absorption or bioavailability:
  - To limit severe adverse GI effects, the patient is expected to be on a diet with ≤20% energy from fat during therapy.
  - Administration 2 hours after last meal of the day is recommended, to reduce risk of GI effects.
  - Ethanol may increase adverse hepatic effects.
  - Grapefruit juice may increase drug exposure and adverse effects.

Recommendations

Gastric	• Do not administer by enteral access device. • Use an alternative therapy.
Postpyloric	• Do not administer by enteral access device. • Use an alternative therapy.
Other	• Consider supplementation with essential and conditionally essential fatty acids and vitamin E.

Lorazepam

Product Availability

Solid	• Tablet: 0.5 mg, 1 mg, 2 mg (Ativan® [Valeant]; others)
Liquid	• Oral solution concentrate: 2 mg/mL (various)

Physicochemical (drug)

Molecular weight: • 321.17	Permeability: • LogP 2.39 • LogD 2.39 (pH 7.4)	Water solubility: • 0.08 mg/mL
pKa: • 1.3, 11.5	Classification: • BCS Class 1; BDDCS Class 1	

Pharmaceutical (product)

Solid	• Tablet disperses in water (20 mL) in about 1 minute.
Liquid	• Oral solution: ○ pH n/a ○ Osmolality n/a ○ Viscosity n/a ○ Dose requires dilution in at least 30 mL of diluent (eg, water). ○ May contain polyethylene glycol ○ Store solution at 2°C–8°C.

Pharmacokinetic (patient)

Absorption	• Specific site not known; t_{max} ~2 hours after an oral dose • Bioavailability ~93%
Transport	• Plasma protein binding ~91% • V_d ~1.3 L/kg
Metabolism	• Undergoes conjugation via UGT2B7/2B15 to inactive metabolites, eliminated renally • Cl ~8–10 mL/min/kg

Enteral Administration and Nutrition Considerations

Compatibility, Stability, and Bioavailability Considerations
- In aqueous solution, lorazepam has optimal stability at pH 5.[1]
- An extemporaneously compounded oral suspension (1 mg/mL) prepared from tablets (2 mg) in sterile water and then in OraSweet/OraPlus, stored in amber glass bottles at 4°C or 22°C, remained stable (HPLC analysis) for 91 days (refrigerated) and 63–91 days (room temperature; varying by manufacturer tablet).[2]
- An oral suspension (1 mg/mL) prepared from drug powder in SyrSpend SF PH4 and stored in low-actinic, light-resistant bottles at 2°C–8°C or 20°C–25°C remained stable for 60 days.[3]

Drug-Nutrition Interactions
- Drug may influence nutrition status directly or indirectly:
  - Weight gain or loss
  - CNS: drowsiness, ataxia, fatigue, confusion, anterograde amnesia, visual disturbance
  - GI: dry mouth, glossitis, altered taste, nausea
  - Other: weakness
- Influence of malnutrition or obesity on drug disposition:
  - Weight-normalized volume of distribution was no different in obesity, although drug clearance was increased.[4]
- Influence of food on oral absorption or bioavailability:
  - Food may increase the clearance of the drug.

Recommendations

Gastric	• Crush and/or disperse tablet in water just prior to administration. • Alternative: Dilute concentrated liquid in at least 30 mL of water just prior to administration. • No need to hold EN beyond the time required to flush-administer-flush.
Postpyloric	• As above. • Monitor for any unexpected change in effect.

References

1. Carvalho Ferreira D, Nogueira Prista LV, Ramos Morgado RM, et al. Stability of lorazepam in aqueous solutions: pH effects. *Rev Port Farm.* 1992;42:26–30.
2. Lee W-ME, Lugo RA, Rusho WJ, et al. Chemical stability of extemporaneously prepared lorazepam suspension at two temperatures. *J Pediatr Pharmacol Ther.* 2004;9:254–258.
3. Polonini HC, Silva SL, Cunha CN, et al. Compatibility of cholecalciferol, haloperidol, imipramine hydrochloride, levodopa/carbidopa, lorazepam, minocycline hydrochloride, tacrolimus monohydrate, terbinafine, tramadol hydrochloride and valsartan in SyrSpend SF PH4 oral suspensions. *Pharmazie.* 2016;71:185–191.
4. Abernathy DR, Greenblatt DJ, Divoll M, et al. Enhanced glucuronide conjugation of drugs in obesity: studies of lorazepam, oxazepam, and acetaminophen. *J Lab Clin Med.* 1983;101:873–880.

Lorcaserin Hydrochloride

Product Availability

Solid	• Tablet:
	   ○ Immediate-release: 10 mg (salt) (Belviq® [Eisai])
	   ○ Sustained-release: 20 mg (salt) (Belviq® XR [Eisai])

Physicochemical (drug)

Molecular weight: • 195.69 (salt 232.15)	Permeability: • LogP 3.0 • LogD n/a	Water solubility: • 400 mg/mL
pKa: • 10.1	Classification: • BCS Class 1; BDDCS Class n/a	

Pharmaceutical (product)

Solid	• Immediate-release tablets are film-coated. • Do not crush the sustained-release product.

Pharmacokinetic (patient)

Absorption	• Specific site not known; t_{max} ~1.5–2 hours after an oral dose • Bioavailability n/a
Transport	• Plasma protein binding ~70% • V_d ~280 liters
Metabolism	• Extensive hepatic metabolism to several inactive metabolites via several CYP isoenzymes and UGTs, with most eliminated renally • Cl ~19 L/h

Enteral Administration and Nutrition Considerations

Compatibility, Stability, and Bioavailability Considerations
- No data are available.

Drug-Nutrition Interactions
- Drug may influence nutrition status directly or indirectly:
  - Weight loss
  - CNS: agitation and other mental status disturbances (as part of serotonin syndrome or an NMS-like reaction), confusion, fatigue
  - GI: dry mouth, nausea, vomiting, diarrhea, constipation
- No data on the influence of malnutrition or obesity on drug disposition.
- Influence of food on oral absorption or bioavailability:
  - A high-fat meal may have increased bioavailability by ~17% in a single-dose study of the sustained-release tablet, but no food effect is observed at steady state.

Recommendations

Gastric	• Avoid administration via an enteral access device. • No need to hold EN beyond the time required to flush-administer-flush.
Postpyloric	• As above. • Monitor for any unexpected change in effect.

Losartan Potassium

Product Availability

Solid	• Tablet: 25 mg, 50 mg, 100 mg (Cozaar® [Merck]; others)

Physicochemical (drug)

Molecular weight: • 422.92	Permeability: • LogP 4.10 (calc) • LogD 3.84 (pH 6.5) 3.85 (pH 7.4)	Water solubility: • 336 mg/mL
pKa: • 3.15	Classification: • BCS Class 2 or 3; BDDCS Class 2	

Pharmaceutical (product)

Solid	• Tablet products are film-coated. • Tablet disperses in water after crushing.

Pharmacokinetic (patient)

Absorption	• Specific site not known; t_{max} ~1 hour after an oral dose • Bioavailability ~33%
Transport	• Substrate for P-glycoprotein efflux • Plasma protein binding ~98% • V_d ~34 liters (parent), ~12 liters (active metabolite)
Metabolism	• This prodrug is activated to a carboxylic acid (via CYP2C9) and also metabolized via CYP3A4 to inactive(s) • Cl ~600 mL/min

Enteral Administration and Nutrition Considerations

Compatibility, Stability, and Bioavailability Considerations

- An extemporaneously compounded oral liquid (2.5 mg/mL) has a pH of 4.71.
- An oral liquid (2.5 mg/mL) prepared from tablets (50 mg) in purified water with OraSweet/OraPlus (1:1) and stored in amber polyethylene terephthalate bottles at 2°C–8°C can be stored for up to 4 weeks, although stability was not reported; osmolality and viscosity of the preparation were not reported.[1]
- According to the manufacturer, the above extemporaneous suspension yields similar bioavailability to the tablet with oral administration.
- Based on animal data, P-glycoprotein may be influenced by circadian rhythm, which could affect bioavailability.[2]

Drug-Nutrition Interactions

- Drug may influence nutrition status directly or indirectly:
  - CNS: dizziness
  - GI: gastritis, diarrhea

- ○ Metabolic: hyperkalemia, hypoglycemia, anemia
- ○ Other: pain (back, legs), muscle cramps
- No data on the influence of malnutrition or obesity on drug disposition.
- Influence of food on oral absorption or bioavailability:
  - ○ Although food may decrease the rate of oral absorption, oral bioavailability is not altered.

Recommendations

Gastric	• If there is no therapeutic alternative (eg, irbesartan), crush and disperse the tablet in water prior to administration. • No need to hold EN beyond the time required to flush-administer-flush.
Postpyloric	• As above. • Monitor for any unexpected change in effect.

References

1. Allen LV. Losartan potassium 2.5 mg/mL oral liquid. *Int J Pharm Compd.* 2007;11:248.
2. Okyar A, Dressler C, Hanafy A, et al. Circadian variations in exsorptive transport: in situ intestinal perfusion data and in vivo relevance. *Chronobiol Int.* 2012;29:443–453.

Lovastatin

Product Availability

Solid	• Tablet:
	o Immediate-release: 10 mg, 20 mg, 40 mg (various)
	o Extended-release: 20 mg, 40 mg, 60 mg (Altoprev® [Covis Pharma])

Physicochemical (drug)

Molecular weight: • 404.55	Permeability: • LogP 4.26 • LogD 4.26 (pH 7.4)	Water solubility: • <0.001 mg/mL (25°C)
pKa: • 13.5	Classification: • BCS Class 2; BDDCS Class 2	

Pharmaceutical (product)

Solid	• Tablets may be film-coated.
	• Do not crush the extended-release product.

Pharmacokinetic (patient)

Absorption	• Specific site not known; t_{max} ~2–3 hours after an oral dose (immediate-release) • Bioavailability <10% (immediate-release)
Transport	• Substrate for P-glycoprotein efflux (as is the active metabolite) • Plasma protein binding ≥90%, mostly to albumin • V_d n/a
Metabolism	• This prodrug requires hydrolysis to the active mevinolinic acid. • Requires intestinal epithelial CYP3A activity, with most excreted in bile • Cl n/a

Enteral Administration and Nutrition Considerations

Compatibility, Stability, and Bioavailability Considerations
- The drug in immediate-release tablet is sensitive to light.
- Several techniques have been attempted commercially to improve solubility, dissolution, and bioavailability:
  - o Preparation of a nanostructured lipid carrier remained stable (no aggregation, precipitation, or phase separation) for 6 months at refrigeration and allowed for increased oral bioavailability in an animal model.[1]
  - o Nanocrystals improve dissolution and bioavailability in an animal model, with the additional differences based on the shape of the crystal (rod better than sphere).[2]

Drug-Nutrition Interactions
- Drug may influence nutrition status directly or indirectly:
  - CNS: headache, fatigue
  - GI: anorexia, stomatitis, taste disturbance, nausea, vomiting, dyspepsia, abdominal pain, diarrhea, elevated transaminases (may be >3 times upper normal), rare hepatitis and pancreatitis
  - Metabolic: elevated HbA1c
  - Other: myalgia, elevated creatine kinase, or severe myopathy
- No data on the influence of malnutrition or obesity on drug disposition.
- Influence of food on oral absorption or bioavailability:
  - Food improves oral bioavailability.
  - Grapefruit juice may increase oral bioavailability.[3]

Recommendations

Gastric	• Crush and disperse immediate-release tablet in water just prior to administration. • No need to hold EN beyond the time required to flush-administer-flush.
Postpyloric	• As above. • Monitor for any unexpected change in effect.

References

1. Zhou J, Zhou D. Improvement of oral bioavailability of lovastatin by using nanostructured lipid carriers. *Drug Design Dev Ther.* 2015;9:5269–5275.
2. Guo M, Fu Q, Wu C, et al. Rod shaped nanocrystals exhibit superior in vitro dissolution and in vivo bioavailability over spherical like nanocrystals: a case study of lovastatin. *Colloids Surf B Biointerf.* 2015;128:410–418.
3. Kantola T, Kivisto KT, Neuvonen PJ. Grapefruit juice increases serum concentrations of lovastatin and lovastatin acid. *Clin Pharmacol Ther.* 1998;63:397–402.

Meclizine Hydrochloride

Product Availability

Solid	• Tablet: 12.5 mg, 25 mg, 50 mg (various)

Physicochemical (drug)

Molecular weight:	Permeability:	Water solubility:
• 390.96 (salt 481.89)	• LogP 5.8	• 1 mg/mL
	• Log D n/a	
pKa:	**Classification:**	
• 8.2	• BCS Class n/a; BDDCS Class 1	

Pharmaceutical (product)

Solid	• Tablets may be film-coated.

Pharmacokinetic (patient)

Absorption	• Specific site not known; t_{max} ~1 hour after an oral dose
	• Bioavailability n/a
Transport	• Plasma protein binding n/a
	• V_d ~6.5 L/kg
Metabolism	• Metabolized in large part by CYP2D6 with excretion in feces and urine
	• Cl ~140 mL/h/kg (will vary with CYP2D6 metabolizer phenotype)

Enteral Administration and Nutrition Considerations

Compatibility, Stability, and Bioavailability Considerations
- The immediate-release tablet is sensitive to light.
- A suspension formulation resulted in faster absorption than the tablet in healthy volunteers with no significant difference in oral bioavailability.[1]
- An orally disintegrating formulation under development exhibited more rapid dissolution (1.4-fold) than conventional tablets.[2]

Drug-Nutrition Interactions
- Drug may influence nutrition status directly or indirectly:
  - CNS: drowsiness, fatigue, blurred vision
  - GI: dry mouth
- No data on the influence of malnutrition or obesity on drug disposition.
- No known influence of food on oral absorption or bioavailability.

Recommendations

Gastric	• Crush and/or disperse tablet in water just prior to administration. • No need to hold EN beyond the time required to flush-administer-flush.
Postpyloric	• As above. • Monitor for any unexpected change in effect.

References

1. Wang Z, Lee B, Pearce D, et al. Meclizine metabolism and pharmacokinetics: formulation on its absorption. *J Clin Pharmacol.* 2012;52:1343–1349.
2. Vemula SK, Vangala M. Formulation development and characterization of meclizine hydrochloride sublimated fast dissolving tablets. *Inter Sch Res Notices.* 2014;2014:281376. doi: 10.1155/2014/281376.

Meloxicam

Product Availability

Solid	• Tablet: 7.5 mg, 15 mg (Mobic® [Boehringer-Ingelheim]; others) • Capsule: 5 mg, 10 mg (Vivlodex® [Iroko Pharms])
Liquid	• Oral suspension: discontinued

Physicochemical (drug)

Molecular weight: • 351.41	Permeability: • LogP 3.02 • LogD 0.10 (pH 7.4)	Water solubility: • 0.012 mg/mL
pKa: • 4.08	Classification: • BCS Class 2; BDDCS Class 2	

Pharmaceutical (product)

Solid	• Tablets may be film-coated.

Pharmacokinetic (patient)

Absorption	• Specific site not known; t_{max} ~6 hours after an oral dose • Bioavailability ~89%
Transport	• Plasma protein binding ~99%, mostly to albumin • V_d ~10 liters
Metabolism	• Extensively metabolized, via CYP2C9 more so than CYP3A4, with enterohepatic recirculation • Cl ~9 mL/min

Enteral Administration and Nutrition Considerations

Compatibility, Stability, and Bioavailability Considerations
- Extemporaneously compounded oral suspensions (0.25 mg/mL, 0.5 mg/mL, 1 mg/mL) prepared in deionized water and stored in amber glass bottles remained stable (HPLC analysis) for 28 days whether stored at 3°C–5°C or 20°C–24°C.[1]
- In a single-dose (15 mg) crossover study, a suspension formulation exhibited bioequivalence with the tablet formulation under fasting conditions in healthy male volunteers.[2]
- Nanosuspension formulations under development revealed significantly enhanced dissolution compared with simple drug.[3]
- A nanocrystal formulation in development displayed enhanced dissolution and increased bioavailability (5-fold) in an animal model.[4]
- Amorphous solid dispersion formulations under study identified one that maintained physicochemical properties (without recrystallization) and exhibited improved dissolution and increased oral bioavailability (2.4-fold) compared with the conventional crystalline product in an animal model.[5]

- Drug formulations in development using self-emulsifying delivery systems revealed better dissolution than powdered drug or commercial tablets and exhibited increased bioavailability (1.3-fold) in an animal model.[6]

Drug-Nutrition Interactions
- Drug may influence nutrition status directly or indirectly:
  - CNS: dizziness, headache, nervousness, fatigue, confusion, amblyopia
  - GI: stomatitis, anorexia, nausea, vomiting, dyspepsia, epigastric pain, ulceration, bleeding, bloating, constipation or diarrhea, LFT elevations including rare jaundice or hepatitis
  - Metabolic: peripheral edema, azotemia, hyperkalemia (associated with renal impairment)
- No data on the influence of malnutrition or obesity on drug disposition.
- No known influence of food on oral absorption or bioavailability.

Recommendations

Gastric	• In the absence of a therapeutic alternative, consider preparing a suspension with known stability prior to administration. • No need to hold EN beyond the time required to flush-administer-flush.
Postpyloric	• As above. • Monitor for any unexpected change in effect.

References

1. Hawkins MG, Karriker MJ, Wiebe V, et al. Drug distribution and stability in extemporaneous preparations of meloxicam and carprofen after dilution and suspension at two storage temperatures. *J Am Vet Med Assoc.* 2006;229:968–974.
2. Helmy SA, El Bedaiwy HM. Effect of the formulation on the bioequivalence of meloxicam: tablet and suspension. *Drug Res.* 2013;63:331–337.
3. Ambrus R, Kocbek P, Kristl J, et al. Investigation of preparation parameters to improve the dissolution of poorly water-soluble meloxicam. *Int J Pharm.* 2009;381:153–159.
4. Ochi M, Kawachi T, Toita E, et al. Development of nanocrystal formulation of meloxicam with improved dissolution and pharmacokinetic behaviors. *Int J Pharm.* 2014;474: 151–156.
5. Ochi M, Kimura K, Kanda A, et al. Physicochemical and pharmacokinetic characterization of amorphous solid dispersion of meloxicam with enhanced dissolution property and storage stability. *AAPS PharmSciTech.* 2016;17:932–939.
6. Agarwal V, Alayoubi A, Siddiqui A, Nazzal S. Powdered self-emulsified lipid formulations of meloxicam as solid dosage forms for oral administration. *Drug Dev Ind Pharm.* 2013; 39:1681–1689.

Memantine Hydrochloride

Product Availability

Solid	• Tablet: 5 mg, 10 mg (Namenda® [Forest Labs]; others) • Capsule: Extended-release: 7 mg, 14 mg, 21 mg, 28 mg (Namenda® XR [Forest Labs])
Liquid	• Oral solution: 10 mg/5 mL (Namenda® [Forest Labs]; others)

Physicochemical (drug)

Molecular weight: • 179.31 (salt 215.77)	Permeability: • LogP 3.28 • LogD n/a	Water solubility: • 35 mg/mL
pKa: • 10.3	Classification: • BCS Class n/a; BDDCS Class 3	

Pharmaceutical (product)

Solid	• Tablets may be film-coated. • Do not crush extended-release product

Liquid	• Oral solution:
	   o pH 3.5–4.5
	   o Osmolality n/a
	   o Viscosity n/a
	   o Do not mix with any other liquid.
	   o May contain sorbitol (500 mg/5 mL) and propylene glycol
	   o Store at controlled room temperature.

Pharmacokinetic (patient)

Absorption	• Specific site not known; t_{max} ~3–8 hours after an oral dose (immediate-release) • Bioavailability ~40%–50% • Tablet and oral solution considered bioequivalent.
Transport	• Plasma protein binding ~45% • V_d ~9–11 L/kg
Metabolism	• More than half of an administered dose is eliminated unchanged along with metabolites in the urine. • Cl ~7 L/h/kg

Enteral Administration and Nutrition Considerations

Compatibility, Stability, and Bioavailability Considerations
- An aqueous solution has a pH of 3.5–4.5.
- An extemporaneously compounded formulation (0.166 mg/mL) prepared from crushed tablets in deionized water and packaged in glass prescription bottles experienced minimal drug loss (GC-MS analysis) over 28 days when stored at 2°C, but it was not stable at room temperature (25°C).[1]

- Incorporating memantine with lipoic acid in a solid lipid nanoparticle formulation under study revealed in vitro stability under simulated GI fluid conditions that may improve drug delivery.[2]

Drug-Nutrition Interactions

- Drug may influence nutrition status directly or indirectly:
  - CNS: dizziness, confusion, headache, fatigue
  - GI: vomiting, constipation
  - Other: pain (including back pain)
- No data on the influence of malnutrition or obesity on drug disposition.
- No known influence of food on oral absorption or bioavailability.

Recommendations

Gastric	• Crush and disperse tablet in water prior to administration. • No need to hold EN beyond the time required to flush-administer-flush.
Postpyloric	• As above. • Monitor for any unexpected change in effect.

References

1. Yamreudeewong W, Teixeira MG, Mayer GE. Stability of memantine in an extemporaneously prepared oral liquid. *Int J Pharm Compd.* 2006;10:316–317.
2. Laserra S, Basit A, Sozio P, et al. Solid lipid nanoparticles loaded with lipoyl-memantine codrug: preparation and characterization. *Int J Pharm.* 2015;485:183–191.

Metformin Hydrochloride

Product Availability

Solid	• Tablet:
	  ○ Immediate-release: 500 mg, 850 mg, 1000 mg (Glucophage® [Bristol Myers Squibb]; others)
	  ○ Extended-release: 500 mg, 750 mg, 1000 mg (Glucophage® XR [Bristol Myers Squibb]; others)

Liquid	• Oral solution: 500 mg/5 mL (Riomet® [Sun Pharm])

Physicochemical (drug)

Molecular weight: • 129.17 (salt 165.63)	Permeability: • LogP –1.43 • Log D –5.41 (pH 7.4)	Water solubility: • 500 mg/mL
pKa: • 12.4	Classification: • BCS Class 3; BDDCS Class 3	

Pharmaceutical (product)

Solid	• Tablets may be film-coated and do not disperse in water, but they may disperse after crushing. • Do not crush extended-release product. • Depending on the manufacturer, the extended-release tablet matrix may appear intact in stool following oral administration.

Liquid	• Oral solution:
	  ○ pH 6.68 (a 1% aqueous solution)
	  ○ Osmolality n/a
	  ○ Viscosity n/a
	  ○ May contain xylitol; cherry-flavored
	  ○ Store at controlled room temperature.

Pharmacokinetic (patient)

Absorption	• Specific site not known, but the effective permeability at the proximal and distal small bowel is similar; t_{max} ~2.5 hours after an oral dose (immediate-release, in fasted state) • Absorption is saturable, slow, and incomplete. • Bioavailability ~50%–60%
Transport	• Widely distributed, concentrating in GI tissues • Substrate for organic cation transporter (OCT3) uptake • Limited plasma protein-binding, but some (~5%) binding to RBCs • V_d ~654 liters
Metabolism	• Does not undergo significant metabolism, with unchanged drug eliminated renally (glomerular filtration, proximal tubular secretion) • Cl ~700–1500 mL/min

Enteral Administration and Nutrition Considerations

Compatibility, Stability, and Bioavailability Considerations

- An extemporaneously compounded aqueous preparation (100 mg/mL) in a complex vehicle can be given a 6-month BUD when stored at controlled room temperature, although stability and osmolality were not reported.[1]
- Microemulsion formulations under study improved bioavailability even with dilution prior to administration.[2]
- Oral bioavailability was increased several months following gastric bypass compared to controls.[3]

Drug-Nutrition Interactions

- Drug may influence nutrition status directly or indirectly:
  - Potential for decreasing thiamin absorption and vitamin B_{12} concentrations; although these effects may not be clinically significant, consider monitoring during long-term therapy.
  - Weight loss or stabilization
  - CNS: headache, agitation
  - GI: taste disturbance, nausea, vomiting, abdominal bloating, cramping, diarrhea
  - Metabolic: hypoglycemia, rare lactic acidosis
  - Other: musculoskeletal pain
- No data on the influence of malnutrition or obesity on drug disposition.
- Influence of food on oral absorption or bioavailability:
  - Food may reduce oral bioavailability of immediate-release tablet by ~10%–20%, but taking drug with or after food reduces adverse GI effects.
  - Food may increase oral bioavailability of the oral solution by ~20%.

Recommendations

Gastric	• Crush and disperse immediate-release tablet in water prior to administration. • Alternative: Dilute oral solution in water prior to administration. • Administer consistently with respect to EN; no need to hold EN beyond the time required to flush-administer-flush.
Postpyloric	• As above. • Monitor for any unexpected change in effect.

References

1. Allen LV. Metformin hydrochloride 100-mg/mL oral liquid. *Int J Pharm Compd.* 2007;11:155.
2. Li Y, Song J, Tian N, et al. Improving bioavailability of metformin hydrochloride using water-in-oil microemulsions and analysis of phase behavior after dilution. *Int J Pharm.* 2014;473:316–325.
3. Padwal RS, Gabr RQ, Sharma AM, et al. Effect of gastric bypass surgery on the absorption and bioavailability of metformin. *Diabetes Care.* 2011;34:1295–1300.

Methadone Hydrochloride

Product Availability

Solid	• Tablet:
	○ Immediate-release: 5 mg, 10 mg (various)
	○ Dispersible: 40 mg (various)
Liquid	• Oral solution:
	○ Standard: 5 mg/5 mL, 10 mg/5 mL (various)
	○ Concentrated: 10 mg/mL (various)

Physicochemical (drug)

Molecular weight:	Permeability:	Water solubility:
• 309.46 (salt 345.91)	• LogP 3.93	• 120 mg/mL
	• LogD 2.07 (pH 7.4)	
pKa:	**Classification:**	
• 8.25	• BCS Class n/a; BDDCS Class 1	

Pharmaceutical (product)

Solid	• Tablets may disperse in water (20 mL) within 5 minutes.
	• Dispersible tablet intended for oral suspension, with the 40 mg dispersed in 120 mL water at room temperature within 1 minute.
Liquid	• Oral solution:
	○ pH:
	■ 1% aqueous solution 4.5–6.5
	■ standard 1.0–4.0
	■ concentrated 1.0–6.0
	○ Osmolality n/a
	○ Viscosity n/a
	○ Oral concentrate solution is intended to be diluted in 30 mL water before administration.
	○ May contain propylene glycol and sucrose; unflavored or cherry-flavored
	○ Store at controlled room temperature.

Pharmacokinetic (patient)

Absorption	• Specific site not known; t_{max} ~1–5 hours after an oral dose
	• Bioavailability varies widely: ~36%–100% (average ~80%)
Transport	• Substrate for P-glycoprotein efflux
	• Plasma protein binding ~85%–90%
	• V_d ~3.6 L/kg
Metabolism	• Extensively metabolized to inactive metabolites via CYP3A4, CYP2B6, CYP2C19, and possibly also CYP2C9 and CYP2D6, with drug and metabolites excreted primarily in feces
	• Cl ~3.2–8.5 L/h

Enteral Administration and Nutrition Considerations

Compatibility, Stability, and Bioavailability Considerations
- Solutions of methadone are most stable at low pH.[1]
- Drug preparations have been administered through an enteral access device.[2]
- Methadone is compatible when diluted (0.2, 0.8, 1, 1.5, 5 mg/mL) in deionized water or several beverages intended for oral administration without significant drug loss (HPLC analysis) by 8 days when refrigerated.[3-6]
- Methadone solutions prepared as above supports bacterial growth if kept at room temperature, even though they include a preservative (Na-benzoate).[5]
- Drug was inadequately absorbed in a patient with multiple small bowel enterocutaneous fistulas.[7]
- To reduce the risk for illicit parenteral administration, a tablet formulation under study has exhibited significantly reduced drug solubility but still maintains pharmacokinetic properties, including oral bioavailability.[8]

Drug-Nutrition Interactions
- Drug may influence nutrition status directly or indirectly:
  - CNS: sedation, confusion
  - GI: constipation
- No data on the influence of malnutrition or obesity on drug disposition.
- Influence of food on oral absorption or bioavailability:
  - Grapefruit juice may increase oral bioavailability.[9]

Recommendations

Gastric	• Dilute an oral solution as needed prior to administration. • No need to hold EN beyond the time required to flush-administer-flush.
Postpyloric	• As above. • Monitor for any unexpected change in effect.

References

1. Bamio-Nuez A, Artalejo-Orgega B, Fauli Trillo C, et al. Influence of pH on the stability of methadone hydrochloride in oral solutions. *Farm Clin.* 1989;6:618–622.
2. de Conno F, Groff L, Brunelli C, et al. Clinical experience with oral methadone administration in the treatment of pain in 196 advanced cancer patients. *J Clin Oncol.* 1996;14:2836–2842.
3. Sochasky C, Johannesson B, Isaacs E, et al. Methadone stability in lemonade. *Can J Hosp Pharm.* 1987;40:188.
4. Allen LV, Stiles ML. Methadone lemonade. *US Pharmacist.* 1988;13:86–88.
5. Lauriault G, LeBelle MJ, Lodge BA, et al. Stability of methadone in four vehicles for oral administration. *Am J Hosp Pharm.* 1991;48:1252–1256.
6. Donnelly R. Chemical stability of methadone concentrate and powder diluted in orange-flavored drink. *Int J Pharm Compd.* 2004;8:489–491.

7. Viswesh VV. Unpredictable absorption of oral opioid medications in a quadriplegic patient with chronic enterocutaneous fistulas. *J Pain Palliat Care Pharmacother.* 2012;26: 254–256.
8. Vinson RK. Pharmacokinetics of a new immediate-release methadone tablet formulation with decreased in vitro solubility. *Clin Drug Investig.* 2012;32:487–495.
9. Benmebarek M, Devaud C, Gex-Fabry M, et al. Effects of grapefruit juice on the pharmacokinetics of the enantiomers of methadone. *Clin Pharmacol Ther.* 2004;76: 55–63.

Methocarbamol

Product Availability

Solid	• Tablet: 500 mg, 750 mg (various)

Physicochemical (drug)

Molecular weight:	Permeability:	Water solubility:
• 241.24	• LogP 0.61	• 25 mg/mL (20°C)
	• LogD n/a	
pKa:	**Classification:**	
• 13	• BCS Class n/a; BDDCS Class n/a	

Pharmaceutical (product)

Solid	• Some products are film-coated.

Pharmacokinetic (patient)

Absorption	• Specific site not known; t_{max} ~1–2 hours after an oral dose
	• Bioavailability ~70%–83%
Transport	• Widely distributed
	• Plasma protein binding ~46%–50%
	• V_d at least 1 L/kg
Metabolism	• Extensively metabolized (dealkylation, hydroxylation, and conjugation) and rapidly excreted in urine
	• Cl ~0.2–0.8 L/h/kg

Enteral Administration and Nutrition Considerations

Compatibility, Stability, and Bioavailability Considerations
• No data are available.

Drug-Nutrition Interactions
• Drug may influence nutrition status directly or indirectly:
  o CNS: headache, drowsiness, dizziness, blurred vision
  o GI: anorexia, metallic taste
• No data on the influence of malnutrition or obesity on drug disposition.
• No known influence of food on oral absorption or bioavailability.

Recommendations

Gastric	• Crush and/or disperse non-film-coated tablet in water prior to administration.
	• No need to hold EN beyond the time required to flush-administer-flush.
Postpyloric	• As above.
	• Monitor for any unexpected change in effect.

Methotrexate Sodium

Product Availability

Solid	• Tablet: 2.5 mg, 5 mg, 7.5 mg, 10 mg, 15 mg (base) (various)
Liquid	• Oral solution: 2.5 mg/mL (base) (various)

Physicochemical (drug)

Molecular weight: • 454.45 (salt 498.41)	Permeability: • LogP −1.85 • LogD −2.52 (pH 7.4)	Water solubility: • 0.45 mg/mL
pKa: • 4.7	Classification: • BCS Class 3; BDDCS Class 3	

Pharmaceutical (product)

Solid	• Some brands may be film-coated. • The tablet may disperse in water. • Do not crush (cytotoxicity).

Liquid	• Oral solution:
	     o pH n/a
	     o Osmolality n/a
	     o Viscosity n/a
	     o May contain sucralose
	     o Refrigerate or store at controlled room temperature for up to 60 days.

Pharmacokinetic (patient)

Absorption	• Specific site not known; t_{max} ~1–5 hours after an oral dose • Variable and saturable absorption • Bioavailability <50%
Transport	• Substrate for P-glycoprotein, MRP2, and BCRP efflux • Substrate for proton-coupled folate transporter uptake and OATP uptake • Plasma protein binding ~50%, mostly to albumin • V_d ~0.4–0.8 L/kg
Metabolism	• Can form polyglutamates (active) that can be hydrolyzed back to the parent drug or hydroxylated and excreted primarily in the urine. • Enterohepatic recirculation is also possible. • Cl ~2.1 mL/min/kg

Enteral Administration and Nutrition Considerations

Compatibility, Stability, and Bioavailability Considerations
- The drug is not stable at pH <6.6.
- An extemporaneously compounded oral formulation (2 mg/mL) prepared from the injectable product (25 mg/mL) with sodium bicarbonate, OraSweet, and sterile water, stored in amber glass bottles at 4°C or 25°C (relative humidity <60%), was stable for up to 120 days.[1]
- An improvement in oral bioavailability (1.28-fold) can be achieved by splitting the single dose into two doses, 8 hours apart, as reported in patients with rheumatoid arthritis receiving 25–30 mg doses.[2]
- At 1 year following bariatric surgery (gastric bypass), oral bioavailability decreased significantly (66%) compared to preoperative values.[3]

Drug-Nutrition Interactions
- Drug may influence nutrition status directly or indirectly:
  o CNS: headache, drowsiness, fatigue, visual disturbances
  o GI: stomatitis, glossitis, gingivitis, pharyngitis, anorexia, nausea, vomiting, abdominal distress, GI bleed, diarrhea, pancreatitis, transaminase elevations, rare hepatotoxicity
  o Metabolic: azotemia, uric acidemia, hypogammaglobulinemia, osteoporosis
  o Other: arthralgia, myalgia
- Influence of malnutrition or obesity on drug disposition:
  o The elimination half-life is prolonged in undernourished patients, likely due to reduced clearance rather than altered volume of distribution.[4]
- Influence of food on oral absorption or bioavailability:
  o Food may delay the absorption but without significant influence on oral bioavailability.
  o Administration of folate or its analogues reduced drug absorption early in the small bowel.[5]

Recommendations

Gastric	• Disperse tablet in a closed syringe prior to administration. • Discard enteral syringe as cytotoxic waste. • No need to hold EN beyond the time required to flush-administer-flush.
Postpyloric	• As above. • Monitor for any unexpected change in effect.

References
1. Vrignaud S, Briot T, Launay A, et al. Design and stability study of paediatric oral solution of methotrexate 2 mg/mL. *Int J Pharm*. 2015;487:270–273.

2. Hoekstra M, Haagsma C, Neef C, et al. Splitting high-dose oral methotrexate improves bioavailability: a pharmacokinetic study in patients with rheumatoid arthritis. *J Rheumatol.* 2006;33:481–485.
3. Aron-Wisnewsky J, Lemaitre F, Clement K, et al. Pharmacokinetics of immunomodulatory treatments after Roux-en-Y bypass in obese patients. *J Clin Pharmacol.* 2013;53:779–784.
4. Rajeswari R, Shetty PA, Gothoskar BP, Akolkar PN, Gokhale SV. Pharmacokinetics of methotrexate in adult Indian patients and its relationship to nutritional status. *Cancer Treat Rep.* 1984;68:727–732.
5. Yokooji T, Mori N, Murakami T. Site-specific contribution of proton-couple folate transporter/haem carrier protein 1 in the intestinal absorption of methotrexate in rats. *J Pharm Pharmacol.* 2009;61:911–918.

Methylphenidate Hydrochloride

Product Availability

Solid	• Tablet:
	  ○ Immediate-release: 5 mg, 10 mg, 20 mg (Ritalin® [Novartis]; others)
	  ○ Chewable: 2.5 mg, 5 mg, 10 mg (various)
	  ○ Orally disintegrating: 8.6 mg, 17.3 mg, 25.9 mg (Cotempla® XR-ODT [Neos])
	  ○ Extended-release: 10 mg, 20 mg (various)
	  ○ Extended-release: 18 mg, 27 mg, 36 mg, 54 mg (Concerta® [Janssen]; others)
	• Capsule: Extended-release: 10 mg, 15 mg, 20 mg, 30 mg, 40 mg, 50 mg, 60 mg (Aptensio® XR [Rhodes]; others)

Liquid	• Oral solution: 5 mg/5 mL, 10 mg/5 mL (various)

Physicochemical (drug)

Molecular weight: • 233.31 (salt 269.77)	Permeability: • LogP 1.80 • LogD –0.28 (pH 7.4)	Water solubility: • 100 mg/mL
pKa: • 8.8	Classification: • BCS Class 4; BDDCS Class 1	

Pharmaceutical (product)

Solid	• Immediate-release tablet may disperse in water (20 mL) within 5 minutes. • Capsules contain varying proportions of immediate- and extended-release granules, depending on the manufacturer. • Some extended-release tablets also contain immediate-release granules. • Do not crush modified-release tablet or capsule. • The orally disintegrating tablet should not be crushed or chewed as it also contains extended-release granules.

Liquid	• Oral solution:
	  ○ pH n/a
	  ○ Osmolality n/a
	  ○ Viscosity n/a
	  ○ May contain glycerin and polyethylene glycol; grape-flavored
	  ○ Store at controlled room temperature.

Pharmacokinetic (patient)

Absorption	• Specific site not known; t_{max} ~1–2 hours after an oral dose (immediate-release) • Bioavailability ~30% (10%–52%)

Transport	• Plasma protein binding ~10%–33%
	• V_d varies by enantiomer: ~2.65 L/kg (D-), ~1.80 L/kg (L-)
Metabolism	• Substantial first-pass metabolism by carboxylesterases (1A1)
	• Cl varies by enantiomer: ~0.4 L/h/kg (D-), ~0.7 L/h/kg (L-)

Enteral Administration and Nutrition Considerations

Compatibility, Stability, and Bioavailability Considerations

- Aqueous solutions are expected to be most stable at pH 3–4; otherwise, the drug is subject to ester hydrolysis.[1]
- A manufacturer-recommended, extemporaneously compounded oral liquid prepared from tablets in a vehicle that includes 70% sorbitol can be provided a BUD of 28 days; however, no stability, viscosity, or osmolality data are available.[1]
- Although gastric banding did not influence the absorption of methylphenidate, gastric bypass may significantly alter bioavailability. Therapeutic efficacy of the immediate-release product was reduced within 2 weeks in a patient following gastric bypass, and changes in formulation and increased doses were of limited benefit, with the patient eventually requiring use of the transdermal product; another patient exhibited drug toxicity within 2 weeks of the bariatric surgery.[2,3]

Drug-Nutrition Interactions

- Drug may influence nutrition status directly or indirectly:
  - Weight loss
  - CNS: insomnia, restlessness, tremor
  - GI: dry mouth, decreased appetite, nausea, abdominal pain
- No data on the influence of malnutrition or obesity on drug disposition.
- Influence of food on oral absorption or bioavailability:
  - High-fat meals can increase oral bioavailability of immediate-release products by ~20%–25%, and extended-release orally disintegrating tablets by ~16%.
  - Extended-release products may not be bioequivalent when administered in the fed state.[4]

Recommendations

Gastric	• If there is no therapeutic alternative (eg, transdermal product), disperse immediate-release tablet in water prior to administration.
	• Alternative: Dilute oral solution prior to administration.
	• No need to hold EN beyond the time required to flush-administer-flush.
Postpyloric	• As above.
	• Monitor for any unexpected change in effect.

References

1. Woods DJ. *Formulation in Pharmacy Practice.* Dunedin, New Zealand: Health-Care Otago; 1993:1–104.
2. Ludvigsson M, Haenni A. Methylphenidate toxicity after Roux-en-Y gastric bypass. *Surg Obes Relat Dis.* 2016;12:e55–e57.
3. Azran C, Langguth P, Dahan A. Impaired oral absorption of methylphenidate after Roux-en-Y gastric bypass. *Surg Obes Relat Dis.* 2017;13:1245–1247.
4. Haessler F, Tracik F, Dietrich H, Stammer H, Klatt J. A pharmacokinetic study of two modified-release methylphenidate formulations under different food conditions in healthy volunteers. *Int J Clin Pharmacol Ther.* 2008;46:466–476.

Methylprednisolone

Product Availability

Solid	• Tablet: 2 mg, 4 mg, 8 mg, 16 mg, 32 mg (Medrol® [Pharmacia]; others)

Physicochemical (drug)

Molecular weight: • 374.48	Permeability: • LogP 1.50 • LogD 2.18 (pH 7.4)	Water solubility: • 0.12 mg/mL (20°C) • Salts used for injectable products are more soluble.
pKa: • 12.6	Classification: • BCS Class n/a; BDDCS Class 1	

Pharmaceutical (product)

Solid	• Some products may disperse in water (20 mL) in about 1 minute. • 4 mg methylprednisolone ≈ 5 mg prednisone

Pharmacokinetic (patient)

Absorption	• Specific site not known; t_{max} ~1.5–2.5 hours after an oral dose • Bioavailability ~82%
Transport	• Substrate for P-glycoprotein efflux • Plasma protein binding ~78% • V_d ~1.2 L/kg
Metabolism	• Metabolized by CYP3A • Cl ~6.2 mL/min/kg

Enteral Administration and Nutrition Considerations

Compatibility, Stability, and Bioavailability Considerations
- The sodium-succinate salt (used for the injectable product) undergoes ester hydrolysis the least at pH ~3.5, whereas acyl migration occurs especially at pH 3.4–7.4

Drug-Nutrition Interactions
- Drug may influence nutrition status directly or indirectly:
  ○ CNS: headache, dizziness, fatigue
  ○ GI: nausea, vomiting, dyspepsia, abdominal pain, diarrhea
  ○ Metabolic: glucose intolerance, reduced bone mineral density with long-term systemic use
  ○ Other: arthralgia, myalgia
- Influence of malnutrition or obesity on drug disposition:
  ○ Body weight–normalized volume of distribution is lower in obesity, as is total clearance, which suggests that dosing should be based on a lean body weight.[1]

- Influence of food on oral absorption or bioavailability:
  - Grapefruit juice may increase oral bioavailability.[2]

Recommendations

Gastric	• Disperse tablet in water just prior to administration.
	• No need to hold EN beyond the time required to flush-administer-flush.
Postpyloric	• As above.
	• Monitor for any unexpected change in effect

References

1. Dunn TE, Ludwig EA, Slaughter RL, et al. Pharmacokinetics and pharmacodynamics of methylprednisolone in obesity. *Clin Pharmacol Ther.* 1991;49:536–549.
2. Varis T, Kivisto KT, Neuvonen PJ. Grapefruit juice can increase the plasma concentrations of oral methylprednisolone. *Eur J Clin Pharmacol.* 2000;56:489–493.

Metoclopramide Hydrochloride

Product Availability

Solid	• Tablet:
	   ○ Immediate-release: 5 mg, 10 mg (base) (Reglan® [Ani Pharms]; others)
	   ○ Orally disintegrating: 5 mg, 10 mg (base) (Metozolv® ODT [Salix Pharms]; others)

Liquid	• Oral solution: 5 mg/5 mL (base) (various)

Physicochemical (drug)

Molecular weight: • 299.80 (salt 336.26)	Permeability: • LogP 2.62 • LogD 0.32 (pH 7.4)	Water solubility: • 1430 mg/mL
pKa: • 0.6, 9.4	Classification: • BCS Class 3; BDDCS Class 3	

Pharmaceutical (product)

Solid	• Tablets do not disperse easily in water, but they can be crushed. • Orally dissolving tablet may contain mannitol and acesulfame-K.

Liquid	Oral solution:
	• pH 2.0–5.5
	• Osmolality 8350 mOsm/kg
	   ○ Two brands were evaluated:[1]
	     ■ pH 2.74 and 5180 mOsm/kg (calculated based on measurement of 1:10 dilution with sterile water)
	     ■ pH 2.83 and 4660 mOsm/kg (calculated based on measurement of 1:10 dilution with sterile water)
	• Viscosity low
	• May contain saccharin and sorbitol
	• Maintain at controlled room temperature with limited exposure to light.

Pharmacokinetic (patient)

Absorption	• Specific site not known; t_{max} ~0.5–2 hours after an oral dose (immediate-release) • Bioavailability variable ~30%–100% (~75%)
Transport	• Plasma protein binding ~13%–30%, mostly to albumin • V_d 2.2–3.5 L/kg
Metabolism	• Undergoes glucuronic acid and sulfate conjugation with renal excretion • Cl ~11 mL/min/kg

Enteral Administration and Nutrition Considerations

Compatibility, Stability, and Bioavailability Considerations
- Metoclopramide hydrochloride is most stable in the pH range 2–9.
- The admixture of the oral solution (1:1) with EN formulas was visually compatible for TwoCal HN and Vivonex TEN, but it was incompatible (increased granular particle formation) with Enrich; there was no evaluation of the pH, viscosity, or osmolality changes of the formula or the stability of the drug.[2]
- Commercial solution combined (1:1) with Osmolite 1.2, under simulated clinical conditions, would clog an 8 Fr feeding tube and may clog a 20 Fr feeding tube, depending on the product.[1]

Drug-Nutrition Interactions
- Drug may influence nutrition status directly or indirectly:
  o CNS: restlessness, fatigue, headache, confusion, extrapyramidal reactions (eg, acute dystonic reactions)
  o GI: xerostomia, nausea, diarrhea
  o Metabolic: fluid retention
- No data on the influence of malnutrition or obesity on drug disposition.
- No known influence of food on oral absorption or bioavailability.

Recommendations

Gastric	• Crush and disperse tablet in water prior to administration.
	• Alternative: Dilute solution with water prior to administration.
	• No need to hold EN beyond the time required to flush-administer-flush.
Postpyloric	• Crush and disperse tablet in water prior to administration.
	• Monitor for any unexpected change in effect.

References

1. Klang M, McLymont V, Ng N. Osmolality, pH, and compatibility of selected oral liquid medications with an enteral nutrition product. *JPEN J Parenter Enteral Nutr.* 2013;37:689–694.
2. Burns PE, McCall L, Wirsching R. Physical compatibility of enteral formulas with various common medications. *J Am Diet Assoc.* 1988;88:1094–1096.

Metoprolol

Product Availability

Solid	• Tablet:
	  o Immediate-release (tartrate): 25 mg, 50 mg, 75 mg, 100 mg (salt) (various)
	  o Extended-release (succinate): 25 mg, 50 mg, 100 mg, 200 mg (salt) (Toprol® XL [Aralez Pharms]; others)

Physicochemical (drug)

Molecular weight: • 267.37	Permeability: • LogP 1.88 or 2.20 • LogD 0.16 (pH 7.4); −1.57 (pH 6.5, calc); −0.67 (pH 7.4, calc)	Water solubility (tartrate): • ≥1000 mg/mL (25°C)
pKa: • 9.68	Classification: • BCS Class 1; BDDCS Class 1	

Pharmaceutical (product)

Solid	• Immediate-release tablet does not disperse well in water without crushing first. • Do not crush the extended-release tablet.

Pharmacokinetic (patient)

Absorption	• Despite higher ileal permeability, 80% of oral dose is absorbed in the upper 50 cm of the small bowel;[1,2] t_{max} ~1.5 hours after an oral dose (immediate-release) • Bioavailability variable ~40%–50%
Transport	• Substrate for P-glycoprotein efflux • Plasma protein binding ~11%–12% to albumin • V_d ~4.2 L/kg
Metabolism	• Extensive first-pass metabolism via CYP2D6 (variable depending on metabolizer phenotype) to 3 major metabolites excreted renally • Cl ~50 L/h

Enteral Administration and Nutrition Considerations

Compatibility, Stability, and Bioavailability Considerations
- A 10% aqueous solution of metoprolol has a pH of 6–7.
- The official USP oral solution or oral suspension (10 mg/mL) using metoprolol tartrate powder will have a pH of 3.6–4.6 and can have a BUD of 60 days when stored in a tight, light-resistant bottle at room temperature or at refrigeration.

- An extemporaneously compounded oral suspension (10 mg/mL) prepared from tablets (100 mg) in 3 vehicles (OraSweet/OraPlus [1:1], OraSweet SF/OraPlus [1:1], or cherry syrup/simple syrup [1:4]) and stored in amber polyethylene terephthalate plastic bottles remained stable (HPLC analysis) at 60 days.[3]
- An aqueous preparation (5 mg/mL) made from tablets (50 mg) and stored in amber glass bottles remained stable (HPLC analysis) for 16 days at 25°C.[4]
- An oral suspension (10 mg/mL) prepared from tablets and additional components and stored in amber glass bottles resulted in minimal drug loss (HPLC analysis) in 28 days (21°C–25°C) and in 60 days (5°C–7°C).[5]
- Another oral liquid preparation (1.25 mg/mL) made from tablets diluted with deionized water and sorbitol, stored in amber polyethylene terephthalate plastic bottles at 4°C–8°C or 22°C–26°C, resulted in variable and inconclusive stability findings (HPLC analysis).[6]
- After taking both CYP2D6 metabolizer phenotype and age into consideration, the remaining variability of the drug's oral bioavailability may be related to a saturable absorption step.[7]
- Oral bioavailability of immediate-release drug was increased by approximately one-third in patients following gastric bypass compared with their preoperative values.[8]

Drug-Nutrition Interactions
- Drug may influence nutrition status directly or indirectly:
  - CNS: dizziness, insomnia, tiredness, depression
  - GI: gastric upset, nausea, abdominal pain, diarrhea
  - Metabolic: dysglycemia
  - Other: musculoskeletal pain
- Influence of malnutrition or obesity on drug disposition
  - Body weight–normalized volume of distribution and the total clearance are both higher in obesity.[9]
- Influence of food on oral absorption or bioavailability:
  - Food may increase the oral bioavailability of the tartrate salt.

Recommendations

Gastric	• If no therapeutic alternative is available, crush and disperse immediate-release tablet in water prior to administration. • Consider administration in close proximity to EN (ie, no need to hold EN beyond the time required to flush-administer-flush).
Postpyloric	• As above. • Monitor for any unexpected change in effect.

References

1. Zur M, Cohen N, Agbaria R, Dahan A. The biopharmaceutics of successful controlled release drug product: segmental-dependent permeability of glipizide vs metoprolol throughout the intestinal tract. *Int J Pharmaceut*. 2015;489:304–310.
2. Jobin G, Cortot A, Godbillon J, et al. Investigation of drug absorption from the gastrointestinal tract of man: metoprolol in the stomach, duodenum and jejunum. *Br J Clin Pharmacol*. 1985;19:97S–105S.
3. Allen LV, Erickson MA. Stability of labetalol hydrochloride, metoprolol tartrate, verapamil hydrochloride, and spironolactone with hydrochlorothiazide in extemporaneously compounded oral liquids. *Am J Health-Syst Pharm*. 1996;53:2304–2309.
4. Gupta VD, Maswoswe J. Quantitation of metoprolol tartrate and propranolol hydrochloride in pharmaceutical dosage forms: stability of metoprolol in aqueous mixture. *Int J Pharm Compd*. 1997;1:125–127.
5. Peterson GM, Meaney MF, Reid CA. Stability of extemporaneously prepared mixtures of metoprolol and spironolactone. *Aust J Hosp Pharm*. 1989;19:344–346.
6. Yamreudeewong W, Dolence EK, Pahl D. Stability of two extemporaneously prepared oral metoprolol and carvedilol liquids. *Hosp Pharm*. 2006;41:254–259.
7. Fukao M, Ishida K, Horie A, et al. Variability of bioavailability and intestinal absorption mechanisms of metoprolol. *Drug Metab Pharmacokinet*. 2014;29:162–167.
8. Gesquiere I, Darwich AS, Van der Schueren B, et al. Drug disposition and modelling before and after gastric bypass: immediate and controlled-release metoprolol formulations. *Br J Clin Pharmacol*. 2015;80:1021–1030.
9. Galletti F, Fasano ML, Ferrara LA, et al. Obesity and beta-blockers: influence of body fat on their kinetics and cardiovascular effects. *J Clin Pharmacol*. 1989;29:212–216.

Metronidazole

Product Availability

Solid	• Tablet:
	  ○ Immediate-release: 250 mg, 500 mg (various)
	  ○ Extended-release: 750 mg (Flagyl® ER [Searle]; others)
	• Capsule: 375 mg (Flagyl® [Searle]; others)

Physicochemical (drug)

Molecular weight: • 171.16	Permeability: • LogP –0.02 or 0.75 • LogD 0.14 (pH 7.4)	Water solubility: • 10 mg/mL (20°C)
pKa: • 2.6	Classification: • BCS Class 1; BDDCS Class 1	

Pharmaceutical (product)

Solid	• Some tablet products are film-coated; with exposure precautions, they could be crushed but would disperse poorly with fragments blocking syringe tip. • Non-film-coated tablet may disperse in water (20 mL) within 5 minutes. • Do not crush the extended-release tablet.

Pharmacokinetic (patient)

Absorption	• Absorbed in proximal intestine; t_{max} ~1–2 hours after an oral dose (immediate-release) • Bioavailability is variable (~80%–90%).
Transport	• Widely distributed • Plasma protein binding <20% • V_d ~0.51–1.1 L/kg
Metabolism	• About 30%–60% of a dose is metabolized (hydroxylation, side-chain oxidation, glucuronic acid conjugation) and excreted mainly in the urine. • Cl ~1.3 mL/min/kg

Enteral Administration and Nutrition Considerations

Compatibility, Stability, and Bioavailability Considerations
- A saturated aqueous solution would have a pH of 5.8.[1]
- Metronidazole should be protected from light to maintain stability.
- Drug decomposition is independent of pH between pH 3.9 and 6.6, with a maximum stability at pH 5.1–5.6; however, the rate increases with higher pH (especially pH >8).[2,3]
- The official USP oral suspension (50 mg/mL) prepared from metronidazole benzoate powder in OraBlend is expected to have a pH of 3.6–4.6 with a BUD of 90 days, stored at controlled room temperature.

- An oral liquid preparation (10 mg/mL) made from tablets diluted in water or syrup, stored in amber glass bottles at 25°C, underwent significant decomposition with 16%–37% loss (HPLC analysis) in 28 days.[4]
- The same preparation using bulk metronidazole powder (5 mg/mL) resulted in no drug loss after 60 days.[4]
- An extemporaneously compounded oral liquid (10 mg/mL) prepared from tablets in OraPlus or OraPlus/OraSweet (1:1) and stored in amber glass bottles at 25°C remained stable (HPLC analysis) for up to 90 days.[5]
- A more concentrated oral suspension (15 mg/mL) prepared from tablets in simple syrup and in chocolate syrup underwent accelerated decomposition at elevated temperature, providing an estimated stability (HPLC analysis) of ~4 days (25°C) or ~200 days (refrigerated), with subsequent bioavailability of 97% compared with intact tablets in a group of adult subjects.[6]
- Another oral suspension (15 mg/mL) using 2 suspending agents among other components in distilled water was estimated by accelerated decomposition at elevated temperature to remain stable (HPLC analysis) for at least 90 days at 25°C.[1]
- An oral suspension (50 mg/mL) prepared from powder and diluted in OraSweet/OraPlus (1:1), OraSweet SF/OraPlus (1:1), or cherry syrup/ simple syrup (1:4) and stored in clear polyethylene terephthalate plastic bottles at 5°C and 25°C remained stable (HPLC analysis) for 60 days.[7]
- An oral liquid formulation added to 200 mL of an EN product (Precitene, Novartis) exhibited no visible incompatibilities (no phase separation or evident particle growth) in 24 hours.[8]

Drug-Nutrition Interactions
- Drug may influence nutrition status directly or indirectly:
  - CNS: headache, vertigo, ataxia, confusion
  - GI: anorexia, dry mouth, metallic taste, glossitis, stomatitis, nausea, abdominal discomfort, diarrhea, rare pancreatitis
  - Other: peripheral neuropathy
- No data on the influence of malnutrition or obesity on drug disposition.
- Influence of food on oral absorption or bioavailability:
  - Food may delay absorption of immediate-release solids, without a change in oral bioavailability. However, food may reduce the bioavailability of a suspension.

Recommendations

Gastric	• If no therapeutic alternative is available, disperse non-film-coated immediate-release tablet in water prior to administration.
	• No need to hold EN beyond the time required to flush-administer-flush.
	• Consider administering within 60 minutes of an intermittent EN administration to reduce GI complaints.

Postpyloric	• Not recommended.
Other	• As with all antimicrobials, consider parenteral alternative for acutely ill patients to ensure therapeutic concentrations.

References

1. Alexander KS, Vangala SSKS, Dollimore D. The formulation development and stability of metronidazole suspension. *Int J Pharm Compd.* 1997;1:200–205.

2. Suresh P, Gupta BK. pH and stability of metronidazole benzoate suspensions. *J Instit Chem.* 1993;65:22–23.

3. Wang DP, Yeh MK. Degradation kinetics of metronidazole in solution. *J Pharm Sci.* 1993;82:95–98.

4. Mathew M, Das Gupta V, Bethea C. The development of oral liquid dosage forms of metronidazole. *J Clin Pharm Ther.* 1993;18:291–294.

5. Mathew M, Das Gupta V, Bethea C. Stability of metronidazole in solutions and suspensions. *J Clin Pharm Ther.* 1994;19:27–29.

6. Irwin DB, Dupuis LL, Prober CG, et al. The acceptability, stability and relative bioavailability of an extemporaneous metronidazole suspension. *Can J Hosp Pharm.* 1987;40:42–46.

7. Allen LV, Erickson MA. Stability of ketoconazole, metolazone, metronidazole, procainamide hydrochloride, and spironolactone in extemporaneously compounded oral liquids. *Am J Health-Syst Pharm.* 1996;53:2073–2078.

8. Ortega de la Cruz C, Fernandez Gallardo LC, Damas Fernandez-Figares M, et al. Physicochemical compatibility of drugs with enteral nutrition. *Nutr Hosp.* 1993;8: 105–108.

Minocycline Hydrochloride
Product Availability

Solid	• Tablet:
	    ○ Immediate-release: 50 mg, 75 mg, 100 mg (base) (various)
	    ○ Extended-release: 55 mg, 65 mg, 80 mg, 105 mg, 115 mg,
	       135 mg (base) (various)
	• Capsule:
	    ○ Immediate-release: 50 mg, 75 mg, 100 mg (base) (Dynacin®
	      [Medicis]; others)
	    ○ Pellet-containing: 50 mg, 100 mg (base) (Minocin® [Precision
	      Derm]; others)
	    ○ Extended-release: 45 mg, 90 mg, 135 mg (base) (Ximino®
	      [Sun Pharm])

Physicochemical (drug)

Molecular weight: • 457.49 (salt 493.94)	Permeability: • LogP 0.05 • LogD 0.04 (pH 7.4)	Water solubility: • 52 mg/mL (25°C)
pKa: • 8.3	Classification: • BCS Class n/a; BDDCS Class 1	

Pharmaceutical (product)

Solid	• Most immediate-release tablet products are film-coated to protect from risk of esophageal irritation/ulceration with oral administration. • Do not crush the extended-release tablet. • Do not crush extended-release capsule contents. • Do not open, chew, or crush contents of pellet-containing capsule.

Pharmacokinetic (patient)

Absorption	• Specific site not known; t_{max} ~1–3 hours after an oral dose (immediate-release, fasting) • Bioavailability ~90%–100% (fasting)
Transport	• Plasma protein binding ~55%–76% • V_d ~4.5 L/kg
Metabolism	• Partial metabolism to at least 6 metabolites with elimination in urine and feces • Cl ~9.1 mL/min/kg

Enteral Administration and Nutrition Considerations
Compatibility, Stability, and Bioavailability Considerations
- A 10 mg/mL aqueous solution would have a pH of 3.5–4.5.
- Minocycline can be hygroscopic, is subject to surface oxidation, and is light-sensitive.
- An extemporaneously compounded oral formulation (10 mg/mL) prepared from drug powder in SyrSpend SF PH4, stored in low-actinic, light-resistant bottles at 2°C–8°C or 20°C–25°C, remained stable (HPLC analysis) for 60 days.[1]

Drug-Nutrition Interactions
- Drug may influence nutrition status directly or indirectly:
  - CNS: vestibular reactions (dizziness, vertigo, ataxia, headache, fatigue)
  - GI: stomatitis, glossitis, nausea, vomiting, diarrhea
  - Metabolic: azotemia, hyperphosphatemia
- No data on the influence of malnutrition or obesity on drug disposition.
- Influence of food on oral absorption or bioavailability:
  - Although the influence is variable, food (and/or milk) can decrease oral bioavailability (by ~6%–27%)
  - Divalent (eg, calcium, magnesium) or trivalent (eg, aluminum, iron) cation–containing products may reduce oral bioavailability.

Recommendations

Gastric	• Disperse immediate-release capsule contents in water just prior to administration. • No need to hold EN beyond the time required to flush-administer-flush.
Postpyloric	• Not recommended.
Other	• As with all antimicrobials, consider parenteral alternative for acutely ill patients to ensure therapeutic concentrations.

Reference
1. Polonini HC, Silva SL, Cunha CN, et al. Compatibility of cholecalciferol, haloperidol, imipramine hydrochloride, levodopa/carbidopa, lorazepam, minocycline hydrochloride, tacrolimus monohydrate, terbinafine, tramadol hydrochloride and valsartan in SyrSpend SF PH4 oral suspensions. *Pharmazie.* 2016;71:185–191.

Mirtazapine

Product Availability

Solid	• Tablet:
	  ○ Immediate-release: 15 mg, 30 mg, 45 mg (Remeron® [Organon]; others)
	  ○ Orally disintegrating: 15 mg, 30 mg, 45 mg (Remeron® SolTab [Organon]; others)

Physicochemical (drug)

Molecular weight: • 265.36	Permeability: • LogP 2.9 • LogD n/a	Water solubility: • 0.5 mg/mL
pKa: • 6.6	Classification: • BCS Class 1; BDDCS Class 1	

Pharmaceutical (product)

Solid	• Immediate-release tablet products are film-coated. • Orally disintegrating tablet products may not disperse completely in water; may contain mannitol and aspartame.

Pharmacokinetic (patient)

Absorption	• Specific site not known; t_{max} ~2 hours after an oral dose • Bioavailability ~50%
Transport	• Plasma protein binding ~85% • V_d ~4.5 L/kg
Metabolism	• Metabolism by hydroxylation, demethylation, and glucuronic acid conjugation to at least 6 metabolites, with elimination in urine and feces • Cl ~9.1 mL/min/kg

Enteral Administration and Nutrition Considerations

Compatibility, Stability, and Bioavailability Considerations
• CYP2D6 metabolizer phenotype and sex each can influence oral bioavailability.[1]

Drug-Nutrition Interactions
• Drug may influence nutrition status directly or indirectly:
  ○ Increased appetite, weight gain
  ○ CNS: sedation, dizziness
  ○ GI: nausea, vomiting, diarrhea
  ○ Metabolic: hyponatremia, hypertriglyceridemia
• No data on the influence of malnutrition or obesity on drug disposition.
• No known influence of food on oral absorption or bioavailability.

Recommendations

Gastric	• Crush and/or disperse tablet in water just prior to administration. • No need to hold EN beyond the time required to flush-administer-flush.
Postpyloric	• Not recommended.

Reference

1. Borobia AM, Novalbos J, Guerra-López P, et al. Influence of sex and CYP2D6 genotype on mirtazapine disposition, evaluated in Spanish healthy volunteers. *Pharmacol Res.* 2009;59:393–398.

Montelukast Sodium

Product Availability

Solid	• Tablet:
	o Immediate-release: 10 mg (base) (Singulair® [Merck]; others)
	o Chewable: 4 mg, 5 mg (base) (Singulair® [Merck]; others)
	o Granules: 4 mg/packet (base) (Singulair® [Merck]; others)

Physicochemical (drug)

Molecular weight: • 568.20 (salt 608.17)	Permeability: • LogP 8.47 (calc) • LogD n/a	Water solubility: • 0.0005 mg/mL (25°C)
pKa: • 2.8, 5.7	Classification: • BCS Class 1; BDDCS Class 2	

Pharmaceutical (product)

Solid	• Immediate-release tablet products are often film-coated; they may disperse in water but may need to be crushed first. • Chewable tablet may contain mannitol and aspartame; cherry-flavored. • Granules should not be crushed, chewed, or mixed with liquid.

Pharmacokinetic (patient)

Absorption	• Specific site not known; t_{max} ~3–4 hours after an oral dose (immediate-release, fasted) • Bioavailability ~58%–66%
Transport	• Plasma protein binding >99% • V_d ~8–11 liters
Metabolism	• Extensively metabolized to at least 6 metabolites, including a hydroxyl metabolite and sulfoxide metabolites (via CYP3A4 and CYP2C9); excreted through the bile • Cl ~45 mL/min

Enteral Administration and Nutrition Considerations

Compatibility, Stability, and Bioavailability Considerations
- Nanostructured lipid carrier drug formulations under study using a mixture of LCTs and MCTs revealed significantly increased bioavailability (more than 100-fold), in part by reducing CYP3A4 and CYP2C9 metabolism, in an animal model.[1]

Drug-Nutrition Interactions
- Drug may influence nutrition status directly or indirectly:
  - o CNS: headache, fatigue
  - o GI: nausea, dyspepsia, abdominal pain, diarrhea, elevated transaminases
  - o Other: dental pain

- No data on the influence of malnutrition or obesity on drug disposition.
- Influence of food on oral absorption or bioavailability:
  - Grapefruit juice increased oral drug absorption and bioavailability compared with water in a crossover study conducted in healthy volunteers.[2]

Recommendations

Gastric	• Crush and/or disperse tablet in water just prior to administration. • No need to hold EN beyond the time required to flush-administer-flush.
Postpyloric	• As above. • Monitor for any unexpected change in effect.

References

1. Patil-Gadhe A, Pokharkar V. Montelukast-loaded nanostructured lipid carriers: part I oral bioavailability improvement. *Eur J Pharm Biopharm.* 2014;88:160–168.
2. Cingi C, Toroz SZ, Gürbüz MK, et al. Effect of grapefruit juice on bioavailability of montelukast. *Laryngoscope.* 2013;123:816–819.

Moxifloxacin Hydrochloride

Product Availability

| Solid | • Tablet: 400 mg (base) (Avelox® [Bayer]; others) |

Physicochemical (drug)

Molecular weight: • 401.44 (salt 437.90)	Permeability: • LogP –0.08 (calc) • Log D –0.53 (pH 7; calc)	Water solubility: • 27.5–33 mg/mL
pKa: • 6.4, 9.5	Classification: • BCS Class 1; BDDCS Class 3	

Pharmaceutical (product)

| Solid | • Tablet is film-coated. |

Pharmacokinetic (patient)

Absorption	• Specific site not known; t_{max} ~1–2 hours after an oral dose • Bioavailability ~90%
Transport	• Plasma protein binding ~40% • V_d ~2 L/kg
Metabolism	• Metabolized by conjugation (sulfate, glucuronic acid) • Cl ~2.3 mL/min/kg

Enteral Administration and Nutrition Considerations

Compatibility, Stability, and Bioavailability Considerations

- Moxifloxacin can be hygroscopic, easily absorbing moisture from the environment.
- An aqueous solution at 2 mg/mL has a pH of 3.9–4.6.
- An extemporaneously compounded oral liquid (20 mg/mL) made from tablets (with coating particles removed by sieve) diluted in OraSweet/OraPlus (1:1) and stored in amber plastic bottle at 23°C–25°C for 90 days exhibited little loss (HPLC analysis); osmolality and viscosity were not reported.[1]
- Compared to IV dosing, switching to enteral administration (equivalent dose tablet dispersed in 20 mL water and flushed through the feeding tube [EAD not described]) resulted in mean bioavailability reduction of 21% (8%–33%) in four critically ill patients; whether patients received EN was not reported.[2]
- Absolute oral bioavailability was no different than expected (~90%) compared with IV administration in a crossover study of 12 patients who previously underwent gastric bypass; however, regardless of route of administration, the concentrations were greater than expected (~50%) compared with healthy subjects, possibly because of increased enterohepatic recirculation.[3]

- The powder (from crushed 400 mg tablet) dispersed in 50 mL water and administered through a nasogastric tube (12 Fr, 100 cm long, polyurethane) followed by a 200 mL water flush, as reported in an open-label, randomized, controlled, crossover study in 12 healthy volunteers, resulted in a mean 9% reduction in bioavailability compared with the intact tablet taken by mouth with 250 mL water.[4]
- The powder (from crushed 400 mg tablet) dispersed in 50 mL water and administered through a nasogastric tube (12 Fr, 100 cm long, polyurethane) with EN (Isosource at 100 mL/h) held only for drug administration (from 30 minutes before until 2 hours after the dose), as reported in an open-label, randomized, controlled, crossover study in 12 healthy volunteers, resulted in a mean 9% reduction in bioavailability compared with the intact tablet taken by mouth with 250 mL water.[4]

Drug-Nutrition Interactions
- Drug may influence nutrition status directly or indirectly:
  - CNS: headache, dizziness, agitation, anxiety, insomnia, confusion, depression, blurry vision
  - GI: anorexia, bad taste, oral pain, vomiting, abdominal discomfort, diarrhea (including *Clostridium difficile*–associated), LFT elevations and rare hepatotoxicity
  - Metabolic: hyperamylasemia, hypoglycemia, crystalluria
  - Other: peripheral neuropathy (sensory or sensorimotor), tendonitis, arthralgia, weakness
- Influence of malnutrition or obesity on drug disposition:
  - The volume of distribution and clearance are not significantly different in obesity, suggesting that dosing should not be based on total body weight.[5]
- Influence of food on oral absorption or bioavailability:
  - No known influence of food, including a high-fat meal or yogurt, on oral bioavailability.
  - Products containing divalent and trivalent cations may reduce oral bioavailability, leading to recommendations to separate drug administration (by 4 hours before, 8 hours after these products).

Recommendations

Gastric	<ul><li>If there is no therapeutic alternative, crush and disperse tablet in water prior to administration.</li><li>Consider holding EN for at least 2 hours before and after drug administration.</li></ul>
Postpyloric	<ul><li>As above.</li><li>Monitor for any unexpected change in effect.</li></ul>
Other	<ul><li>As with all antimicrobials, consider parenteral alternative for acutely ill patients to ensure therapeutic concentrations.</li></ul>

References

1. Hutchinson DJ, Johnson CE, Klein KC. Stability of extemporaneously prepared moxifloxacin oral suspensions. *Am J Health-Syst Pharm.* 2009;66:665–667.
2. De Smet J, Colpaert K, De Paepe P, et al. Switch from intravenous to enteral moxifloxacin in critically ill patients: a pilot study. *Scand J Infect Dis.* 2012;44:874–878.
3. De Smet J, Colin P, De Paepe P, et al. Oral bioavailability of moxifloxacin after Roux-en-Y gastric bypass surgery. *J Antimcrob Chemother.* 2012;67:226–229.
4. Burkhardt O, Stass H, Thuss U, et al. Effects of enteral feeding on the oral bioavailability of moxifloxacin in healthy volunteers. *Clin Pharmacokinet.* 2005;44:969–976.
5. Kees MG, Weber S, Kees F, et al. Pharmacokinetics of moxifloxacin in plasma and tissue of morbidly obese patients. *J Antimicrob Chemother.* 2011;66:2330–2335.

Nabumetone

Product Availability

Solid	• Tablet: 500 mg, 750 mg (various)

Physicochemical (drug)

Molecular weight: • 228.29	Permeability: • LogP 3.08 • LogD 3.38 (pH 7.4)	Water solubility: • 0.015 mg/mL
pKa: • n/a	Classification: • BCS Class 2; BDDCS Class 2	

Pharmaceutical (product)

Solid	• Tablet products are typically film-coated.

Pharmacokinetic (patient)

Absorption	• Specific site not known; t_{max} ~2–4 hours after an oral dose • Bioavailability ~80%
Transport	• Plasma protein binding ~99%, mostly as the active metabolite • V_d ~50–55 liters
Metabolism	• Extensive first-pass metabolism as the prodrug is activated to 6-methoxy-2-naphthylacetic acid (6MNA) by oxidation and to other metabolites then all excreted in the urine • Cl ~20–30 mL/min

Enteral Administration and Nutrition Considerations

Compatibility, Stability, and Bioavailability Considerations
  • An aqueous dispersion may have a pH of 3.5–4.5.

Drug-Nutrition Interactions
  • Drug may influence nutrition status directly or indirectly:
    ○ CNS: dizziness, headache, fatigue
    ○ GI: dry mouth, gastritis, mucosal inflammation/ulceration, perforation, abdominal pain, diarrhea or constipation, elevated transaminases
    ○ Metabolic: fluid retention, edema
  • No data on the influence of malnutrition or obesity on drug disposition.
  • Influence of food on oral absorption or bioavailability:
    ○ Food including milk increased oral bioavailability compared to the fasting state without influencing the conversion to 6MNA.[1]

Recommendations

Gastric	• Consider a therapeutic alternative (eg, naproxen).
Postpyloric	• As above.

Reference

1. von Shrader HW, Buscher G, Dierdorf D, Mügge H, Wolf D. Nabumetone—a novel anti-inflammatory drug: the influence of food, milk, antacids, and analgesics on bioavailability of single oral doses. *Int J Clin Pharmacol Ther Toxicol.* 1983;21:311–321.

Naproxen / Naproxen Sodium

Product Availability

Solid	• Tablet: Naproxen: o Immediate-release: 250 mg, 375 mg, 500 mg (Naprosyn® [Atnahs Pharma]; others) o Enteric-coated: 375 mg, 500 mg (various) • Tablet: Naproxen sodium: o Immediate-release: 200 mg (base) (Aleve® [Bayer]; others); 250 mg, 500 mg (base) (Anaprox® [Atnahs Pharma]; others) o Extended-release: 375 mg, 500 mg, 750 mg (base) (Naprelan® [Alvogen]; others) • Capsule: Naproxen sodium: 200 mg (base) (various)
Liquid	• Oral suspension: Naproxen: 125 mg/5 mL (Naprosyn® [Atnahs Pharma]; others)

Physicochemical (drug)

Molecular weight: • 230.27 (salt 252.25)	Permeability: • LogP 3.18 • LogD 1.70 (pH 7.4), 0.47 (pH 6.5, calc)	Water solubility: • 0.115 mg/mL
pKa: • 4.15	Classification: • BCS Class 2; BDDCS Class 2	

Pharmaceutical (product)

Solid	• If not film-coated, some tablets may disperse in water (20 mL) within 5 minutes. • Non-enteric-coated tablets may be crushed and dispersed in water. • Do not break, chew, or crush extended-release or enteric-coated tablets.
Liquid	• Oral suspension: o pH 2.2–3.7 o Osmolality n/a o Viscosity n/a o May contain sucrose, sorbitol, and sodium (39 mg/5 mL) o Maintain at controlled room temperature in light-resistant container.

Pharmacokinetic (patient)

Absorption	• Specific site not known, but within proximal small intestine; t_{max} ~1–2 hours after an oral dose (immediate-release or suspension) • Bioavailability variable, ~95%

Transport	• Plasma protein binding ~99%
	• V_d ~0.16 L/kg
Metabolism	• Extensive hepatic metabolism to 6-desmethyl naproxen via CYP1A2 and CYP2C9, subsequently conjugated prior to renal excretion
	• Cl ~0.13 mL/min/kg

Enteral Administration and Nutrition Considerations

Compatibility, Stability, and Bioavailability Considerations
- The sodium salt is freely soluble in water at neutral pH, whereas the solubility of the acid form in water is pH-dependent—freely soluble at high pH, but practically insoluble at low pH.
- Extemporaneously compounded oral suspensions (25 mg/mL) were prepared from naproxen tablets (250 mg) in OralMix or OralMix SF. When stored in amber glass or polyethylene terephthalate plastic bottles at 4°C or 25°C, or in amber plastic syringes at 25°C, the suspensions had a pH of 4.30–4.39. All preparations remained stable (HPLC analysis) under study conditions for 91 days.[1]
- An extemporaneously compounded oral suspension (25 mg/mL) prepared from naproxen powder in SyrSpend SF PH4, stored in low-actinic bottles at 2°C–8°C or 20°C–25°C, remained stable (HPLC analysis) for 90 days.[2]
- A self-emulsifying and stable drug formulation improved both dissolution and oral bioavailability in an animal model compared to the suspension product.[3]
- A fast-dissolving oral formulation under study using micronized drug particles improved dissolution and increased oral bioavailability in an animal model.[4]

Drug-Nutrition Interactions
- Drug may influence nutrition status directly or indirectly:
  o CNS: headache, drowsiness, vertigo, tinnitus
  o GI: stomatitis, nausea, heartburn, abdominal pain, GI bleed, constipation, colitis, diarrhea
  o Metabolic: peripheral edema, hyperkalemia, dysglycemia
  o Other: myalgia, muscle cramps and weakness
- No data on the influence of malnutrition or obesity on drug disposition.
- Influence of food on oral absorption or bioavailability:
  o Food may delay oral absorption (greater influence on extended-release, than immediate-release) but without significant influence on oral bioavailability.[5]
  o Concurrent food intake may decrease GI intolerance.
  o Concurrent administration of DHA (docosahexaenoic acid) increased drug bioavailability (~1.3-fold) and analgesic effect in an animal model.[6]

Recommendations

Gastric	• If there is no therapeutic alternative, disperse capsule contents in water just prior to administration. • No need to hold EN beyond the time required to flush-administer-flush.
Postpyloric	• As above. • Monitor for any unexpected change in effect.

References

1. Ensom MHH, Décarie D, Lingertat-Walsh K. Stability of extemporaneously compounded naproxen 25 mg/mL suspension in glass and plastic bottles and plastic syringes. *Can J Hosp Pharm.* 2015;68:489–491.
2. Polonini HC, Loures S, de Araujo EP, et al. Stability of allopurinol, amitriptyline hydrochloride, carbamazepine, domperidone, isoniazid, ketoconazole, lisinopril, naproxen, paracetamol (acetaminophen), and sertraline hydrochloride in SyrSpend SF PH4 oral suspensions. *Int J Pharm Compd.* 2016;20:426–434.
3. Penjuri SCB, Saritha D, Ravouru N, Poreddy SR. Development of self emulsifying formulations of poorly soluble naproxen for enhanced drug delivery. *Recent Pat Drug Deliv Formul.* 2016;10:235–244.
4. García-Herrero V, Torrado C, García-Rodríguez JJ, et al. Improvement of the surface hydrophilic properties of naproxen particles with addition of hydroxypropylmethyl cellulose and sodium dodecyl sulphate: in vitro and in vivo studies. *Int J Pharm.* 2017; 529:381–390.
5. Laurora I, Wang Y. Pharmacokinetics profile for extended-release versus immediate-release oral naproxen sodium after single and multiple dosing under fed and fasting conditions: two randomized, open-label trials. *Int J Clin Pharmacol Ther.* 2016;54: 750–760.
6. Arroyo-Lira AG, Rodríguez-Ramos F, Ortiz MI, et al. Supra-additive interaction of docosahexaenoic acid and naproxen and gastric safety on the formalin test in rats. *Drug Dev Res.* 2017;78:332–339.

Nebivolol Hydrochloride

Product Availability

Solid	• Tablet: 2.5 mg, 5 mg, 10 mg, 20 mg (base) (Bystolic® [Forest Labs]; others)

Physicochemical (drug)

Molecular weight: • 405.44 (salt 441.90)	Permeability: • LogP 3.2 • LogD n/a	Water solubility: • 0.041 mg/mL
pKa: • 8.22	Classification: • BCS Class 2; BDDCS Class n/a	

Pharmaceutical (product)

Solid	• Tablet may be crushed for dispersion in water.

Pharmacokinetic (patient)

Absorption	• Specific site not known; t_{max} <1–2 hours after an oral dose • Bioavailability variable (12%–96%) based on CYP2D6 metabolizer phenotype
Transport	• Possible substrate for P-glycoprotein • Plasma protein binding ~98%, mostly to albumin • V_d ≥~9 L/kg
Metabolism	• Extensive hepatic metabolism of the parent by glucuronidation, and N-dealkylation and oxidation via CYP2D6; the proportion ultimately excreted via urine and feces depends on CYP2D6 phenotype • Cl varies by CYP2D6 metabolizer phenotype.

Enteral Administration and Nutrition Considerations

Compatibility, Stability, and Bioavailability Considerations
- A fast-dissolving formulation under development exhibited greater (at least 2-fold) in vitro drug release than conventional tablets.[1]
- Incorporating nebivolol into a solid lipid nanoparticle formulation under study revealed improved in vitro stability in GI fluid conditions that may improve drug transport.[2]

Drug-Nutrition Interactions
- Drug may influence nutrition status directly or indirectly:
  o CNS: headache, fatigue, dizziness
  o GI: nausea, abdominal pain, diarrhea
  o Metabolic: peripheral edema, hypercholesterolemia

- Influence of malnutrition or obesity on drug disposition:
  - Body weight–normalized volume of distribution is unchanged in obesity, and, although total clearance may be higher, therapeutic effect is unchanged.[3]
- No known influence of food on oral absorption or bioavailability.

Recommendations

Gastric	• If there is no therapeutic alternative, crush and disperse tablet in water just prior to administration. • No need to hold EN beyond the time required to flush-administer-flush.
Postpyloric	• Not recommended.

References

1. Sipos E, Szabó ZI, Rédai E, et al. Preparation and characterization of nanofibrous sheets for enhanced oral dissolution of nebivolol hydrochloride. *J Pharm Biomed Anal.* 2016;129:224–228.
2. Ustundag-Okur N, Yurdasiper A, Gundogdu E, Gokce EH. Modification of solid lipid nanoparticles loaded with nebivolol hydrochloride for improvement of oral bioavailability in treatment of hypertension: polyethylene glycol versus chitosan oligosaccharide lactate. *J Microencapsul.* 2016;33:30–42.
3. Cheymol G, Woestenborghs R, Snoeck E, et al. Pharmacokinetic study and cardiovascular monitoring of nevibolol in normal and obese subjects. *Eur J Clin Pharmacol.* 1997;51: 493–498.

Niacin (Nicotinic Acid)

Product Availability

Solid	• Tablet:
	    ○ Immediate-release: 500 mg (Niacor® [Upsher-Smith]; others)
	    ○ Extended-release: 500 mg, 750 mg, 1000 mg (Niaspan® [Kos]; others)

Physicochemical (drug)

Molecular weight: • 123.11	Permeability: • LogP 0.36 • LogD −2.87 (pH 7.4)	Water solubility: • 16.7 mg/mL
pKa: • 4.75	Classification: • BCS Class 3; BDDCS Class 1	

Pharmaceutical (product)

Solid	• Some tablet products are film-coated. • Do not break or crush extended-release product. • Products are not necessarily bioequivalent and therefore are not interchangeable.

Pharmacokinetic (patient)

Absorption	• Specific site not known; t_{max} ~30–60 minutes after an oral dose (immediate-release) • Bioavailability ~60%–75%
Transport	• Distributes initially to liver, adipose tissue, and kidneys • V_d n/a
Metabolism	• Rapid metabolism (amidation pathway) to nicotinamide, nicotinamide adenine dinucleotide, and additional nicotinamide derivatives, and (glycine conjugation pathway) to nicotinuric acid, then excreted in urine • Cl n/a

Enteral Administration and Nutrition Considerations

Compatibility, Stability, and Bioavailability Considerations
- A saturated aqueous solution is expected to have pH ~2.7.

Drug-Nutrition Interactions
- Drug may influence nutrition status directly or indirectly:
  - CNS: headache including migraines
  - GI: nausea, vomiting, abdominal pain, diarrhea, abnormal LFTs, rare hepatotoxicity
  - Metabolic: hyperglycemia, hypophosphatemia
  - Other: myalgia, myopathy, rhabdomyolysis

- No data on the influence of malnutrition or obesity on drug disposition.
- Influence of food on oral absorption or bioavailability:
  - Take with food, preferably a low-fat meal or snack; avoid taking with spicy foods, alcohol, and hot beverages.

Recommendations

Gastric	• Crush and/or disperse immediate-release tablet in water prior to administration. • No need to hold EN beyond the time required to flush-administer-flush.
Postpyloric	• As above. • Monitor for any unexpected change in effect.

Nifedipine

Product Availability

Solid	• Tablet: Extended-release: 30 mg, 60 mg, 90 mg (Procardia® XL [Pfizer]; Adalat® CC [Alvogen]; others) • Capsule: Immediate-release: 10 mg (Procardia® [Pfizer]; others)

Physicochemical (drug)

Molecular weight: • 346.34	Permeability: • LogP 2.20 • LogD 2.80 (pH 7.4)	Water solubility: • 0.006 mg/mL
pKa: • 3.9	Classification: • BCS Class 2; BDDCS Class 2	

Pharmaceutical (product)

Solid	• Immediate-release soft-gelatin capsule is filled with viscous liquid; do not attempt to aspirate liquid with needle and syringe (incomplete dose extraction, further drug loss when transferring to enteral syringe). • Do not chew or crush the modified-release tablet; solid matrix may appear in stool following oral administration.

Pharmacokinetic (patient)

Absorption	• Predominant site may be the stomach; t_{max} ~0.5–2 hours after an oral dose (immediate-release) • Bioavailability ~45%–75%
Transport	• Substrate for P-glycoprotein efflux • Concentration-dependent plasma protein binding ~92%–98% • V_d ~0.62–0.77 L/kg
Metabolism	• Extensive metabolism to inactives (via CYP3A4), mostly excreted in the urine with some via bile • Cl ~450–700 mL/min

Enteral Administration and Nutrition Considerations

Compatibility, Stability, and Bioavailability Considerations
- Nifedipine is very light-sensitive, decomposing to form pyridine homologs, more so with the amorphous than the crystalline form.[1,2]
- Preparation requires a dimly lit environment, avoiding fluorescent light to prevent drug decomposition.[3]
- Some previously commercially available oral formulations remained stable exposed to artificial light.[4]

- Pure drug powder is preferred over capsule liquid contents for extemporaneous compounding.[3]
- Crushed tablets (10 mg extended-release), diluted with lactose (1:500) in a minimal light environment and stored in waxed/sealed powder paper packets covered in black plastic bags, still resulted in 8% drug loss (HPLC analysis) during preparation.[5]
- A less-controlled environment results in >20% drug loss (HPLC analysis) in less than 24 hours.[4]
- An extemporaneously compounded oral solution (10 mg/mL) prepared from drug powder in a mixture of glycerin and propylene glycol, stored in amber glass bottles or amber polypropylene oral syringes at 22°C–25°C, then exposed to fluorescent light (bottles and syringes) unprotected or wrapped in aluminum foil (syringes), remained stable (HPLC analysis) for 35 days (bottles), 14 days (protected syringes), or <7 days (unprotected).[6]
- An extemporaneously compounded oral suspension (4 mg/mL) prepared from drug powder in SyrSpend SF PH4, stored in low-actinic plastic at 2°C–8°C or controlled room temperature, remained stable (HPLC analysis) for 92 days.[7]
- An extemporaneously compounded oral suspension (1 mg/mL) prepared from pure drug powder or crushed tablets (extended-release) with 1% hydroxypropyl methylcellulose, stored in vials and oral syringes, maintained stability (HPLC analysis) at room temperature or under refrigeration for 1 month, as long as the preparation was protected from light. Light exposure resulted in 25% drug loss in 3 hours. Suspension pH and viscosity were reported as 6.94 and 8.2–12.0 mPa·s after 28 days refrigerated.[8,9]
- Novel formulations in development with incorporation of lipid can improve drug dissolution and oral bioavailability.[10–13]

Drug-Nutrition Interactions

- Drug may influence nutrition status directly or indirectly:
  - CNS: weakness, tremor
  - GI: nausea, heartburn, abdominal cramps
  - Metabolic: peripheral edema
  - Other: muscle cramps
- No data on the influence of malnutrition or obesity on drug disposition.
- Influence of food on oral absorption or bioavailability:
  - Food (low-fat meal more so than high-fat meal) may decrease the rate of absorption from immediate-release formulations but without a significant influence on oral bioavailability.[2]
  - Grapefruit juice may increase oral bioavailability.

Recommendations

Gastric	• If there is no therapeutic alternative (eg, amlodipine), can consider preparing an extemporaneous suspension with stability cautions. • No need to hold EN beyond the time required to flush-administer-flush. • Monitor for any unexpected change in effect.
Postpyloric	• Not recommended.

References

1. Sousa LA, Beezer A, Clapham D, et al. The use of photocalorimetry to assess the photostability of nifedipine solutions. *J Pharm Pharmacol.* 2010;62:1214–1215.
2. Gajendran J, Krämer J, Shah VP, et al. Biowaiver monographs for immediate-release solid oral dosage forms: nifedipine. *J Pharm Sci.* 2015;104:3289–3298.
3. McCluskey SV, Brunn GJ. Nifedipine in compounded oral and topical preparations. *Int J Pharm Compd.* 2011;15:166–169.
4. Grundy JS, Kherani R, Foster RT. Photostability determination of commercially available nifedipine oral dosage formulations. *J Pharm Biomed Anal.* 1994;12:1529–1535.
5. Helin MM, Kontra KM, Naaranlahti TJ, et al. Content uniformity and stability of nifedipine in extemporaneously compounded oral powders. *Am J Health-Syst Pharm.* 1998;55:1299–1301.
6. Dentinger PJ, Swenson CF, Anaizi NH. Stability of nifedipine in an extemporaneously compounded oral solution. *Am J Health-Syst Pharm.* 2003;60:1019–1022.
7. Geiger CM, Sorenson B, Whaley P. Stability assessment of 10 active pharmaceutical ingredients compounded in SyrSpend SF. *Int J Pharm Compd.* 2015;19:420–427.
8. Helin-Tanninen M, Naaranlahti T, Kontra K, et al. Enteral suspension of nifedipine for neonates, part 1: formulation of nifedipine suspension for hospital use. *J Clin Pharm Ther.* 2001;26:49–57.
9. Helin-Tanninen M, Naaranlahti T, Kontra K, et al. Enteral suspension of nifedipine for neonates, part 2: stability of an extemporaneously compounded nifedipine suspension. *J Clin Pharm Ther.* 2001;26:59–66.
10. Weerapol Y, Limmatvapirat S, Kumpugdee-Vollrath M, Sriamornsak P. Spontaneous emulsification of nifedipine-loaded self-nanoemulsifying drug delivery system. *AAPS PharmSciTech.* 2014;16:435–443.
11. Weerapol Y, Limmatvapirat S, Jansakul C, Takeuchi H, Sriamornsak P. Enhanced dissolution and oral bioavailability of nifedipine by spontaneous emulsifying powders: effect of solid carriers and dietary state. *Eur J Pharm Biopharm.* 2015;91:25–34.
12. Jannin V, Chevrier S, Michenaud M, et al. Development of self emulsifying lipid formulations of BCS class II drugs with low to medium lipophilicity. *Int J Pharm.* 2015; 495:385–392.
13. Ali MA, Kataoka N, Ranneh AH, et al. Enhancing the solubility and oral bioavailability of poorly water-soluble drugs using monoolein cubosomes. *Chem Pharm Bull.* 2017;65: 42–48.

Nitrofurantoin

Product Availability

Solid	• Capsule: 25 mg, 50 mg, 75 mg, 100 mg (various)
Liquid	• Oral suspension: 25 mg/5 mL (various)

Physicochemical (drug)

Molecular weight: • 238.16	Permeability: • LogP –0.47 • Log D –0.19 (pH 7.4)	Water solubility: • 0.19 mg/mL • 0.37 mg/mL (pH 7.2)
pKa: • 3.5, 7.8	Classification: • BCS Class 4; BDDCS Class 4	

Pharmaceutical (product)

Solid	• Capsule contents (granules) disperse poorly in water (20 mL); some products' granules may also block syringe tip. • Capsule contains the macrocrystalline form of drug; some products contain a proportion as the monohydrate.

Liquid	• Oral suspension:
	  o pH 4.5–6.5
	  o Osmolality n/a
	  o Viscosity can be significant.
	  o Suspension contains the microcrystalline form.
	  o May contain glycerin and sorbitol
	  o Store at controlled room temperature; use product within 30 days.
	  o Shake very well prior to measuring out the dose.

Pharmacokinetic (patient)

Absorption	• Specific site not known; t_{max} ~1–4 hours after an oral dose (immediate-release) • Macrocrystalline form (capsule) has slower dissolution than either the monohydrate or the microcrystalline form (suspension). • Bioavailability ~87%
Transport	• Substrate for BCRP efflux • Plasma protein binding ~20%–60% • V_d ~0.58 L/kg
Metabolism	• Partially metabolized, with most drug eliminated unchanged in the urine • Cl ~9.9 mL/min/kg

Enteral Administration and Nutrition Considerations

Compatibility, Stability, and Bioavailability Considerations
- Although nitrofurantoin remains stable at pH 5.4–9.9, the drug can undergo reversible hydrolysis at more acidic pH.
- An oral suspension (10 mL) added to 15–240 mL of EN formula (Ensure, Ensure Plus, or Osmolite) was physically compatible (no phase separation or particle growth) on visual inspection.[1]
- An oral suspension (10 mL) added to 15–240 mL of EN formula (Ensure HN, Ensure Plus HN, Osmolite HN, or Vital) was physically compatible (no phase separation or particle growth) on visual inspection.[2]
- An oral suspension (10 mL) combined with 10 mL of EN (Enrich, TwoCal HN or Vivonex T.E.N.) was physically compatible (no phase separation or particle growth) on visual inspection.[3]
- No data were reported on the pH, osmolality, or viscosity of the above-described admixtures; drug stability was not evaluated.

Drug-Nutrition Interactions
- Drug may influence nutrition status directly or indirectly:
  ○ CNS: dizziness, headache, asthenia
  ○ GI: anorexia, nausea, vomiting, diarrhea or constipation, cholestasis, pancreatitis
  ○ Other: peripheral neuropathy, arthralgia, myalgia
- No data on the influence of malnutrition or obesity on drug disposition.
- Influence of food on oral absorption or bioavailability:
  ○ Although the influence of food on oral absorption may vary with formulation, it is best to take with food to enhance GI tolerance.
  ○ Food slows gastric emptying and allows better dissolution and significantly improves oral bioavailability of the macrocrystalline form.

Recommendations

Gastric	• If there is no therapeutic alternative, dilute oral suspension with water (at least 1:1) just prior to administration. • No need to hold EN beyond the time required to flush-administer-flush.
Postpyloric	• As above. • Monitor for any unexpected change in effect.
Other	• As with all antimicrobials, consider parenteral alternative for acutely ill patients to ensure therapeutic concentrations.

References

1. Cutie AJ, Altman E, Lenkel L. Compatibility of enteral products with commonly employed drug additives. *JPEN J Parenter Enteral Nutr.* 1983;7:186–191.
2. Altman E, Cutie AJ. Compatibility of enteral products with commonly employed drug additives. *Nutr Supp Serv.* 1984;4:8–17.
3. Burns PE, McCall L, Wirsching R. Physical compatibility of enteral formulas with various common medications. *J Am Diet Assoc.* 1988;88:1094–1096.

Nortriptyline Hydrochloride

Product Availability

Solid	• Capsule: 10 mg, 25 mg, 50 mg, 75 mg (base) (Pamelor® [Mallinckrodt]; others)
Liquid	• Oral solution: 10 mg/5 mL (base) (various)

Physicochemical (drug)

Molecular weight: • 263.39 (salt 299.84)	Permeability: • LogP 4.04 • LogD 1.69 (pH 7.4)	Water solubility: • 0.02 mg/mL
pKa: • 9.73	Classification: • BCS Class 2; BDDCS Class 1	

Pharmaceutical (product)

Solid	• Capsule contents may disperse in water (20 mL).

Liquid	• Oral solution:
	   o pH 2.5–4.0
	   o Osmolality n/a
	   o Viscosity n/a
	   o May contain ethanol and sorbitol
	   o Store at controlled room temperature.

Pharmacokinetic (patient)

Absorption	• Specific site not known; t_{max} ~2–4 hours after an oral dose • Bioavailability ~60%
Transport	• Plasma protein binding ~93% • V_d ~21 L/kg
Metabolism	• Metabolism via CYP2D6 to 10-hydroxy and N-demethyl metabolites, with subsequent glucuronidation • Cl ~30.6 L/h

Enteral Administration and Nutrition Considerations

Compatibility, Stability, and Bioavailability Considerations
- The drug appeared to have adequate oral bioavailability in a patient with short bowel syndrome (5–6 feet of small bowel).[1]

Drug-Nutrition Interactions
- Drug may influence nutrition status directly or indirectly:
  - CNS: confusion, ataxia, blurred vision
  - GI: dry mouth, stomatitis, anorexia, nausea, vomiting, abdominal cramps, constipation
  - Metabolic: dysglycemia, SIADH
  - Other: peripheral neuropathy

- Influence of malnutrition or obesity on drug disposition:
  - Poor antidepressant response is more likely at higher BMI, but that is not likely related to altered volume of distribution or clearance.[2]
- No known influence of food on oral absorption or bioavailability.

Recommendations

Gastric	• Disperse capsule contents in water prior to administration. • Alternative: Dilute solution in water (at least 1:1) just prior to administration. • No need to hold EN beyond the time required to flush-administer-flush.
Postpyloric	• As above. • Monitor for any unexpected change in effect.

References

1. Broyles JE, Brown RO, Self TH, Frederick RC, Luther RW. Nortriptyline absorption in short bowel syndrome. *JPEN J Parenter Enteral Nutr.* 1990;14:326–327.
2. Uher R, Mors O, Hauser J, et al. Body weight as a predictor of antidepressant efficacy in the GENDEP project. *J Affect Disord.* 2009;118:147–154.

Olanzapine

Product Availability

Solid	• Tablet:
	  ○ Immediate-release: 2.5 mg, 5 mg, 7.5 mg, 10 mg, 15 mg, 20 mg (Zyprexa® [Lilly]; others)
	  ○ Orally disintegrating: 5 mg, 10 mg, 15 mg, 20 mg (Zyprexa® Zydis [Lilly]; others)

Physicochemical (drug)

Molecular weight: • 312.44	Permeability: • LogP 3.00 • LogD n/a	Water solubility: • 0.01 mg/mL
pKa: • 4.0, 7.2, 14.2	Classification: • BCS Class 2; BDDCS Class 2	

Pharmaceutical (product)

Solid	• Some immediate-release tablet products are film-coated. • Orally disintegrating tablet products can disperse in water; they may contain aspartame. • Immediate-release and orally disintegrating tablet products are considered bioequivalent.

Pharmacokinetic (patient)

Absorption	• Specific site not known; t_{max} ~5–8 hours after an oral dose • Bioavailability ~60%
Transport	• Substrate for P-glycoprotein efflux • Plasma protein binding ~93%, mostly to albumin and α_1-acid glycoprotein • V_d ~16.4 L/kg
Metabolism	• Extensively metabolized via CYP1A2 and CYP2D6 and glucuronidation, then excreted in urine and feces • Cl ~12–47 L/h

Enteral Administration and Nutrition Considerations

Compatibility, Stability, and Bioavailability Considerations
- The drug products need to be well protected from light and moisture.
- An oral suspension formulation (10 mg/5 mL) was shown to be bioequivalent to the orally disintegrating tablet (10 mg) in a single-dose crossover study conducted in 18 healthy male volunteers (BMI 18.6–26.2 kg/m^2).[1]
- Another fast-dissolving solid dispersion exhibited faster dissolution and greater oral bioavailability in human volunteers.[2]

- A solid microcrystalline dispersion formulation enhanced drug dissolution.[3]
- A nanostructured lipid carrier formulation significantly increased in vitro permeability compared with conventional tablets.[4]

Drug-Nutrition Interactions
- Drug may influence nutrition status directly or indirectly:
  - Increased appetite and weight gain (no difference between conventional tablets and orally disintegrating tablets)[5]
  - CNS: somnolence, asthenia, tremor, abnormal gait
  - GI: dry mouth, nausea, dysphagia, vomiting, abdominal pain, dyspepsia, constipation, transaminase elevations, rare pancreatitis
  - Metabolic: hyperglycemia, dyslipidemia, hyperprolactinemia
  - Other: pain (joints, back, extremities)
- No data on the influence of malnutrition or obesity on drug disposition.
- No known influence of food on oral absorption or bioavailability.

Recommendations

Gastric	• Crush and disperse tablet in water prior to administration. • Alternative: Disperse orally disintegrating tablet in water just prior to administration. • No need to hold EN beyond the time required to flush-administer-flush.
Postpyloric	• As above. • Monitor for any unexpected change in effect.

References

1. Singhal R, Thakkar V, Srivastava A. Evaluation of bioequivalence of two oral formulations of olanzapine. *Indian J Pharm Sci.* 2011;73:678–682.
2. Maher EM, Ali AMA, Salem HF, Abdelrahman AA. In vitro/in vivo evaluation of an optimized fast dissolving oral film containing olanzapine co-amorphous dispersion with selected carboxylic acids. *Drug Deliv.* 2016;23:3088–3100.
3. de Mohac LM, de Fátima Pina M, Raimi-Abraham BT. Solid microcrystalline dispersion films as a new strategy to improve the dissolution rate of poorly water soluble drugs: a case study using olanzapine. *Int J Pharm.* 2016;508:42–50.
4. Mendes M, Soares HT, Arnaut LG, et al. Can lipid nanoparticles improve intestinal absorption? *Int J Pharm.* 2016;515:69–83.
5. Kusumi I, Honda M, Uemura K, et al. Effect of olanzapine orally disintegrating tablet versus oral standard tablet on body weight in patients with schizophrenia: a randomized open-label trial. *Prog Neuro-Psychopharmacol Biol Psych.* 2012;36:313–317.

Olmesartan Medoxomil

Product Availability

Solid	• Tablet: 5 mg, 20 mg, 40 mg (Benicar® [Daiichi Sankyo]; others)

Physicochemical (drug)

Molecular weight: • 446.51 (medoxomil 558.60)	Permeability: • LogP 5.9 • LogD n/a	Water solubility: • 2 mg/mL
pKa: • 0.9, 4.9, 5.6, 13.9	Classification: • BCS Class n/a; BDDCS Class 1	

Pharmaceutical (product)

Solid	• Do not crush tablet (pregnancy exposure risk). • Although the tablet may be film-coated, it may disperse in water after a long period of time.

Pharmacokinetic (patient)

Absorption	• Specific site not known; t_{max} ~1–2 hours after an oral dose • Bioavailability ~28%
Transport	• Substrate for P-glycoprotein efflux • Plasma protein binding ~99% • V_d ~0.36 L/kg
Metabolism	• This prodrug is acted upon by esterases (ester hydrolysis at gut mucosa) to release the active olmesartan, which does not seem to undergo further metabolism before biliary and renal excretion. • Cl ~0.31 mL/min/kg

Enteral Administration and Nutrition Considerations

Compatibility, Stability, and Bioavailability Considerations

- As described in the product's prescribing information, an extemporaneous oral suspension (2 mg/mL) prepared using 20 mg tablets in purified water further diluted in OraSweet/OraPlus (2:1), stored in amber polyethylene terephthalate bottles, remains stable for up to 4 weeks at 2°C–8°C.
- A nanosuspension formulation revealed that the saturation solubility and dissolution rate are significantly greater than the aqueous suspension or commercial tablet that suggest improved bioavailability.[1]
- Nanoparticle and nanosuspension formulations under study enhanced dissolution and increased oral bioavailability compared with a conventional suspension in an animal model.[2]
- Nanostructured lipid carrier formulations under study remained stable in simulated gastric fluids and allowed increased oral bioavailability compared with the free drug in an animal model.[3,4]

- A nanoemulsion formulation studied in an animal model revealed not only better oral bioavailability compared to an aqueous suspension but also better tissue distribution.[5]
- Drug formulations in development using self-microemulsification improved dissolution, in situ permeability, and oral bioavailability in an animal model.[6,7]

Drug-Nutrition Interactions
- Drug may influence nutrition status directly or indirectly:
  - CNS: headache, dizziness
  - GI: sprue-like enteropathy (villous atrophy, diarrhea, weight loss)
  - Metabolic: hyperglycemia, hyperkalemia
- No data on the influence of malnutrition or obesity on drug disposition.
- No known influence of food on oral absorption or bioavailability.

Recommendations

Gastric	• If there is no therapeutic alternative, disperse tablet in water prior to administration. • No need to hold EN beyond the time required to flush-administer-flush.
Postpyloric	• As above. • Monitor for any unexpected change in effect.

References

1. Thakkar HP, Patel BV, Thakkar SP. Development and characterization of nanosuspensions of olmesartan medoxomil for bioavailability enhancement. *J Pharm Bioallied Sci.* 2011;3:426–434.
2. Butreddy A, Dudhipala N, Veerabrahama K. Development of olmesartan medoxomil lipid-based nanoparticles and nanosuspension: preparation, characterization and comparative pharmacokinetic evaluation. *Artif Cells Nanomed Biotechnol.* 2018;46:126–137.
3. Kaithwas V, Dora CP, Kushwah V, Jain S. Nanostructured lipid carriers of olmesartan medoxomil with enhanced oral bioavailability. *Colloids Surf B Biointerfaces.* 2017;154:10–20.
4. Nooli M, Chella N, Kulhari H, Shastri NR, Sistla R. Solid lipid nanoparticles as vesicles for oral delivery of olmesartan medoxomil: formulation, optimization and in vivo evaluation. *Drug Dev Ind Pharm.* 2017;43:611–617.
5. Gorain B, Choudhury H, Tekade RK, et al. Comparative biodistribution and safety profiling of olmesartan medoxomil oil-in-water oral nanoemulsion. *Regul Toxicol Pharmacol.* 2016;82:20–31.
6. Lee BS, Kang MJ, Choi WS, et al. Solubilized formulation of olmesartan medoxomil for enhancing oral bioavailability. *Arch Pharm Res.* 2009;32:1629–1635.
7. Kang MJ, Kim HS, Jeon HS, et al. In situ intestinal permeability and in vivo absorption characteristics of olmesartan medoxomil in self-microemulsifying drug delivery system. *Drug Dev Ind Pharm.* 2012;38:587–596.

Omeprazole

Product Availability

Solid	• Tablet: Delayed-release (omeprazole magnesium): 20 mg (base) (Prilosec® OTC [AstraZeneca]; others) • Capsule: ○ Immediate-release: 20 mg, 40 mg (Zegerid® [Santarus]) ○ Delayed-release: 10 mg, 20 mg, 40 mg (Prilosec® [AstraZeneca]; others)
Liquid	• Powder for oral suspension: 20 mg per packet (Zegerid® OTC [Bayer]), 20 mg, 40 mg per packet (Zegerid® [Santarus]) • Omeprazole magnesium delayed-release granules for oral suspension: 2.5 mg, 10 mg per packet (Prilosec® [Covis Pharma])

Physicochemical (drug)

Molecular weight: • 345.42	Permeability: • LogP 2.23 • LogD 2.23 (pH 7.4)	Water solubility: • 0.5 mg/mL
pKa: • 4.2, 9.0	Classification: • BCS Class n/a; BDDCS Class 1	

Pharmaceutical (product)

Solid	• Immediate-release capsule contents can disintegrate in water; capsules contain sodium bicarbonate (1.1 g/capsule). • Delayed-release capsules and tablets contain enteric-coated granules. These products should not be crushed; although they may disperse in water, they may occlude enteral syringe tips.
Liquid	• Powder for suspension contains sodium bicarbonate (1.68 g per packet); prepared in 15–30 mL water. • Granules for suspension are enteric-coated with a bioavailability ~87% of the capsule granules; prepared in 15–30 mL water. • No data are available on pH, osmolality, or viscosity of reconstituted suspensions.

Pharmacokinetic (patient)

Absorption	• Proximal to mid-small intestine; t_{max} ~30 minutes after an oral dose (immediate-release, fasted) or ~3 hours after an oral dose (delayed-release) • Bioavailability ~75%
Transport	• Substrate for P-glycoprotein efflux • Plasma protein binding ~95% • V_d ~0.3 L/kg
Metabolism	• Extensively metabolized via CYP2C19 and CYP3A4 to multiple metabolites excreted in the urine • Cl ~0.5–0.6 L/min

Enteral Administration and Nutrition Considerations

Compatibility, Stability, and Bioavailability Considerations

- Omeprazole is hygroscopic and must be protected from moisture exposure.
- Drug will dissolve in alkaline solutions and has maximum stability at pH 11.[1,2]
- A 2% solution of the sodium salt of omeprazole has a pH of 10.3–11.3.
- Decomposition occurs at pH <7.8, especially in the presence of citric acid.[1–3]
- The official USP oral suspension formulation (2 mg/mL) is expected to have a pH of 7.5–8.5 and can be provided a BUD of 45 days under refrigeration.
- An extemporaneously compounded oral suspension (2 mg/mL) prepared from drug powder in reconstituted SyrSpend SF Alka, stored in a bottle at 2°C–8°C, remained stable (HPLC analysis) for up to 92 days.[4]
- An oral liquid (2 mg/mL) prepared from capsule contents (20 mg) dissolved (not crushed) in 8.4% sodium bicarbonate, remained stable (HPLC analysis) for 14 days at room temperature and 30 days at 4°C; findings were similar whether stored in a vial or amber oral syringes.[5,6]
- The 2 mg/mL oral suspension stored in amber plastic prescription bottles and stored at 3°C–5°C remained stable at 45 days.[7]
- That 2 mg/mL preparation has been used successfully in clinical practice following administration via nasogastric tube.[8,9]
- A 4 mg/mL preparation was administered successfully through a gastrostomy tube (15 Fr) in 10 inpatients while EN was on hold.[10]
- Oral suspensions (0.6, 1.2, 2, 3, 4 mg/mL) prepared from commercially available omeprazole powder and stored in polypropylene tubes at 4°C in the dark remained stable (HPLC analysis) for 28 days; at room temperature the 2, 3, and 4 mg/mL preparations remained stable for 7 days; suspension viscosity was reported as remaining stable for 7 days, varying from ~20 to ~200 mPa·s from lowest to highest concentrations.[11]
- Although not necessary for enteral administration, flavoring the extemporaneously compounded formulation caused foam formation that interfered with dosing accuracy, and may interfere with drug assay.[12]
- Water and apple juice have been used separately as vehicles to suspend capsule granules; when administered through a 14 Fr nasogastric tube, a mean of 53% of granules were delivered distally; when administered through 16 Fr gastroduodenal tubes (polyurethane and silicone), and followed by 10–20 mL flush of the same vehicle, a mean of 61% of granules were delivered distally and numerous samples resulted in a clogged tube.[13,14]
- Oral suspensions administered by nasogastric, duodenal or jejunal access had similar efficacy.[8,15]
- Although the rate of drug absorption may be altered following gastric bypass, the oral bioavailability is not significantly altered.[16]

Drug-Nutrition Interactions
- Drug may influence nutrition status directly or indirectly:
  - CNS: lethargy, fatigue
  - GI: dry mouth, nausea, prolonged gastric emptying, abdominal pain, diarrhea (including *Clostridium difficile*–associated)
  - Metabolic: hypomagnesemia
  - Other: increased risk of osteoporosis-related fracture; muscle weakness and cramps
- Influence of malnutrition or obesity on drug disposition:
  - An animal model suggests increased drug exposure in protein-energy malnutrition related to decreased total drug clearance (including CYP activity).[17]
- Influence of food on oral absorption or bioavailability:
  - Food may delay the oral absorption and may reduce bioavailability by up to 24%.[18]
  - Administration of liquid protein solutions should be separated by 2 hours from omeprazole suspension administration to prevent a gas-producing reaction.[19]

Recommendations

Gastric	• If there is no therapeutic alternative (eg, esomeprazole), use the powder for oral suspension (or a suspension compounded from capsule contents in sodium bicarbonate), but dilute further with water just prior to administration.
	• Consider holding continuous EN for 1 hour before and after drug administration; also hold liquid protein administration for at least 1 hour before and after drug administration.
Postpyloric	• As above.
	• Monitor for any unexpected change in effect.

References

1. Mathew M, Gupta VD, Bailey RE. Stability of omeprazole solutions at various pH values as determined by high-performance liquid chromatography. *Drug Dev Industr Pharm.* 1995;21:965–971.
2. El-Badry M, Taha E, Alanazi FK, et al. Study of omeprazole stability in aqueous solution: influence of cyclodextrins. *J Drug Deliv Sci Tech.* 2009;19:347–351.
3. Ekpe A, Jacobsen T. Effect of various salts on the stability of lansoprazole, omeprazole, and pantoprazole as determined by high-performance liquid chromatography. *Drug Dev Industr Pharm.* 1999;25:1057–1065.
4. Whaley PA, Voudrie MA, Sorenson B. Stability of omeprazole in SyrSpend SF Alka (reconstituted). *Int J Pharm Compd.* 2012;16:164–166.
5. Quercia RA, Fan C, Liu X, et al. Stability of omeprazole in an extemporaneously prepared oral liquid. *Am J Health-Syst Pharm.* 1997;54:1833–1836.
6. DiGiacinto JL, Olsen KM, Bergman KL, et al. Stability of suspension formulations of lansoprazole and omeprazole stored in amber-colored plastic oral syringes. *Ann Pharmacother.* 2000;34:600–605.

7. Johnson CE, Cober MP, Ludwig JL. Stability of partial doses of omeprazole-sodium bicarbonate oral suspension. *Ann Pharmacother.* 2007;41:1954–1961.

8. Phillips JP, Metzler MH, Palmieri TL, et al. A prospective study of simplified omeprazole suspension for the prophylaxis of stress-related mucosal damage. *Crit Care Med.* 1996;24: 1793–1800.

9. Carrol M, Trudeau W. Nasogastric administration of omeprazole for control of gastric pH (abstract). *Proceedings of the 10th World Congress of Gastroenterology, Los Angeles, CA, 1994.*

10. Boussery K, De Smet J, De Cock P, et al. Pharmacokinetics of two formulations of omeprazole administered through a gastrostomy tube in patients with severe neurodevelopmental problems. *Br J Clin Pharmacol.* 2011;72:990–996.

11. Burnett JE, Balkin ER. Stability and viscosity of a flavored omeprazole oral suspension for pediatric use. *Am J Health-Syst Pharm.* 2006;63:2240–2247.

12. Chuong MC, Taglieri CA, Kerr SG. To flavor or not to flavor extemporaneous omeprazole liquid. *Int J Pharm Compd.* 2017;21:500–512.

13. Dunn A, White CM, Reddy P, et al. Delivery of omeprazole and lansoprazole granules through a nasogastric tube in vitro. *Am J Health-Syst Pharm.* 1999;56:2327–2330.

14. Messaouik D, Sauto-Miranda V, Bagel-Boithias S, et al. Comparative study and optimization of the administration mode of three proton pump inhibitors by nasogastric tube. *Int J Pharm.* 2005;299:65–72.

15. Phillips JP, Olsen KM, Rebuck JA, et al. A randomized pharmacokinetic and pharmacodynamics cross-over study of duodenal or jejunal administration compared to nasogastric administration of omeprazole suspension in patients at risk for stress ulcers. *Am J Gastroenterol.* 2001;96:367–372.

16. Tandra S, Chalasani N, Jones DR, et al. Pharmacokinetic and pharmacodynamics alterations in Roux-en-Y gastric bypass recipients. *Ann Surg.* 2013;258:262–269.

17. Lee DY, Lee I, Lee MG. Effects of cysteine on the pharmacokinetic parameters of omeprazole in rates with protein-calorie malnutrition. *JPEN J Parenter Enteral Nutr.* 2007;31:37–46.

18. Cornish P. "Avoid the crush": hazards of medication administration in patients with dysphagia or a feeding tube. *CMAJ.* 2005;172:871–872.

19. Freeman KL, Trezevant MS. Interaction between liquid protein solution and omeprazole suspension. *Am J Health-Syst Pharm.* 2009;66:1901–1902.

Ondansetron Hydrochloride

Product Availability

Solid	• Tablet:
	 o Immediate-release: 4 mg, 8 mg, 24 mg (base) (Zofran®
	  [Novartis]; others)
	 o Orally disintegrating: 4 mg, 8 mg (base) (Zofran® ODT
	  [Novartis]; others)
	 o Oral soluble film: 4 mg, 8 mg (base) (Zuplenz® [Midatech
	  Pharma])

Liquid	• Oral solution: 4 mg/5 mL (base) (Zofran® [Novartis]; others)

Physicochemical (drug)

Molecular weight: • 293.37 (salt 329.83)	Permeability: • LogP 2.72 (calc) • LogD 2.12 (pH 7.4)	Water solubility: • 5.7 mg/mL
pKa: • 7.4	Classification: • BCS Class 1; BDDCS Class 1	

Pharmaceutical (product)

Solid	• Orally disintegrating tablet and soluble film are prepared as the base.

Liquid	• Oral solution:
	 o pH 3.73
	 o Osmolality 2935 mOsm/kg (calculated based on
	  measurement of 1:5 dilution with sterile water)[1]
	 o Viscosity n/a
	 o May contain xylitol or sorbitol; strawberry-flavored
	 o Store at controlled room temperature and protect from
	  light.

Pharmacokinetic (patient)

Absorption	• Specific site not known; t_{max} ~1–1.5 hours after an oral dose • Bioavailability ~56%
Transport	• Substrate for P-glycoprotein efflux • Plasma protein binding ~70%–76% • V_d ~160 liters
Metabolism	• Extensively metabolized (via CYP1A2, CYP2D6, CYP3A4) and metabolites excreted in urine • Cl ~0.3 L/h/kg

Enteral Administration and Nutrition Considerations

Compatibility, Stability, and Bioavailability Considerations
- An aqueous solution of ondansetron hydrochloride has a pH of ~4.5, with precipitation of free base at pH >5.7–7.[2-4]
- The official USP oral suspension (1 mg/mL) formulation using powder or crushed tablet is expected to have a pH of 3.6–4.6 and is provided a BUD of 42 days under refrigeration.
- An extemporaneously compounded oral suspension (0.8 mg/mL) made from crushed tablets suspended in OraPlus and then diluted with cherry syrup USP, Syrpalta, OraSweet, or OraSweet SF, stored in amber plastic vials at 4°C, remained stable (HPLC analysis) for 42 days; of note, these preparations had an osmolality of 2438–3328 mOsm/kg, but viscosity was not reported.[5]
- The commercial solution combined (1:1) with Osmolite 1.2, under simulated clinical conditions, would result in clogging of both an 8 Fr and a 20 Fr feeding tube.[1]
- Although not recommended, dilution of 4 mL of the ondansetron injection (2 mg/mL) in orange juice or Coca-Cola to final concentrations of 267 and 67 mg/mL remained stable for 30–60 minutes. Osmolality, viscosity, and bioavailability were not reported.[6]
- Dilution of 2, 4, or 6 mL of the ondansetron injection (2 mg/mL) in a number of different oral fluids (eg, apple juice, Kool-Aid, Sprite, Diet Coke, Lipton tea) to final concentrations of 32.8, 64.5, and 95.2 mg/mL remained stable for 72 hours at room temperature or refrigerated (apple juice, Kool-Aid), remained stable for 48 hours (Sprite, Diet Coke), or exhibited a turbid precipitate (Lipton tea). Osmolality, viscosity, and bioavailability were not reported.[7]
- Solid self-nanoemulsifying granules under study demonstrated faster dissolution than pure drug and increased oral bioavailability in an animal model.[8]

Drug-Nutrition Interactions
- Drug may influence nutrition status directly or indirectly:
  - CNS: headache, dizziness
  - GI: abnormal taste, heartburn, abdominal cramps, constipation or diarrhea, transaminase elevations
- No data on the influence of malnutrition or obesity on drug disposition.
- Influence of food on oral absorption or bioavailability:
  - Food may enhance oral bioavailability.

Recommendations

Gastric	• Disperse orally dissolving tablet in water just prior to administration. • Alternative: Dilute oral solution in water (at least 1:1) prior to administration. • No need to hold EN beyond the time required to flush-administer-flush.
Postpyloric	• As above. • Monitor for any unexpected change in effect.

References

1. Klang M, McLymont V, Ng N. Osmolality, pH, and compatibility of selected oral liquid medications with an enteral nutrition product. *JPEN J Parenter Enteral Nutr.* 2013;37: 689–694.
2. MacKinnon JWM, Collin DT. The chemistry of ondansetron. *Eur J Cancer Clin Oncol.* 1989;25(Suppl 1):S61.
3. Leak RE, Woodford JD. Pharmaceutical development of ondansetron injection. *Eur J Cancer Clin Oncol.* 1989;25(Suppl 1):S67–S69.
4. Jarosinski PF, Hirschfield S. Precipitation of ondansetron in alkaline solutions. *N Engl J Med.* 1991;325:1315–1316.
5. Williams CL, Sanders PL, Laizure SC, et al. Stability of ondansetron hydrochloride in syrups compounded from tablets. *Am J Hosp Pharm.* 1994;51:806–809.
6. Graham CL, Dukes GE, Fox JL, et al. Stability of ondansetron hydrochloride injection in extemporaneously prepared oral solutions. *Am J Hosp Pharm.* 1993;50:106–108.
7. Yamreudeewong W, Danthi SN, Hill RA, et al. Stability of ondansetron hydrochloride injection in various beverages. *Am J Health-Syst Pharm.* 1995;52:2011–2014.
8. Beg S, Jena SS, Patra CN, et al. Development of solid self-nanoemulsifying granules (SSNEGs) of ondansetron hydrochloride with enhanced bioavailability potential. *Colloids Surf B Biointerfaces.* 2013;101:414–423.

Oseltamivir Phosphate

Product Availability

Solid	• Capsule: 30 mg, 45 mg, 75 mg (base) (Tamiflu® [Roche]; others)
Liquid	• Powder for oral suspension: 6 mg/mL (base) (Tamiflu® [Roche]; others)

Physicochemical (drug)

Molecular weight: • 312.4 (salt 410.40)	Permeability: • LogP 0.36, 2.13 (calc) • LogD n/a	Water solubility (salt): • 588 mg/mL (25°C)
pKa: • 7.75	Classification: • BCS Class 3; BDDCS Class 1	

Pharmaceutical (product)

Solid	• Capsule contents may disperse easily in water.

Liquid	• Oral suspension (reconstituted):
	  o pH 3–5
	    ▪ pH 3.86 (a 6 mg/mL product)
	  o Osmolality n/a
	  o Viscosity n/a
	  o May contain saccharin, sorbitol; tutti-frutti-flavored
	  o Store at 2°C–8°C for up to 17 days; it may be stable for up to 10 days at 25°C; do not freeze.
	  o Shake well prior to measuring each dose for administration.

Pharmacokinetic (patient)

Absorption	• Absorption similar in stomach and proximal jejunum; t_{max} ~2–3 hours after an oral dose • Bioavailability ~80% (prodrug base), ~4% (active carboxylate)
Transport	• Plasma protein binding ~42% (prodrug base), ~3% (active carboxylate) • V_d ~23–26 liters
Metabolism	• >90% of the prodrug is hydrolyzed to the active oseltamivir carboxylate by hepatic esterases, and subsequently excreted in urine. • Cl ~18 L/h

Enteral Administration and Nutrition Considerations

Compatibility, Stability, and Bioavailability Considerations
   • An extemporaneously compounded oral suspension (15 mg/mL) prepared from capsule contents using one of several vehicles (cherry

syrup, OraSweet SF) and stored in amber glass or amber polyethylene terephthalate plastic prescription bottles can be given a BUD of 5 days (room temperature) or 5 weeks (refrigerated); osmolality and viscosity were not reported.[1]

- An extemporaneously compounded oral suspension (15 mg/mL) prepared from capsule contents in one of three different vehicles (SyrSpend SF, SyrSpend SF [for reconstitution], or cherry syrup), stored in low-actinic plastic bottles at 2°C–8°C, remained stable (HPLC analysis) for 30 days; osmolality and viscosity were not reported.[2]

- An oral liquid preparation of oseltamivir made from capsule contents with sodium benzoate in purified water had minimal drug loss at 84 days whether stored at 6°C or 25°C, but the preparation required inclusion of anhydrous citric acid to maintain drug stability (HPLC analysis) and prevent calcium and magnesium phosphate precipitates.[3]

- The reconstituted commercial suspension is considered bioequivalent to the capsule formulation in healthy adults.[4]

- Capsule contents dispersed in water and administered through a nasogastric tube (tube diameter/length and flushing protocol not reported) via enteral syringe to 14 patients receiving ECMO resulted in interesting pharmacokinetic profiles; mean drug exposure was comparable to that in ambulatory patients and well above effective concentrations, but with considerable variability in these critically ill patients; specifically, there was a delay in absorption and significantly greater volume of distribution.[5]

- The administration of oseltamivir (1.5–6.5 mg/kg) by nasogastric tube (drug preparation and tube description not provided) to children during an influenza pandemic resulted in elevated concentrations far exceeding the therapeutic levels, although formal pharmacokinetic data were not evaluated.[6]

- A unique prodrug of oseltamivir carboxylate linked to valine under study is a substrate for PEPT1 uptake, with enhanced permeability and rapid intracellular hydrolysis to the parent drug, which is expected to have superior bioavailability.[7,8]

Drug-Nutrition Interactions
- Drug may influence nutrition status directly or indirectly:
  o CNS: headache, vertigo
  o GI: nausea, vomiting, diarrhea
- Influence of malnutrition or obesity on drug disposition:
  o Increased clearance of the parent drug may account for the reduced drug exposure in obesity, although this effect is not considered clinically significant enough to alter standard dosing because therapeutic concentrations are maintained.[9]

- Influence of food on oral absorption or bioavailability:
  - ○ A high-fat meal may reduce oral bioavailability compared to the fasted state, although the effect is not clinically significant.
  - ○ Despite the limited influence of food on oral bioavailability, it may improve GI tolerance to the drug.

Recommendations

Gastric	• Disperse capsule contents in water (75 mL) just prior to administration. • No need to hold EN beyond the time required to flush-administer-flush.
Postpyloric	• As above. • Monitor for any unexpected change in effect.

References

1. Winiarski AP, Infeld MH, Tscherne R, et al. Preparation and stability of extemporaneous oral liquid formulations of oseltamivir using commercially available capsules. *J Am Pharm Assoc.* 2007;47:747–755.
2. Voudrie MA, Allen DB. Stability of oseltamivir phosphate in SyrSpend SF, cherry syrup, and SyrSpend SF (for reconstitution). *Int J Pharm Compd.* 2010;14:82–85.
3. Albert K, Bockshorn J. Chemical stability of oseltamivir in oral solutions. *Pharmazie.* 2007;62:678–682.
4. Lennon S, Barrett J, Kirkpatrick C, Rayner C. Oseltamivir oral suspension and capsules are bioequivalent for the active metabolite in healthy adult volunteers. *Int J Clin Pharmacol Ther.* 2009;47:539–548.
5. Mulla H, Peek GJ, Harvey C, et al. Oseltamivir pharmacokinetics in critically ill adults receiving extracorporeal membrane oxygenation support. *Anaesth Intensive Care.* 2013;41:66–73.
6. Giraud C, Manceau S, Oualha M, et al. High levels and safety of oseltamivir carboxylate plasma concentrations after nasogastric administration in critically ill children in a pediatric intensive care unit. *Antimicrob Agent Chemother.* 2011;55:433–435.
7. Gupta D, Gupta SV, Dahan A, et al. Increasing oral absorption of polar neuraminidase inhibitors: a prodrug transporter approach applied to oseltamivir analogue. *Mol Pharm.* 2013;10:512–522.
8. Incecayir T, Sun J, Tsume Y, et al. Carrier-mediated prodrug uptake to improve the oral bioavailability of polar drugs: an application to an oseltamivir analogue. *J Pharm Sci.* 2016;105:925–934.
9. Thorne-Humphrey LM, Goralski KB, Slayter KL, et al. Oseltamivir pharmacokinetics in morbid obesity (OPTIMO trial). *J Antimicrob Chemother.* 2011;66:2083–2091.

Oxybutynin

Product Availability

Solid	• Tablet:
	   ○ Immediate-release: 5 mg (various)
	   ○ Extended-release: 5 mg, 10 mg, 15 mg (various)

Liquid	• Oral solution: 5 mg/5 mL (various)

Physicochemical (drug)

Molecular weight: • 357.50	Permeability: • LogP 4.87 (calc) • LogD n/a	Water solubility: • 0.8 mg/mL
pKa: • 6.96	Classification: • BCS Class 1; BDDCS Class 1	

Pharmaceutical (product)

Solid	• Immediate-release tablet may be crushed and dispersed in water (it does not disperse well without crushing). • Do not chew or crush extended-release tablet; the inert tablet shell may remain intact into feces following oral administration.

Liquid	• Oral solution:
	   ○ pH n/a
	   ○ Osmolality n/a
	   ○ Viscosity n/a
	   ○ May contain glycerin, sorbitol, and sucrose; raspberry-flavored
	   ○ Store at controlled room temperature.

Pharmacokinetic (patient)

Absorption	• Specific site not known; t_{max} ~1 hour after an oral dose (immediate-release) • Bioavailability ~6%
Transport	• Plasma protein binding n/a • V_d ~1.3 L/kg
Metabolism	• Extensive first-pass metabolism, mostly via CYP3A4 to desethyl-oxybutynin and inactive phenylcyclohexylglycolic acid • Cl ~8.1 mL/min/kg

Enteral Administration and Nutrition Considerations

Compatibility, Stability, and Bioavailability Considerations
• Aqueous solubility and stability is pH-dependent.
• Oxybutynin is most stable in acidic solutions and poorly soluble at pH >6.

- Liquid preparations (0.125 mg/mL) intended for irrigation made from commercial tablets either crushed or allowed to dissolve in tap water (pH 8.6) or 0.9% NaCl (pH 6.3) were not stable (GC analysis) at room temperature for 1 week or 3 weeks, respectively.[1]

Drug-Nutrition Interactions
- Drug may influence nutrition status directly or indirectly:
  - CNS: dizziness, confusion, dry eyes, blurred vision
  - GI: dry mouth, altered taste, abdominal pain, constipation more likely than diarrhea
- No data on the influence of malnutrition or obesity on drug disposition.
- Influence of food on oral absorption or bioavailability:
  - Although food may delay oral absorption, it may increase oral bioavailability (especially of the solution) by ~25%.
  - A high-fat meal can increase the rate of absorption.

Recommendations

Gastric	• If there is no therapeutic alternative (eg, transdermal system), dilute the liquid preparation in water (at least 1:1) prior to administration. • No need to hold EN beyond the time required to flush-administer-flush.
Postpyloric	• As above. • Monitor for any unexpected change in effect.

Reference

1. Wan J, Rickman C. The durability of intravesical oxybutynin solutions over time. *J Urol.* 2007;178:1768–1770.

Oxycodone Hydrochloride

Product Availability

Solid	• Tablet:
	  ○ Immediate-release: 5 mg, 7.5 mg, 10 mg, 15 mg, 20 mg, 30 mg (salt) (various)
	  ○ Extended-release: 10 mg, 15 mg, 20 mg, 30 mg, 40 mg, 60 mg, 80 mg (salt) (Oxycontin® [Purdue]; others)
	• Capsule: 5 mg (salt) (various)

Liquid	• Oral solution:
	  ○ Standard: 5 mg/5 mL (various)
	  ○ Concentrate: 100 mg/5 mL (various)

Physicochemical (drug)

Molecular weight: • 315.37 (salt 351.83)	Permeability: • LogP 0.3 • LogD 1.65 (pH 7.4)	Water solubility: • 100–167 mg/mL
pKa: • 8.3	Classification: • BCS Class 4; BDDCS Class 1	

Pharmaceutical (product)

Solid	• Do not chew or crush modified-release products. • Avoid crushing or dispersing tablets (immediate- or extended-release) for enteral access device administration (clogging risk).

Liquid	• Oral solution (standard):
	  ○ pH 1.4–4.0
	  ○ Osmolality n/a
	  ○ Viscosity n/a
	  ○ May contain glycerin and sorbitol; raspberry-flavored
	  ○ Store at controlled room temperature.

Pharmacokinetic (patient)

Absorption	• Specific site not known; t_{max} ~1 hour after an oral dose (immediate-release) • Bioavailability can be variable: ~42% (immediate-release), ~60%–87% (controlled-release)
Transport	• Plasma protein binding ~45% • V_d ~2.6 L/kg
Metabolism	• Extensively metabolized to noroxycodone (via CYP3A) and oxymorphone and noroxymorphine (via CYP2D6) and subsequently conjugated with glucuronic acid; excreted mainly in urine • Cl ~0.8 L/min but can be quite variable

Enteral Administration and Nutrition Considerations

Compatibility, Stability, and Bioavailability Considerations
- Drug was inadequately absorbed in a patient with multiple small bowel enterocutaneous fistulas.[1]

Drug-Nutrition Interactions
- Drug may influence nutrition status directly or indirectly:
  - CNS: sedation, confusion
  - GI: constipation
- No data on the influence of malnutrition or obesity on drug disposition.
- No known influence of food on oral absorption or bioavailability.

Recommendations

Gastric	• If there is no therapeutic alternative, dilute the standard oral solution in water (at least 1:1) prior to administration. • No need to hold EN beyond the time required to flush-administer-flush.
Postpyloric	• As above. • Monitor for any unexpected change in effect.

Reference

1. Viswesh VV. Unpredictable absorption of oral opioid medications in a quadriplegic patient with chronic enterocutaneous fistulas. *J Pain Palliat Care Pharmacother.* 2012;26: 254–256.

Pantoprazole Sodium

Product Availability

Solid	• Tablet: 20 mg, 40 mg (base) (Protonix® [Pfizer]; others)
Liquid	• Granules for oral suspension: 40 mg/packet (Protonix® [Pfizer])

Physicochemical (drug)

Molecular weight:	Permeability:	Water solubility:
• 383.38 (salt 405.35)	• LogP 2.11 (calc)	• 0.5 mg/mL
	• LogD n/a	
pKa:	Classification:	
• 3.92, 8.19	• BCS Class n/a; BDDCS Class 1	

Pharmaceutical (product)

Solid	• Do not crush, chew, or split tablet or granules for suspension.
	• Granules can be dissolved in 8.4% sodium bicarbonate solution in preparation for enteral delivery into the stomach.
Liquid	• Oral suspension (reconstituted):
	○ pH n/a
	○ Osmolality n/a
	○ Viscosity n/a
	○ Store at controlled room temperature.
	○ Suspension contains granules that clog feeding tubes <16 Fr, but it may be acceptable through tubes ≥16 Fr into the stomach.

Pharmacokinetic (patient)

Absorption	• Small bowel; t_{max} ~2 hours after an oral dose
	• Bioavailability ~77%
Transport	• Substrate for BCRP efflux
	• Plasma protein binding ~98%, mostly to albumin
	• V_d ~11–23.6 liters
Metabolism	• Extensively metabolized by CYP2C19 > CYP3A4, CYP2D6, CYP2C9
	• Cl ~7.6–14 L/h

Enteral Administration and Nutrition Considerations

Compatibility, Stability, and Bioavailability Considerations

- Aqueous drug stability is pH-dependent, with greater degradation at lower pH; maximum stability is at pH ~9.[1]
- Including citric acid, trisodium citrate, and monosodium citrate in a preparation of pantoprazole increased the rate of drug decomposition.[2]
- The official USP suspension (2 mg/mL) prepared from commercial tablets in 8.4% sodium bicarbonate will have a pH between 7.9 and 8.3 and can be given a BUD of 14 days when stored at 2°C–8°C.

- When the USP preparation is prepared using sodium bicarbonate powder and stored in amber polyethylene terephthalate bottles at 2°C–8°C, the drug remains stable (HPLC analysis) for 62 days.[3]
- When the USP preparation is stored in plastic at room temperature (25°C, 60% relative humidity) or refrigerated (5°C), it remains stable (HPLC analysis) for at least 1 day or 2 weeks, respectively, although the preparation's bioavailability is lower than for the tablet.[1]
- Investigators compared (a) a preparation of delayed-release granules (40 mg) added to 5 mL apple juice (Mott's) followed up with additional 5 mL aliquots and then ≤240 mL water administered orally and (b) a preparation of granules added to 10 mL apple juice in a 60 mL syringe followed up with additional aliquots and then ≤240 mL water administered by nasogastric tube (16 Fr). These preparations were bioequivalent in healthy subjects based on drug concentration-time profiles.[4]

Drug-Nutrition Interactions
- Drug may influence nutrition status directly or indirectly:
  - CNS: headache, dizziness
  - GI: vomiting, abdominal pain, atrophic gastritis with long-term use, diarrhea (including an association with *Clostridium difficile*)
  - Metabolic: osteoporosis, hypomagnesemia, vitamin B_{12} malabsorption
  - Other: arthralgia
- No data on the influence of malnutrition or obesity on drug disposition.
- Influence of food on oral absorption or bioavailability:
  - Food may delay the rate of oral absorption but with limited influence on oral bioavailability of tablets, although the effect may be more clinically relevant depending on the brand of tablet.[5]
  - Suspension may be administered 30 minutes before a meal.

Recommendations

Gastric	• If there is no therapeutic alternative (eg, esomeprazole, lansoprazole), prepare a dispersion of tablets in sodium bicarbonate solution prior to administration. • Consider holding EN for 30–60 minutes before drug administration.
Postpyloric	• As above. • Monitor for any unexpected change in effect.

References
1. Ferron GM, Ku S, Abell M, et al. Oral bioavailability of pantoprazole suspended in sodium bicarbonate solution. *Am J Health-Syst Pharm.* 2003;60:1324–1329.
2. Ekpe A, Jacobsen T. Effect of various salts on the stability of lansoprazole, omeprazole, and pantoprazole as determined by high-performance liquid chromatography. *Drug Dev Ind Pharm.* 1999;25:1057–1065.

3. Dentinger PJ, Swenson CF, Anaizi NH. Stability of pantoprazole in an extemporaneously compounded oral liquid. *Am J Health-Syst Pharm.* 2002;59:953–956.

4. Tammara B, Weisel K, Katz A, et al. Bioequivalence among three methods of administering pantoprazole granules in healthy subjects. *Am J Health-Syst Pharm.* 2009; 66:1923–1928.

5. de Campos DR, Vieira NR, Bernasconi G, et al. Bioequivalence of two enteric coated formulations of pantoprazole in healthy volunteers under fasting and fed conditions. *Arzneimitt.* 2007;57:309–314.

Paroxetine Hydrochloride or Mesylate

Product Availability

Solid	• Tablet (immediate-release):
	   ○ Hydrochloride: 10 mg, 20 mg, 30 mg, 40 mg (base) (Paxil®
	     [GSK]; others)
	   ○ Mesylate: 10 mg, 20 mg, 30 mg, 40 mg (base) (Pexeva® [Sebela])
	• Table (extended-release): 12.5 mg, 25 mg, 37.5 mg (base)
	  (Paxil CR® [GSK]; others)
	• Capsule: 7.5 mg (base) (Brisdelle® [Sebela])

Liquid	• Oral suspension: 10 mg/5 mL (base) (Paxil® [GSK]; others)

Physicochemical (drug)

Molecular weight:
• 329.37
  ○ hydrochloride salt 365.83
  ○ mesylate 425.47
	Permeability:
	• LogP 3.6
	• LogD 1.19 (pH 7.4)
		Water solubility:
		• 5.4 mg/mL
		  (hydrochloride)
		• 1000 mg/mL
		  (mesylate)

pKa: • 9.9	Classification: • BCS Class 1; BDDCS Class 1	

Pharmaceutical (product)

Solid	• Most tablet products are film-coated. • Do not crush film-coated or extended-release products. • The extended-release product is also enteric-coated.

Liquid	• Oral suspension (reconstituted):
	  ○ pH n/a
	  ○ Osmolality n/a
	  ○ Modest viscosity
	  ○ May contain glycerin, propylene glycol, saccharin, and
	    sorbitol; orange-flavored
	  ○ Store at controlled room temperature.
	  ○ Shake well before drawing up dose for administration.

Note	• The various salts are not considered bioequivalent.

Pharmacokinetic (patient)

Absorption	Specific site not known; t_{max} ~5 hours after an oral dose (immediate-release, HCl) Bioavailability is low.
Transport	Plasma protein binding ~95% V_d ~17 L/kg
Metabolism	Metabolized at least in part by CYP2D6, with metabolites excreted in urine and feces Cl ~8.6 mL/min/kg

Enteral Administration and Nutrition Considerations

Compatibility, Stability, and Bioavailability Considerations
* No data are available.

Drug-Nutrition Interactions
* Drug may influence nutrition status directly or indirectly:
  ○ Decreases appetite, with possible weight loss
  ○ CNS: asthenia, somnolence, dizziness, tremor
  ○ GI: dry mouth, nausea, constipation or diarrhea, LFT elevations
  ○ Metabolic: anemia, hyponatremia
  ○ Other: arthralgia, myalgia
* No data on the influence of malnutrition or obesity on drug disposition.
* Influence of food on oral absorption or bioavailability:
  ○ Food may increase the rate of absorption but with little influence on oral bioavailability.

Recommendations

Gastric	• If there is no therapeutic alternative (eg, fluoxetine, sertraline), dilute oral suspension in water (at least 1:1) just prior to administration. • No need to hold EN beyond the time required to flush-administer-flush.
Postpyloric	• As above. • Monitor for any unexpected change in effect.

Penicillin V Potassium

Product Availability

Solid	• Tablet: 250 mg, 500 mg (base) (various)
Liquid	• Powder for oral solution: 125 mg/5 mL, 250 mg/5 mL (base) (various)

Physicochemical (drug)

Molecular weight:	Permeability:	Water solubility:
• 350.40 (salt 388.48)	• LogP 2.09 • LogD −1.54 (pH 7.4)	• 667 mg/mL
pKa:	Classification:	
• 2.73	• BCS Class n/a; BDDCS Class 4	

Pharmaceutical (product)

Solid	• Some tablet products are film-coated. • Tablet does not disperse in water.

Liquid	• Oral suspension (reconstituted):
	  ○ pH 5–7.5
	  ○ Osmolality 2995 mOsm/kg (250 mg/5 mL product)[1]
	  ○ Viscosity n/a
	  ○ Store at 2°C–8°C and use within 14 days of reconstitution.
	  ○ Shake well before drawing up dose for administration.

Pharmacokinetic (patient)

Absorption	• Specific site not known; t_{max} ~30–60 minutes after an oral dose • Bioavailability ~60%–73%
Transport	• Substrate for OAT uptake • Plasma protein binding ~75%–89% • V_d ~0.35 L/kg
Metabolism	• Some metabolism to penicilloic acid (inactive), 6-amino-penicillanic acid, and 1 or more hydroxylated metabolites, mostly eliminated in the urine • Cl ~100–200 mL/min

Enteral Administration and Nutrition Considerations

Compatibility, Stability, and Bioavailability Considerations
- Penicillin V is more acid stable than penicillin G.
- The oral liquid reconstituted from powder (250 mg/5 mL) stored at 5°C maintained ≥90% of labeled content (spectrophotometric analysis) by 14 days.[2]

- When repackaged into plastic oral syringes (6 mL) and stored at 4°C or 25°C, an oral liquid (125 mg/5 mL) declined to <90% of labeled amount (spectrophotometric analysis) in less than 12 days (refrigerated) and in 36 hours (room temperature).[3]
- Five mL of the oral solution (250 mg/5 mL) added to and mixed with 15–240 mL EN formulations (Ensure, Ensure Plus, Osmolite, Ensure HN, Ensure Plus HN, Osmolite HN, and Vital) appeared physically compatible without phase separation or granulation, although drug stability was not evaluated.[4,5]

Drug-Nutrition Interactions
- Drug may influence nutrition status directly or indirectly:
  - GI: glossitis, stomatitis, anorexia, nausea, gastric distress, vomiting, diarrhea, enterocolitis with severe abdominal pain (± *Clostridium difficile*), LFT abnormalities
- Influence of malnutrition or obesity on drug disposition:
  - In individuals with protein-energy malnutrition, oral bioavailability and drug clearance are both reduced, compared with normal-weight subjects.[6–8]
  - As a beta-lactam antimicrobial, penicillin is expected to have a much larger volume of distribution in obesity.
- Influence of food on oral absorption or bioavailability:
  - Food may alter the rate of drug absorption but with no influence on oral bioavailability.
  - May interact with EN to cause unpredictable absorption.[9]

Recommendations

Gastric	• If there is no therapeutic alternative (eg, amoxicillin), dilute oral solution in water (at least 1:1) just prior to administration. • Hold EN for 1 hour before and at least 1 hour after drug administration.
Postpyloric	• As above. • Monitor for any unexpected change in effect.
Other	• As with all antimicrobials, consider parenteral alternative for acutely ill patients to ensure therapeutic concentrations.

References

1. Niemiec PW, Vanderveen TW, Morrison JI, et al. Gastrointestinal disorders caused by medication and electrolyte solution osmolality during enteral nutrition. *JPEN J Parenter Enteral Nutr.* 1983;7:387–389.
2. Jaffe JM, Certo NM, Pirakitikulr P, et al. Stability of several brands of ampicillin and penicillin V potassium oral liquids following reconstitution. *Am J Hosp Pharm.* 1976;33:1005–1010.

3. Grogan LJ, Jensen BK, Makoid MC, et al. Stability of penicillin V potassium in unit dose oral syringes. *Am J Hosp Pharm.* 1979;36:205–208.
4. Cutie AJ, Altman E, Lenkel L. Compatibility of enteral products with commonly employed drug additives. *JPEN J Parenter Enteral Nutr.* 1983;7:186–191.
5. Altman E, Cutie AJ. Compatibility of enteral products with commonly employed drug additives. *Nutr Supp Serv.* 1984;4:8–17.
6. Buchanan N, Robinson R, Koornhof HJ, Eyberg C. Penicillin pharmacokinetics in kwashiorkor. *Am J Clin Nutr.* 1979;32:2233–2236.
7. Mehta S, Nain CK, Sharma B, Mathur VS. Disposition of four drugs in malnourished children. *Drug Nutr Interact.* 1982;1:205–211.
8. Bolme P, Eriksson M, Paazlow L, et al. Malnutrition and pharmacokinetics of penicillin in Ethiopian children. *Pharmacol Toxicol.* 1995;76:259–262.
9. Engle KK, Hannawa TE. Techniques for administering oral medication to critical care patients receiving continuous enteral nutrition. *Am J Health-Syst Pharm.* 1999;56:1441–1444.

Phenytoin / Phenytoin Sodium

Product Availability

Solid	• Tablet: Chewable (base): 50 mg (Dilantin® Infatabs [Pfizer]; others) • Capsule (sodium salt): 30 mg, 100 mg, 200 mg, 300 mg (Dilantin® [Pfizer]; others)
Liquid	• Oral suspension (base): 125 mg/5 mL (various)

Physicochemical (drug)

Molecular weight: • 252.28 (salt 274.26)	Permeability: • LogP 2.47 • LogD 2.47 (pH 7.4)	Water solubility: • 0.02 mg/mL (base) • 15 mg/mL (sodium salt)
pKa: • 8.03–8.33 (~8.1)	Classification: • BCS Class 2; BDDCS Class 2	

Pharmaceutical (product)

Solid	• Chewable tablet may be crushed and dispersed in water; it does not disperse easily in water. • Capsule contents can be dispersed in water. • Some phenytoin sodium products are immediate-release whereas others are slow-release.

Liquid	• Oral suspension:
	   o pH 4.9 or 4.49[1,2]
	   o Osmolality 1500 mOsm/kg, or 1725 mOsm/kg, or 3095 mOsm/kg (the latter calculated based on measurement of 1:5 dilution with sterile water)[1–3]; osmolality for a 30 mg/5 mL suspension was 2000 mOsm/kg.[2]
	   o Viscosity is too high for jejunostomy administration.[4]
	   o May contain alcohol, glycerin, and sucrose; orange-vanilla-flavored
	   o Store at controlled room temperature.
	   o Shake well before drawing up dose for preparation.

Note	• 92 mg phenytoin = 100 mg phenytoin sodium • Different oral phenytoin products are not necessarily bioequivalent.

Pharmacokinetic (patient)

Absorption	• Specific site not known; t_{max} ~2–4 hours after an oral dose (immediate-release) • Bioavailability variable
Transport	• Substrate for P-glycoprotein efflux • Plasma protein binding ~95%, mostly to albumin • V_d ~0.64 L/kg

Metabolism	• Saturable hepatic oxidation to 5-hydroxy-phenyl-5-phenyl-hydantoin and other minor metabolites via CYP2C9/19 • Cl varies considerably between patients

Enteral Administration and Nutrition Considerations

Compatibility, Stability, and Bioavailability Considerations

- A saturated aqueous solution of phenytoin sodium has a pH of 11.7.
- An extemporaneously compounded oral suspension (15 mg/mL) prepared from drug powder in SyrSpend SF PH4, stored in low-actinic bottles at controlled room temperature or refrigeration, remained stable (HPLC analysis) for 90 days.[5]
- When 500 mg of suspension was diluted in 10 mL of water, 93% of the drug dose (GC analysis) was delivered to the end of a nasogastric tube sitting in 37°C water bath.[6]
- When phenytoin suspension was diluted (11 mL) before nasogastric tube administration, followed by a 20 mL flush, more than 90% of the dose was delivered (HPLC analysis) to the end of the tube when using either D5%W or 0.9% NaCl; using lactated Ringer's, sterile water for irrigation for dilution and irrigation (or skipping the irrigation step) resulted in 11%–20% drug loss.[7]
- Diluting suspension (12 mL) with deionized water (10–12 mL) resulted in 7.5%–18.5% drug loss (HPLC analysis) when administered through a latex gastrostomy tube (20 Fr, 35.5 cm), compared with losses ≤7% when undiluted.[8]
- Phenytoin delivery through a 20 Fr latex gastrostomy was best with suspension or capsule contents diluted (10 mL deionized water) or irrigation (10 mL deionized water).[9]
- Phenytoin capsule contents mixed in water before administration via nasogastric tube resulted in similar pharmacokinetics to orally administered intact capsule in a small group of hospital patients.[10]
- Administration of a preparation of immediate-release tablets with a blenderized diet via nasogastric tube resulted in higher steady-state serum concentrations than a similar preparation using extended-release capsule contents.[11]
- Administration of the IV formulation of phenytoin sodium through enteral access devices without regard to EN administration, or the IV formulation of the phosphate ester (fosphenytoin) orally, may result in less variability in bioavailability compared with the oral suspension as carried out in healthy subjects.[12,13]
- Phenytoin has greater affinity for casein protein compared with whey protein, with significantly greater loss after filtration (>50% vs <20%) when drug solutions (20 mg/mL) were admixed (1:1) with EN products (Replete, Ultracal) or isolated protein mixture.[14]

- Oral suspension was evaluated at a concentration of 10 mg/L in a variety of solutions (calcium caseinate, sodium caseinate, both, calcium chloride); following admixture, centrifugation, and filtration, the losses were ~20%–50% (HPLC analysis) compared with the distilled water control.[15]
- Phenytoin exhibited significant loss following filtration (~61%–68%) when drug solutions (20 mg/mL) made from tablet, suspension, or pure powder were admixed (1:1) with casein-based EN products (Replete, Ultracal).[14]
- Depending on the solution's pH, the protein binding may increase the solubility of the drug in solution.[16]
- When suspension (5 mL) was added to and thoroughly mixed with 15–240 mL of EN formulations (Ensure, Ensure Plus, Osmolite, Ensure HN, Ensure Plus HN, Osmolite HN, and Vital), it appeared to remain physically compatible, although drug stability was not evaluated.[17,18]
- When suspension (16 mL) was added to and thoroughly mixed with 10 mL of EN formulations (Enrich, TwoCal HN, Vivonex T.E.N), it appeared to remain physically compatible, although drug stability was not evaluated.[19]
- When phenytoin pediatric suspension was added to Osmolite, only 37% of the drug could be recovered following ultrafiltration, compared with 99% recovery when the suspension was added to distilled water of the same pH.[20]
- The contents (100 mg) of a phenytoin sodium capsule diluted in deionized water and then dispersed in 240 mL of enteral formulas (Isocal, Sustacal, Sustacal HC) had no visible physical change after 24 hours at 24°C, with the drug remaining stable (HPLC analysis) prior to ultrafiltration, but only 18%–30% of drug remained following ultrafiltration of the admixtures.[21]
- Adding suspension at 300 mg/L to Ensure, Ensure Plus, or Osmolite resulted in no significant change in physical appearance, osmolality, or viscosity by 12 hours at room temperature, but with highly variable drug concentrations (HPLC analysis) with losses.[3]
- Commercial suspension combined (1:1) with Osmolite 1.2, under simulated clinical conditions, would result in clogging of an 8 Fr, but not a 20 Fr feeding tube.[2]
- Despite the significantly greater aqueous solubility of the sodium salt compared with other salts, oral bioavailability is no different.[22]
- Phenytoin tablet crushed and mixed with pudding (vanilla) resulted in low serum concentrations, whereas serum concentrations are elevated when the tablet was mixed with apple sauce.[23]
- Amorphous solid dispersion formulations under study exhibited improved drug dissolution and solubility compared with pure drug, with the potential to improve oral bioavailability.[24]

- Compared with the commercially available oral suspension, a self-emulsifying formulation under study exhibited improved dissolution, faster absorption, and greater bioavailability in an animal model.[25]
- Oral bioavailability may be reduced following Roux-en-Y gastric bypass, based on steady-state serum concentrations.[26]

Drug-Nutrition Interactions
- Drug may influence nutrition status directly or indirectly:
  - Weight loss, folate deficit, carnitine deficit, and interference with vitamin D metabolism are all possible.
  - CNS: ataxia, confusion, altered vision, headache
  - GI: loss of taste, dysphagia, nausea, vomiting, abdominal pain, constipation
  - Metabolic: osteomalacia
  - Other: sensory peripheral neuropathy
- Influence of malnutrition or obesity on drug disposition:
  - The weight-normalized (and absolute) volume of distribution is increased in obesity, but without significant or consistent differences in total drug clearance, suggesting use of an adjusted body weight greater than total body weight for loading dose, with close therapeutic monitoring.[27-29]
  - Carnitine deficiency may increase drug toxicity.[30]
- Influence of food on oral absorption or bioavailability:
  - Food may reduce the oral bioavailability of some brands of extended-release products.[31]
  - Grapefruit juice has no influence on oral bioavailability.[32]

Recommendations

Gastric	• Dilute suspension with water (at least 1:1) just prior to administration. • Alternative: Disperse capsule contents in water just prior to administration. • Holding EN is not necessary, but could hold EN for 1 hour before and 1 hour after drug administration. • Maintain consistent method of administration, with dose adjustments as needed based on appropriate therapeutic drug monitoring.
Postpyloric	• Avoid. • Monitor for any unexpected change in effect.

References

1. Dickerson RN, Melnik G. Osmolality of oral drug solutions and suspensions. *Am J Hosp Pharm.* 1988;45:832–834.
2. Klang M, McLymont V, Ng N. Osmolality, pH, and compatibility of selected oral liquid medications with an enteral nutrition product. *JPEN J Parenter Enteral Nutr.* 2013;37:689–694.

3. Holtz L, Milton J, Sturek JK. Compatibility of medications with enteral feedings. *JPEN J Parenter Enteral Nutr.* 1987;11:183–186.
4. Rodman DP, Stevenson TL, Ray TR. Phenytoin malabsorption after jejunostomy tube delivery. *Pharmacotherapy.* 1995;15:801–805.
5. Ferreira AO, Polonini HC, Silva SL, et al. Feasibility of amlodipine besylate, chloroquine phosphate, dapsone, phenytoin, pyridoxine hydrochloride, sulfadiazine, sulfasalazine, tetracycline hydrochloride, trimethoprim and zonisamide in SyrSpend SF PH4 oral suspensions. *J Pharm Biomed Anal.* 2016;118:105–112.
6. Ozuna J, Friel P. Effect of enteral tube feeding on serum phenytoin levels. *J Neurosurg Nurs.* 1984;16:289–291.
7. Cacek AT, DeVito JM, Koonce JR. In vitro evaluation of nasogastric administration methods for phenytoin. *Am J Hosp Pharm.* 1986;43:689–692.
8. Splinter MY, Seifert CF, Bradberry JC, et al. Recovery of phenytoin suspension after in vitro administration through percutaneous endoscopic gastrostomy Pezzer catheters. *Am J Hosp Pharm.* 1990;47:373–377.
9. Seifert CF, McGoodwin PL, Allen LV. Phenytoin recovery from percutaneous endoscopic gastrostomy Pezzer catheters after long-term in vitro administration. *JPEN J Parenter Enteral Nutr.* 1993;17:370–374.
10. Lubart E, Berkovitch M, Leibovitz A, et al. Phenytoin blood concentrations in hospitalized geriatric patients: oral versus nasogastric feeding tube administration. *Ther Drug Monitor.* 2010;32:185–188.
11. Panomvana D, Khummuenwal N, Sraium S, et al. Steady-state serum phenytoin concentrations after nasogastric tube administration of immediate-release phenytoin tablets and extended-release phenytoin capsules: an open-label, crossover, clinical trial. *Curr Ther Res Clin Exp.* 2007;68:325–337.
12. Doak KK, Haas CE, Dunnigan KJ, et al. Bioavailability of phenytoin acid and phenytoin sodium with enteral feedings. *Pharmacotherapy.* 1998;18:637–645.
13. Kaucher KA, Acquisto NM, Rao GG, et al. Relative bioavailability of orally administered fosphenytoin sodium injection compared with phenytoin sodium injection in healthy volunteers. *Pharmacotherapy.* 2015;35:482–488.
14. Hennessey DD. Recovery of phenytoin from feeding formulas and protein mixtures. *Am J Health-Syst Pharm.* 2003;60:1850–1852.
15. Smith OB, Longe RL, Altman RE, et al. Recovery of phenytoin from solutions of caseinate salts and calcium chloride. *Am J Hosp Pharm.* 1988;45:365–368.
16. Rosen A, Machera P. The effect of protein on the dissolution of phenytoin. *J Pharm Pharmacol.* 1984;36:723–727.
17. Cutie AJ, Altman E, Lenkel L. Compatibility of enteral products with commonly employed drug additives. *JPEN J Parenter Enteral Nutr.* 1983;7:186–191.
18. Altman E, Cutie AJ. Compatibility of enteral products with commonly employed drug additives. *Nutr Supp Serv.* 1984;4:8–17.
19. Burns PE, McCall L, Wirsching R. Physical compatibility of enteral formulas with various common medications. *J Am Diet Assoc.* 1988;88:1094–1096.
20. Hooks MA, Longe RL, Taylor AT, et al. Recovery of phenytoin from an enteral nutrient formula. *Am J Hosp Pharm.* 1986;43:685–688.
21. Miller SW, Strom JG. Stability of phenytoin in three enteral nutrient formulas. *Am J Hosp Pharm.* 1988;45:2529–2532.
22. Chiang P-C, Wong H. Incorporation of physiologically based pharmacokinetic modeling in the evaluation of solubility requirements for the salt selection process: a case study using phenytoin. *AAPS J.* 2013;15:1109–1118.
23. Jann MW, Bean J, Fidone GS. Interaction of dietary pudding with phenytoin. *Pediatrics.* 1986;78:952–953.

24. Widanapathirana L, Tale S, Reineke TM. Dissolution and solubility enhancement of the highly lipophilic drug phenytoin via interaction with poly(N-isopropylacrylamide-co-vinylpyrrolidone) excipients. *Mol Pharm.* 2015;12:2537–2543.
25. Atef E, Belmonte AA. Formulation and in vitro and in vivo characterization of a phenytoin self-emulsifying drug delivery system (SEDDS). *Eur J Pharm Sci.* 2008;35:257–263.
26. Pournaras DJ, Footitt D, Mahon D, et al. Reduced phenytoin levels in an epileptic patient following Roux-en-Y gastric bypass for obesity. *Obes Surg.* 2011;21:684–685.
27. Abernathy DR, Greenblatt DJ. Phenytoin disposition in obesity: determination of loading dose. *Arch Neurol.* 1985;42:468–471.
28. de Oca GM, Gums JG, Robinson JD. Phenytoin dosing in obese patients: two case reports. *Drug Intell Clin Pharm.* 1988;22:708–710.
29. Olsen KM, Marx MA, Monoghan MS, et al. Phenytoin and plasmapheresis: importance of sampling times and impact of obesity. *Ther Drug Monitor.* 1994;16:624–628.
30. Ling P, Lee DJ, Yoshida EM, Sirrs S. Carnitine deficiency presenting with encephalopathy and hyperammonemia in a patient receiving chronic enteral tube feeding: a case report. *J Med Case Report.* 2012;6:227 (4 pages).
31. Wilder BJ, Leppik I, Hietpas TJ, et al. Effect of food on absorption of Dilantin Kapseals and Mylan extended phenytoin sodium capsules. *Neurology.* 2001;57:582–589.
32. Kumar N, Garg SK, Prabhakar S. lack of pharmacokinetic interaction between grapefruit juice and phenytoin in healthy male volunteers and epileptic patients. *Methods Find Exp Clin Pharmacol.* 1999;21:629–632.

Posaconazole

Product Availability

Solid	• Tablet: 100 mg (Noxafil® [Merck])
Liquid	• Oral suspension: 40 mg/mL (Noxafil® [Schering])

Physicochemical (drug)

Molecular weight:	Permeability:	Water solubility:
• 700.78	• LogP 5.5 • LogD 3.37 (pH 5.5), 4.57 (pH 7.4)	• <0.0001 mg/mL
pKa: • 3.93, 14.83 or 3.6, 4.6	Classification: • BCS Class n/a; BDDCS Class 2	

Pharmaceutical (product)

Solid	• Do not crush or chew tablet (delayed-release).
Liquid	• Oral suspension: o pH 4.52 o Osmolality 2050 mOsm/kg (calculated based on measurement of 1:5 dilution with sterile water)[1] o Viscosity n/a o May contain glycerin and glucose; cherry-flavored o Store at controlled room temperature. o Shake well prior to measuring a dose for administration.
Note	• Tablet and suspension are not interchangeable.

Pharmacokinetic (patient)

Absorption	• Specific site not known; t_{max} ~3 hours (suspension) or ~4–5 hours (tablet) after an oral dose • Saturable absorption • Bioavailability ~54% (tablet, fasting); bioavailability is much more variable for suspension
Transport	• Substrate for P-glycoprotein efflux • Plasma protein binding ~98%, especially to albumin • V_d ~261 liters
Metabolism	• Up to one-third of a dose undergoes glucuronidation via UGT1A4, with the conjugated drug eliminated into feces and urine • Cl ~7.3 L/h

Enteral Administration and Nutrition Considerations

Compatibility, Stability, and Bioavailability Considerations
- Nasogastric tube administration of oral suspension (undiluted) results in a 24% lower bioavailability compared with oral administration.[2]
- Oral suspension (~600–800 mg/d) was less likely to achieve goal serum concentrations compared with oral tablet (~300–400 mg/d) in retrospective analyses and in a prospective study of patients with hematological malignancy (most often acute myeloid leukemia).[3-7]
- The oral bioavailability of the suspension is more likely to be reduced from altered gut pH than is the tablet formulation in healthy subjects.[8,9]
- Subtherapeutic drug concentrations in ~40% patients were most commonly associated with a lack of EN.[10]
- The commercial oral suspension combined (1:1) with Osmolite 1.2, under simulated clinical conditions, would result in no clogging of either an 8 Fr or a 20 Fr feeding tube.[1]

Drug-Nutrition Interactions
- Drug may influence nutrition status directly or indirectly:
  o Decreased appetite, decreased body weight
  o CNS: headache, fatigue
  o GI: anorexia; nausea, vomiting, abdominal pain, and diarrhea; increased AST, ALT, and alkaline phosphatase; cholestasis and rare hepatic failure
  o Metabolic: hypokalemia, edema, hypomagnesemia, hypocalcemia, hyperglycemia
- Influence of malnutrition or obesity on drug disposition:
  o Obese patients may have lower systemic exposure than patients with BMI <30 kg/m^2.[11-13]
- Influence of food on oral absorption or bioavailability:
  o Tablets should be taken with food.
  o Oral suspension should be taken with or following a meal to maximize bioavailability.
  o A high-fat meal (900–1000 kcal, 55%–60% fat) increased oral bioavailability from the tablet formulation 1.5 times.[14]
  o A nonfat meal (461 kcal, 0% fat) increased bioavailability from the oral suspension by 2.6 times, and a high-fat meal (841 kcal, 52% fat) increased bioavailability from the oral suspension by 3.9 times.[15]
  o Oral administration with 240 mL Boost Plus (360 kcal, 34% fat) increased bioavailability from the oral suspension 2.6 times.[16]
  o Varying the volume of Boost Plus between 30 mL and 240 mL, administered orally with the suspension (400 mg), resulted in increased oral bioavailability in a nearly linear fashion from the suspension alone.[17]
  o Ginger ale increased bioavailability from the oral suspension 1.7 times.

Recommendations

Gastric	• If there is no therapeutic alternative, dilute oral suspension with water (at least 1:1) just prior to administration. • No need to hold EN beyond the time required to flush-administer-flush; administer immediately following an intermittent feed.
Postpyloric	• Not recommended. • Monitor for any unexpected change in effect.
Other	• As with all antimicrobials, consider parenteral alternative for acutely ill patients to ensure therapeutic concentrations.

References

1. Klang M, McLymont V, Ng N. Osmolality, pH, and compatibility of selected oral liquid medications with an enteral nutrition product. *JPEN J Parenter Enteral Nutr.* 2013;37: 689–694.
2. Dodds Ashley ES, Varkey JB, Krishna G, et al. Pharmacokinetics of posaconazole administered orally or by nasogastric tube in healthy volunteers. *Antimcrob Agents Chemother.* 2009;53:2960–2964.
3. Durani U, Tosh PK, Barreto JN, et al. Retrospective comparison of posaconazole levels in patients taking the delayed-release tablet versus the oral suspension. *Antimicrob Agents Chemother.* 2015;59:4914–4918.
4. Pham AN, Bubalo JS, Lewis JS. Comparison of posaconazole serum concentrations from haematological cancer patients on posaconazole tablet and oral suspension for treatment and prevention of invasive fungal infections. *Mycoses.* 2016;59:226–233.
5. Belling M, Kanate AS, Shillingburg A, et al. Evaluation of serum posaconazole concentrations in patients with hematological malignancies receiving posaconazole suspension compared to the delayed-release tablet formulation. *Leuk Res Treatment.* 2017;ID 3460892 (6 pages).
6. Suh HJ, Kim I, Cho J-Y, et al. Comparison of plasma concentrations of posaconazole with the oral suspension and tablet in Korean patients with hematologic malignancies. *Infect Chemother.* 2017;49:135–139.
7. Leclerc E, Combarel D, Uzunov M, et al. Prevention of invasive Aspergillus fungal infections with the suspension and delayed-release tablet formulations of posaconazole in patients with haematologic malignancies. *Sci Rep.* 2018;8(1):1681. doi:10.1038/s41598-018-20136-3.
8. Walravens J, Brouwers J, Spriet I, et al. Effect of pH and comedication on gastrointestinal absorption of posaconazole. *Clin Pharmacokinet.* 2011;50:725–734.
9. Kraft WK, Chang PS, van Iersel MLPS, et al. Posaconazole tablet pharmacokinetics: lack of effect of concomitant medications altering gastric pH and gastric motility in healthy subjects. *Antimicrob Agents Chemother.* 2014;58:4020–4025.
10. van der Elst KCM, Brouwers CHS, van den Heuvel ER, et al. Subtherapeutic posaconazole exposure and treatment outcome in patients with invasive fungal disease. *Ther Drug Monit.* 2015;37:766–771.
11. Kuipers S, Bruggemann RJ, de Sevaux RG, et al. Failure of posaconazole therapy in a renal transplant patient with invasive aspergillosis due to Aspergillus fumigatus with attenuated susceptibility to posaconazole. *Antimicrob Agents Chemother.* 2011;55: 3564–3566.
12. Pettis JJ, Hyche SR, Logan KN, et al. Effects of obesity on posaconazole kinetics in a patient with graft versus host disease. *Pharmacol Pharm.* 2013;4:244–247.

13. Miceli MH, Perissinotti AJ, Kauffman CA, Couriel DR. Serum posaconazole levels among haematological cancer patients taking extended release tablets is affected by body weight and diarrhea: single centre retrospective analysis. *Mycoses*. 2015;58:432–436.
14. Kersemaekers WM, Dogterom P, Xu J, et al. Effect of a high-fat meal on the pharmacokinetics of 300-milligram posaconazole in a solid oral tablet formulation. *Antimicrob Agents Chemother*. 2015;59:3385–3389.
15. Courtney R, Wexler D, Radwanski E, et al. Effect of food on the relative bioavailability of two oral formulations of posaconazole in healthy adults. *Br J Clin Pharmacol*. 2003; 57:218–222.
16. Sansone-Parsons A, Krishna G, Calzetta A, et al. Effect of a nutritional supplement on posaconazole pharmacokinetics following oral administration to healthy volunteers. *Antimicrob Agents Chemother*. 2006;50:1881–1883.
17. Krishna G, Ma L, Vickery D, et al. Effect of varying amounts of a liquid nutritional supplement on the pharmacokinetics of posaconazole in healthy volunteers. *Antimicrob Agents Chemother*. 2009;53:4749–4752.

Potassium Chloride

Product Availability

Solid	• Tablet:
	  ○ Immediate-release: 2.5 mEq, 8 mEq, 10 mEq (various)
	  ○ Extended-release: 8 mEq, 10 mEq, 15 mEq, 20 mEq
	  (Klor-Con® [Upsher-Smith]; others)
	• Capsule: Extended-release: 8 mEq, 10 mEq (Micro-K®
	  [Nesher]; others)

Liquid	• Powder for solution: 20 mEq, 25 mEq (Klor-Con® [Upsher-Smith]; others) • Oral solution: 6.7 mEq/5 mL, 10 mEq/5 mL, 13.3 mEq/5 mL (various)

Physicochemical (drug)

Molecular weight: • 74.56 (salt)	Permeability: • LogP –2.14 (calc) • LogD n/a	Water solubility: • 333–357 mg/mL (salt)
pKa: • n/a	Classification: • BCS Class n/a; BDDCS Class 3	

Pharmaceutical (product)

Solid	• Most tablet products are film-coated. • Do not crush film-coated or extended-release products. • Effervescent product may be diluted as per manufacturer instructions.

Liquid	Oral solution:
	• pH varies by product:
	  ○ 7.5–8.5 (aqueous solutions)
	  ○ 3.29 (a 10% KCl product)
	  ○ 6.2 (a KCl elixir)
	  ○ 4.1 (a KCl 10% product)
	  ○ 3.8 (a KCl 20% product)
	  ○ 2.4 (a KCl syrup)
	  ○ 4.7 (KCl granules)
	• Osmolality varies by product:
	  ○ 10% KCl product: ~3000–4350 mOsm/kg;[1,2] 4225 mOsm/
	  kg (calculated based on measurement of 1:5 dilution with
	  sterile water)[3]
	  ○ 1 mEq/mL potassium glucoheptonate product:
	  1998 mOsm/kg;[4] 400 mOsm/kg when diluted 4:1 with
	  water[4]
	• Viscosity n/a

Pharmacokinetic (patient)

Absorption	• Proximal small bowel; t_{max} ~1 hour after an oral dose (immediate-release) • Bioavailability ~70%–90%
Transport	• Not bound to plasma proteins • V_d n/a
Metabolism	• Excreted mainly through the kidneys • Cl ~100–200 mL/min

Enteral Administration and Nutrition Considerations

Compatibility, Stability, and Bioavailability Considerations
- The low pH of many liquid KCl products increases the risk for incompatibility with EN and feeding tube obstruction.
- The admixture of 15 mL KCl elixir (10% or 20%) or KCl syrup with 15–240 mL of EN formulations (Ensure, Ensure Plus, Osmolite) was noted to be physically incompatible on visual inspection, with the latter forming a gelatinous mixture (pH 3.4).[5]
- The admixture of 15 mL KCl elixir with 15–240 mL of EN formulations (Ensure HN, Ensure Plus HN, Osmolite HN, Vital) appeared physically compatible (no granulation, no phase separation) on visual inspection; however, KCl 10%, KCl 20%, and KCl syrups were each physically incompatible with these 4 EN formulations.[6]
- The admixture of KCl elixir (15 mL) with 10 mL of EN formula (Enrich, TwoCal HN, Vivonex T.E.N.) revealed no physical incompatibility on visual inspection.[7]
- A commercial 10% KCl sugar-free solution combined (1:1) with Osmolite 1.2, under simulated clinical conditions, would result in no clogging of either an 8 Fr or a 20 Fr feeding tube.[3]
- Potassium gluconate (20 mEq/15 mL) admixed at equal volumes with several EN formulations (Osmolite, Osmolite HN, Vital) revealed formula thickening with a precipitate forming over time; however, a KCl packet (20 mEq) admixed with these 3 EN formulations appeared physically compatible without thickening or precipitate formation.[8]
- A dose of oral liquid admixed with 200 mL of an EN product (Precitene) appeared physically compatible (no phase separation or particle growth), without a change in viscosity or osmolality.[9]

Drug-Nutrition Interactions
- Drug may influence nutrition status directly or indirectly:
  - GI: nausea, vomiting, abdominal discomfort, diarrhea
  - Metabolic: hyperkalemia
- No data on the influence of malnutrition or obesity on drug disposition.
- Influence of food on oral absorption or bioavailability:
  - No known influence of food on oral bioavailability, but taking the drug with or after meals helps limit GI irritation.

Recommendations

Gastric	• Select a liquid product with pH >4 and dilute with water (at least 3:1) prior to administration.
	• Alternative: Dissolve effervescent or dispersible tablets in at least 60 mL of water prior to administration.
	• No need to hold EN beyond the time required to flush-administer-flush.
Postpyloric	• As above; consider higher dilution (>3:1) for this route.
	• Monitor for any unexpected change in effect.

References

1. Niemiec PW, Vanderveen TW, Morrison JI, et al. Gastrointestinal disorders caused by medication and electrolyte solution osmolality during enteral nutrition. *JPEN J Parenter Enteral Nutr.* 1983;7:387–389.
2. Dickerson RN, Melnik G. Osmolality of oral drug solutions and suspensions. *Am J Hosp Pharm.* 1988;45:832–834.
3. Klang M, McLymont V, Ng N. Osmolality, pH, and compatibility of selected oral liquid medications with an enteral nutrition product. *JPEN J Parenter Enteral Nutr.* 2013;37: 689–694.
4. Fernández Polo A, Cabañas Poy MJ, Clemente Bautista S, et al. Osmolality of oral liquid dosage forms to be administered to newborns in a hospital. *Farm Hosp.* 2007;31: 311–314.
5. Cutie AJ, Altman E, Lenkel L. Compatibility of enteral products with commonly employed drug additives. *JPEN J Parenter Enteral Nutr.* 1983;7:186–191.
6. Altman E, Cutie AJ. Compatibility of enteral products with commonly employed drug additives. *Nutr Supp Serv.* 1984;4:8–17.
7. Burns PE, McCall L, Wirsching R. Physical compatibility of enteral formulas with various common medications. *J Am Diet Assoc.* 1988;88:1094–1096.
8. Fagerman KE, Ballou AE. Drug compatibilities with enteral feeding solutions coadministered by tube. *Nutr Supp Serv.* 1988;8:31–32.
9. Ortega de la Cruz C, Fernández Gallardo LC, Damas Fernández-Figares M, García Martínez E. Compatibilidad físico-química de medicamentos con nutrición enteral. *Nutr Hosp.* 1993;8:105–108.

Pramipexole Dihydrochloride
Product Availability

Solid	• Tablet:
	   o Immediate-release: 0.125 mg, 0.25 mg, 0.5 mg, 0.75 mg,
	     1 mg, 1.5 mg (Mirapex® [Boehringer-Ingelheim]; others)
	   o Extended-release: 0.375 mg, 0.75 mg, 1.5 mg, 2.25 mg, 3 mg,
	     3.75 mg, 4.5 mg (Mirapex® ER [Boehringer-Ingelheim];
	     others)

Physicochemical (drug)

Molecular weight: • 211.33 (salt 284.24)	Permeability: • LogP 1.76 (calc) • LogD –0.77 (pH7)	Water solubility: • ≥20 mg/mL
pKa: • 9.60	Classification: • BCS Class 1; BDDCS Class n/a	

Pharmaceutical (product)

Solid	• Do not crush or chew extended-release tablet.

Pharmacokinetic (patient)

Absorption	• Specific site not known; t_{max} ~2 hours after an oral dose • Bioavailability ~90%
Transport	• Substrate for organic cation transporter (OCT3) uptake • Plasma protein binding ~15% • V_d ~500 liters
Metabolism	• Less than 10% of the drug is metabolized, with the drug excreted in urine. • Cl ~400 mL/min

Enteral Administration and Nutrition Considerations

Compatibility, Stability, and Bioavailability Considerations
• No data are available.

Drug-Nutrition Interactions
• Drug may influence nutrition status directly or indirectly:
   o Weight loss
   o CNS: somnolence, confusion, dyskinesia, visual abnormalities
   o GI: dry mouth, nausea, dysphagia, constipation
   o Other: rare rhabdomyolysis
• No data on the influence of malnutrition or obesity on drug disposition.
• Influence of food on oral absorption or bioavailability:
   o Food may decrease the rate of drug absorption but with no influence
     on oral bioavailability.

Recommendations

Gastric	• Crush and disperse immediate-release tablet in water prior to administration. • No need to hold EN beyond the time required to flush-administer-flush.
Postpyloric	• As above. • Monitor for any unexpected change in effect.

Pravastatin Sodium

Product Availability

Solid	• Tablet: 20 mg, 40 mg, 80 mg (Pravachol® [Bristol Myers Squibb]; others)

Physicochemical (drug)

Molecular weight: • 424.54 (salt 446.52)	Permeability: • LogP 2.18 • LogD –0.23 (pH 7.4)	Water solubility: • >300 mg/mL (25°C)
pKa: • 4.7	Classification: • BCS Class 3; BDDCS Class 3	

Pharmaceutical (product)

Solid	• Uncoated tablet disperses in water; some products may require crushing prior to dispersion.

Pharmacokinetic (patient)

Absorption	• Specific site not known; t_{max} ~1.5 hours following oral dose • Bioavailability ~17%
Transport	• Substrate for MRP2 efflux • Substrate for OATP1B1 uptake • Plasma protein binding ~50% • V_d ~0.46 L/kg
Metabolism	• Does not require hydrolysis like lactone prodrugs (ie, lovastatin, simvastatin), but exhibits extensive first-pass effect as it undergoes isomerization and ring hydroxylation • Cl ~13.5 mL/min/kg

Enteral Administration and Nutrition Considerations

Compatibility, Stability, and Bioavailability Considerations
- A 5% aqueous solution has a pH of 7.2–9.0.
- A simple aqueous suspension prepared from pravastatin tablets in warm (55°C) water disintegrated well.[1]
  o Brand name product dispersed in water within 10 minutes.
  o Some generic products required crushing first to allow for complete dispersion.
  o All aqueous suspensions were delivered through a feeding with nearly 100% recovery at the distal end.
- Extemporaneously compounded oral suspensions (10 mg/mL) prepared from tablets (40 mg) in either (a) simple syrup and 1% methylcellulose (1:10) or (b) OraSweet and OraPlus (1:1), stored in plastic bottles at 4°C or 25°C, remained stable (HPLC analysis) for at least 7 days.[2]

- Given drug instability at gastric pH, delivery into the duodenum, as suggested with enteric-coated formulations in development, may improve bioavailability.[3,4]

Drug-Nutrition Interactions
- Drug may influence nutrition status directly or indirectly:
  - CNS: headache, fatigue
  - GI: anorexia, stomatitis, taste disturbance, nausea, vomiting, dyspepsia, abdominal pain, diarrhea, elevated transaminases (may be >3 times upper normal level), rare hepatitis and pancreatitis
  - Metabolic: elevated HbA1c
  - Other: myalgia, elevated creatine kinase, severe myopathy
- No data on the influence of malnutrition or obesity on drug disposition.
- Influence of food on oral absorption or bioavailability:
  - Food may reduce oral bioavailability by ~35% but without consequence to lipid-lowering effect.
  - In healthy volunteers, orange juice (300 mL before, 100 mL with, and 100 mL after drug administration) increased the oral bioavailability of pravastatin (1.5-fold) compared with water.[5]
  - Grapefruit juice with or within 4 hours of drug administration has no influence on oral bioavailability.[6]

Recommendations

Gastric	• Crush and/or disperse tablet in water prior to administration. • No need to hold EN beyond the time required to flush-administer-flush.
Postpyloric	• As above. • Monitor for any unexpected change in effect.

References

1. Yano K, Ikarashi N, Ito K, et al. Comparison of the pravastatin original and generic drugs in the simple suspension method. *Iryo Yakugaku (Jpn J Pharm Health Care Sci).* 2008;34:699–704.
2. Nahata MC. Stability of levothyroxine, doxycycline, hydrocortisone, and pravastatin in liquid dosage forms stored at two temperatures. *Int J Pharm Compd.* 2015;19:428–431.
3. Tayel SA, El-Nabarawi MA, Tadros MI, Abd-Elsalam WH. Duodenum-triggered delivery of pravastatin sodium via enteric surface-coated nanovesicular spanlastic dispersions: development, characterization and pharmacokinetic assessments. *Int J Pharm.* 2015;483:77–88.
4. Tayel SA, El-Nabarawi MA, Tadros MI, Abd-Elsalam WH. Duodenum-triggered delivery of pravastatin sodium: II. Design, appraisal and pharmacokinetic assessments of enteric surface-decorated nanocubosomal dispersions. *Drug Deliv.* 2016;23:3266–3278.
5. Koitabashi Y, Kumai T, Matsumoto N, et al. Orange juice increased the bioavailability of pravastatin, 3-hydroxy-3-methylglutaryl CoA reductase inhibitor, in rats and healthy human subjects. *Life Sci.* 2006;78:2852–2859.
6. Bailey DG. Fruit juice inhibition of uptake transport: a new type of food-drug interaction. *Br J Clin Pharmacol.* 2010;70:645–655.

Prednisone

Product Availability

Solid	• Tablet:
	   o Immediate-release: 1 mg, 2.5 mg, 5 mg, 10 mg, 20 mg,
	     50 mg (various)
	   o Delayed-release: 1 mg, 2 mg, 5 mg (various)

Liquid	• Oral solution: 5 mg/5 mL (various) • Oral concentrate: 5 mg/mL (various)

Physicochemical (drug)

Molecular weight: • 358.44	Permeability: • LogP 1.46 • LogD 1.46 (pH 7.4)	Water solubility: • 0.133 mg/mL
pKa: • n/a	Classification: • BCS Class 3; BDDCS Class 2	

Pharmaceutical (product)

Solid	• Low-dose immediate-release tablet (<20 mg) may disperse in water (20 mL) within 5 minutes. • Do not crush or chew delayed-release tablet.

Liquid	• Oral:
	   o pH 2.6–3.6 (solution), 3.0–4.5 (concentrate)
	   o Osmolality n/a
	   o Viscosity n/a
	   o Oral concentrate should be diluted prior to administration; it may contain 30% ethanol.

Pharmacokinetic (patient)

Absorption	• Specific site not known; t_{max} ~1–2 hours after an oral dose (immediate-release) • Bioavailability ~80%
Transport	• Substrate for P-glycoprotein efflux • Plasma protein binding ~75% • V_d ~0.97 L/kg
Metabolism	• Rapidly reduced to prednisolone for pharmacologic activity; subsequently hydroxylated and conjugated prior to renal elimination • Cl ~3.6 mL/min/kg

Enteral Administration and Nutrition Considerations

Compatibility, Stability, and Bioavailability Considerations
- A dose of oral liquid admixed with 200 mL of an EN product (Precitene) appeared physically compatible (no phase separation or particle growth), without a change in viscosity or osmolality.[1]

- An extemporaneously compounded oral suspension (0.5 mg/mL) prepared from prednisone powder, first dissolved in ethanol and then diluted with simple syrup, stored in amber bottles at 24°C, remained stable (HPLC analysis) after 84 days.[2]
- An extemporaneously compounded oral liquid (0.5 mg/mL) prepared from drug powder initially dissolved in ethanol and then diluted further resulted in crystallization when the diluting vehicle was water, citrate buffer (pH 4.4), sorbitol (50%), or sucrose (50%), resulting in losses of at least 20% (HPLC analysis). When glycerin (50%) was used as the diluting vehicle, the preparation remained stable for 92 days.[3]
- An extemporaneously compounded oral suspension (5 mg/mL) prepared from tablets in water and simple syrup plus flavoring resulted in similar oral bioavailability as the intact tablet in volunteers.[4]
- An extemporaneously compounded oral suspension (10 mg/mL) prepared from powder (or tablets) in a complex formula that included simple syrup and cherry syrup (2:1), remained easy to redisperse without caking or coalescence and without drug loss (analysis method not reported) after being refrigerated for 2 months.[5]
- A solid dispersion formulation in development improved drug dissolution, which may enhance bioavailability.[6]
- Oral bioavailability is reduced following gastric bypass.[7]

Drug-Nutrition Interactions

- Drug may influence nutrition status directly or indirectly.
  - Increased appetite; decreased vitamin A and vitamin C concentrations
  - CNS: headache, vertigo, insomnia, ocular effects (eg, amblyopia, transient blindness)
  - GI: anorexia, nausea, vomiting, gastritis, abdominal distension, pancreatitis
  - Metabolic: adrenal insufficiency, osteoporotic fracture with long-term use, hyperglycemia, edema, hypokalemia, hypocalcemia, hyperkaluria, hypercalciuria
  - Other: acute myopathy, muscle loss and weakness, poor wound healing, easy bruising
- Influence of malnutrition or obesity on drug disposition:
  - In obesity, body weight–normalized volume of distribution is decreased, whereas total body clearance is increased. Given the increased drug sensitivity in obesity, no dose change is suggested. If using weight-based dosing, consider using total body weight.[8]
- Influence of food on oral absorption or bioavailability:
  - Compared with a full or light meal, the fasted state may reduce oral bioavailability.[9]
  - Grapefruit juice has no influence on oral bioavailability.[10]

Recommendations

Gastric	• Disperse low-dose tablet in water prior to administration. • No need to hold EN beyond the time required to flush-administer-flush.
Postpyloric	• As above. • Monitor for any unexpected change in effect.
Other	• Maintain adequate calcium and vitamin D status when using this medication.

References

1. Ortega de la Cruz C, Fernández Gallardo LC, Damas Fernández-Figares M, García Martínez E. Compatibilidad físico-química de medicamentos con nutrición enteral. *Nutr Hosp*. 1993;8:105–108.
2. Gupta VD, Gibbs CW, Ghanekar AG. Stability of pediatric liquid dosage forms of ethacrynic acid, indomethacin, methyldopate hydrochloride, prednisone, and spironolactone. *Am J Hosp Pharm*. 1978;35:1382–1385.
3. Gupta VD. High-pressure liquid chromatographic evaluation of aqueous vehicles for preparation of prednisolone and prednisone liquid dosage forms. *J Pharm Sci*. 1979;68:908–910.
4. Dupuis LL, Zahn DA, Silverman ED, et al. Palatability and relative bioavailability of an extemporaneous prednisone suspension. *Can J Hosp Pharm*. 1990;43:101–105.
5. Raitt JR, Hotaling WH. Preparation of stable prednisone suspension. *Am J Hosp Pharm*. 1973;30:923–924.
6. Leonardi D, Salomon CJ. Influence of water uptake, gel network, and disintegration time on prednisone release from encapsulated solid dispersions. *Pharm Dev Technol*. 2010;15:184–191.
7. Aron-Wisnewsky J, Lemaitre F, Clement K, et al. Pharmacokinetics of immunomodulatory treatments after Roux-en-Y bypass in obese patients. *J Clin Pharmacol*. 2013;53:779–784.
8. Milsap RL, Plaisance KI, Jusko WJ. Prednisolone disposition in obese men. *Clin Pharmacol Ther*. 1984;36:824–831.
9. Derendorf H, Ruebsamen K, Clarke L, Schaeffler A, Kirwan JR. Pharmacokinetics of modified-release prednisone tablets in healthy subjects and patients with rheumatoid arthritis. *J Clin Pharmacol*. 2013;53:326–333.
10. Hollander AAMJ, van Rooij K, Lentjes EGWM, et al. The effect of grapefruit juice on cyclosporine and prednisone metabolism in transplant patients. *Clin Pharmacol Ther*. 1995;57:318–324.

Pregabalin

Product Availability

Solid	• Tablet: Extended-release: 82.5 mg, 165 mg, 330 mg (Lyrica® CR [Pfizer]; others) • Capsule: Immediate-release: 25 mg, 50 mg, 75 mg, 100 mg, 150 mg, 200 mg, 220 mg, 300 mg (Lyrica® [PF Prism]; others)
Liquid	• Oral solution: 20 mg/mL (Lyrica® [PF Prism]; others)

Physicochemical (drug)

Molecular weight: • 159.23	Permeability: • LogP –0.92 (calc) • LogD –1.35 (pH 7.4)	Water solubility: • 33 mg/mL
pKa: • 4.2, 10.6	Classification: • BCS Class n/a; BDDCS Class 3	

Pharmaceutical (product)

Solid	• Do not crush or chew extended-release tablet. • Capsule contents disperse in water.

Liquid	• Oral solution:
	   o pH ~6.1
	   o Osmolality n/a
	   o Viscosity n/a
	   o May contain sucralose; strawberry-flavored
	   o Store at controlled room temperature, and use within 45 days of opening.

Pharmacokinetic (patient)

Absorption	• Specific site not known; t_{max} ~1 hour after an oral dose (immediate-release, fasted) • Bioavailability may be ≥90% but is significantly lower (~50%–60%) when administered into proximal colon
Transport	• Multiple amino acid transporters (eg, L-type system) are likely involved in drug absorption. • No plasma protein binding • V_d ~0.5 L/kg
Metabolism	• Minimally metabolized and then eliminated by renal excretion • Cl ~5 L/h

Enteral Administration and Nutrition Considerations

Compatibility, Stability, and Bioavailability Considerations
  • Capsule content readily mixes with water and has been administered through nasogastric tube, with resultant serum concentrations in the therapeutic range.[1,2]

- The administration of capsule contents dispersed in water is bioequivalent to the intact capsule in healthy subjects.[3,4]
- In a single-dose crossover study in healthy volunteers, the capsule and solution formulations were bioequivalent.[5]
- The stability or efficacy of the oral liquid product when administered by an enteral access device has not been studied.

Drug-Nutrition Interactions
- Drug may influence nutrition status directly or indirectly:
  o Weight gain
  o CNS: dizziness, somnolence, ataxia, blurred vision
  o GI: dry mouth, vomiting, gastritis, abdominal distension, constipation
  o Metabolic: angioedema, peripheral edema
  o Other: myopathy, creatine kinase elevation
- No data on the influence of malnutrition or obesity on drug disposition.
- Influence of food on oral absorption or bioavailability:
  o Food may slow the rate of drug absorption but without an influence on oral bioavailability.

Recommendations

Gastric	• Disperse capsule content in water prior to administration. • No need to hold EN beyond the time required to flush-administer-flush.
Postpyloric	• As above. • Monitor for any unexpected change in effect.

References

1. Novy J, Rossetti AO. Oral pregabalin as an add-on treatment for status epilepticus. *Epilepsia.* 2010;51:2207–2210.
2. Swisher CB, Doreswamy M, Husain AM. Use of pregabalin for nonconvulsive seizures and nonconvulsive status epilepticus. *Seizure.* 2013;22:116–118.
3. Bockbrader HN, Alvey CW, Corrigan BW, et al. Bioequivalence assessment of a pregabalin capsule and oral solution in fasted healthy volunteers: a randomized crossover study. *Int J Clin Pharmacol Ther.* 2013;51:244–248.
4. Bockbrader HN, Radulovic LL, Posvar EL, et al. Clinical pharmacokinetics of pregabalin in healthy volunteers. *J Clin Pharmacol.* 2010;50:941–950.
5. Bockbrader HN, Alvey CW, Corrigan BW, Radulovic LL. Bioequivalence assessment of a pregabalin capsule and oral solution in fasted healthy volunteers: a randomized, crossover study. *Int J Clin Pharmacol Ther.* 2013;51:244–248.

Promethazine Hydrochloride

Product Availability

Solid	• Tablet: 12.5 mg, 25 mg, 50 mg (various)
Liquid	• Oral solution: 6.25 mg/5 mL (various)

Physicochemical (drug)

Molecular weight: • 284.43 (salt 320.88)	Permeability: • LogP 4.81 • LogD 2.64 (pH 7.4)	Water solubility: • 500 mg/mL
pKa: • 9.1	Classification: • BCS Class 1; BDDCS Class 1	

Pharmaceutical (product)

Solid	• Some tablet products may disperse in water with significant agitation.

Liquid	• Oral solution:
	    o pH 5.2 (5.1–5.3) with an osmolality 3500 mOsm/kg (the 6.25 mg/5 mL product)[1,2]
	    o pH 2.3 with an osmolarity 1407 mOsm/L (a 1 mg/mL product)[3]
	    o Viscosity n/a
	    o May contain maltitol and glucose

Pharmacokinetic (patient)

Absorption	• Specific site not known; t_{max} ~2–3 hours after an oral dose • Bioavailability ~25%
Transport	• Plasma protein binding ~76%–93% • V_d ~970 liters
Metabolism	• Significant hepatic metabolism, with inactive metabolite excreted renally • Cl ~1.2 mL/min

Enteral Administration and Nutrition Considerations

Compatibility, Stability, and Bioavailability Considerations
- Drug is susceptible to oxidation and decomposition from air and light exposure, respectively.
- A 5% or 10% aqueous solution will have a pH of 4.0–5.3.
- Drug stability may improve as pH decreases, but drug is incompatible with alkaline substances, resulting in free drug precipitate.
- Promethazine hydrochloride prepared in simple syrup and preparations using non-sucrose-containing vehicles (including hydrated thickening agents) were stored in amber bottles at elevated temperature conditions (30°C–70°C). Comparatively, the preparation in simple syrup had the best stability (UV spectrophotometric analysis).[4]

- Promethazine liquid diluted in coffee or tea resulted in the formation of an insoluble precipitate.[5]
- Admixture of promethazine solution (10 mL) with 15–240 mL of EN formulas (Ensure, Ensure Plus, Osmolite) appeared physically compatible (no granulation, no phase separation) in each with slightly increased viscosity, and a final pH of 5.8–6.2.[1]
- A dose of oral liquid admixed with 200 mL of an EN product (Precitene) appeared physically compatible (no phase separation or particle growth) but with a significant increase in osmolality to >1200 mOsm/kg.[6]
- When promethazine solution (10 mL) was admixed with 15–240 mL of EN formulas (Ensure HN, Ensure Plus HN, Osmolite HN, Vital), it appeared physically compatible (no granulation, no phase separation) with each.[7]

Drug-Nutrition Interactions
- Drug may influence nutrition status directly or indirectly:
  - CNS: sedation, fatigue, confusion, blurred vision
  - GI: dry mouth, nausea, vomiting, cholestatic jaundice
- No data on the influence of malnutrition or obesity on drug disposition.
- No known influence of food on oral absorption or bioavailability.

Recommendations

Gastric	• Dilute liquid in water (at least 1:1) prior to administration. • No need to hold EN beyond the time required to flush-administer-flush.
Postpyloric	• As above. • Monitor for any unexpected change in effect.

References
1. Cutie AJ, Altman E, Lenkel L. Compatibility of enteral products with commonly employed drug additives. *JPEN J Parenter Enteral Nutr.* 1983;7:186–191.
2. Dickerson RN, Melnik G. Osmolality of oral drug solutions and suspensions. *Am J Hosp Pharm.* 1988;45:832–834.
3. Obladen M, Mutz A. Orale medikation bei frühgeborenen? *Monatsschr Kinderheilkd.* 1985;133:669–674.
4. Iqbal Z, Pasha M. Stability of promethazine-HCl in non-sucrose syrup vehicles and sucrose syrup. *Sci Int.* 1999;11:215–216.
5. Hirsch SR. Precipitation of antipsychotic drugs in interaction with coffee or tea. *Lancet.* 1979;2:1131.
6. Ortega de la Cruz C, Fernández Gallardo LC, Damas Fernández-Figares M, García Martínez E. Compatibilidad físico-química de medicamentos con nutrición enteral. *Nutr Hosp.* 1993;8:105–108.
7. Altman E, Cutie AJ. Compatibility of enteral products with commonly employed drug additives. *Nutr Supp Serv.* 1984;4:8–17.

Propranolol Hydrochloride

Product Availability

Solid	• Tablet: 10 mg, 20 mg, 40 mg, 60 mg, 80 mg (Inderal® [Akrimax Pharms]; others) • Capsule: 60 mg, 80 mg, 120 mg, 160 mg (Inderal® LA [Ani Pharms]; others)
Liquid	• Oral solution: 40 mg/5 mL (various)

Physicochemical (drug)

Molecular weight: • 259.35 (salt 295.81)	Permeability: • LogP 3.48 • LogD 1.20 (pH 7.4)	Water solubility: • 50 mg/mL
pKa: • 9.47	Classification: • BCS Class 1; BDDCS Class 1	

Pharmaceutical (product)

Solid	• Some tablet products may disperse in water (20 mL) within 5 minutes. • Do not open, chew, or crush capsule (modified-release).

Liquid	• Oral solution:
	  ○ pH 3.44
	  ○ Osmolality 8145 mOsm/kg (calculated based on measurement of 1:5 dilution of a reported 20 mg/5 mL product with sterile water)[1]
	  ○ Viscosity n/a
	  ○ May contain maltitol

Note	• Tablet and oral solution are considered bioequivalent. • Tablet and extended-release capsule are not considered bioequivalent.

Pharmacokinetic (patient)

Absorption	• Specific site not known; t_{max} ~1–2 hours after an oral dose (immediate-release) • Bioavailability ~26%
Transport	• Substrate for P-glycoprotein efflux • Plasma protein binding ≥90%, especially to α_1-acid glycoprotein • V_d ~4.3 L/kg
Metabolism	• Significant first-pass hepatic extraction/metabolism (CYP2D6, CYP1A2, CYP2C19) to at least 8 metabolites excreted in the urine • Cl ~16 mL/min/kg

Enteral Administration and Nutrition Considerations

Compatibility, Stability, and Bioavailability Considerations

- A 1% aqueous solution has a pH of 5–6.
- For maximal drug stability, the pH should be 3–4 because the drug undergoes rapid decomposition in more alkaline solutions.[2,3]
- Including preservatives (methyl- and propyl-hydroxybenzoate) in an extemporaneous suspension made from tablets did not prevent bacterial growth, with evidence of drug degradation products (UV spectroscopy, thin-layer chromatography); however, using ethanol as a preservative resulted in a more stable preparation.[2]
- An oral suspension (0.5 mg/mL) prepared from tablets in a simple syrup–containing vehicle, stored in amber glass bottles at 25°C, remained stable (HPLC analysis) for 238 days.[3]
- An extemporaneous preparation (0.25 mg/mL) in a phosphate buffer (pH 7.4) remained stable (HPLC analysis) for 84 hours even at an elevated temperature.[4]
- An extemporaneously compounded oral suspension (1 mg/mL) prepared from 10 mg tablets in a vehicle (PEG 8000 base) and stored in amber glass bottles at 5°C and 25°C remained stable (HPLC analysis) for 4 months.[5]
- An extemporaneously compounded oral suspension (1 mg/mL) prepared from drug powder in SyrSpend SF and stored in non-actinic bottles at room temperature remained stable (HPLC analysis) for 90 days.[6]
- An extemporaneously compounded oral liquid (2 mg/mL, 5 mg/mL) prepared from tablets (40 mg) in OraBlend SF, stored in amber polyvinyl chloride plastic bottles at 4°C or 25°C, remained stable (HPLC analysis) for 120 days without a change in pH or taste, but it became slightly discolored.[7]
- Extemporaneously compounded oral liquid formulations (2 mg/mL, 5 mg/mL) were prepared from tablets or drug powder in OraSweet (72 mPa·s), modified OraSweet (50 mPa·s), or simple syrup with glycerol and sorbitol (62 mPa·s), with pH adjusted to 3 with citric acid, and then stored in amber bottles at 4°C or 25°C and kept out of light. The formulations remained stable (HPLC analysis) for 35 days; although there was no significant change in pH, viscosity generally increased by day 7 but returned near baseline by days 14–35.[8]
- Six different extemporaneous formulations were prepared from 40 mg tablets (varying in suspending agent, preservatives, and flavoring vehicles) and stored in amber glass bottles at 4°C and 30°C for up to 12 weeks. Only a 5 mg/mL formulation that was prepared with citric acid, sodium benzoate, cherry syrup, and distilled water and stored at 4°C remained stable for the duration of the study.[9]

- The admixture of propranolol (from either crushed 40 mg tablets or a 20 mg/5 mL liquid) dispersed in deionized water (10 mL) with 240 mL of EN formulation (Isocal, Sustacal, Sustacal HC) revealed no physical incompatibility (precipitation, phase separation), and the drug remained stable (HPLC analysis) for 24 hours.[10]
- A commercial solution combined (1:1) with Osmolite 1.2, under simulated clinical conditions, would result in no clogging of either an 8 Fr or a 20 Fr feeding tube.[1]

Drug-Nutrition Interactions
- Drug may influence nutrition status directly or indirectly:
  - CNS: lightheadedness, ataxia, hearing loss, depression
  - GI: dry mouth, nausea, vomiting, abdominal cramps, diarrhea, constipation
  - Metabolic: edema, hypoglycemia
  - Other: peripheral neuropathy
- Influence of malnutrition or obesity on drug disposition:
  - Body weight–normalized volume of distribution is lower in obesity; total clearance may also be reduced in obesity, although this finding is not consistent.[11–13]
- Influence of food on oral absorption or bioavailability:
  - Food is expected to increase oral bioavailability.

Recommendations

Gastric	• If there is no therapeutic alternative (eg, atenolol), disperse tablet in water just prior to administration. • Alternative: Dilute oral solution in water (at least 1:1) just prior to administration. • No need to hold EN beyond the time required to flush-administer-flush.
Postpyloric	• As above. • Monitor for any unexpected change in effect.

References

1. Klang M, McLymont V, Ng N. Osmolality, pH, and compatibility of selected oral liquid medications with an enteral nutrition product. *JPEN J Parenter Enteral Nutr.* 2013;37: 689–694.
2. Brown GC, Kayes JB. The stability of suspensions prepared extemporaneously from solid oral dosage forms. *J Clin Pharm.* 1976;1:29–37.
3. Gupta VD, Stewart KR. Stability of propranolol hydrochloride suspension and solution compounded from injection or tablets. *Am J Hosp Pharm.* 1987;44:360–361.
4. Modamio P, Lastra CF, Montejo O, et al. Development and validation of liquid chromatography methods for the quantitation of propranolol, metoprolol, atenolol, and bisoprolol: application in solution stability studies. *Int J Pharm.* 1996;130:137–140.
5. Henry DW, Repta AJ, Smith FM, et al. Stability of propranolol hydrochloride suspension compounded from tablets. *Am J Hosp Pharm.* 1986;43:1492–1495.

6. Geiger CM, Voudrie MA, Sorenson B. Stability of propranolol hydrochloride in SyrSpend SF. *Int J Pharm Compd.* 2012;16:513–515.

7. Ensom MHH, Kendrick J, Rudolph S, et al. Stability of propranolol in extemporaneously compounded suspensions. *Can J Hosp Pharm.* 2013;66:118–124.

8. Muśko M, Sznitowska M. Stability of extemporaneous pediatric oral liquids compounded from tablets and drug substance: use of propranolol and theophylline. *Acta Pol Pharm.* 2013;70:137–145.

9. Ahmed GH, Stewart PJ, Tucker IG. The stability of extemporaneous paediatric formulations of propranolol hydrochloride. *Aust J Hosp Pharm.* 1988;18:312–318.

10. Strom JG, Miller SW. Stability of drugs with enteral nutrient formulas. *DICP Ann Pharmacother.* 1990;24:130–134.

11. Bowman SL, Hudson SA, Simpson G, et al. A comparison of the pharmacokinetics of propranolol in obese and normal volunteers. *Br J Clin Pharmacol.* 1986;21:529–532.

12. Cheymol G, Poirier JM, Barre J, et al. Comparative pharmacokinetics of intravenous propranolol in obese and normal volunteers. *J Clin Pharmacol.* 1987;27:874–879.

13. Poirier JM, Le Jeunne C, Cheymol G, et al. Comparison of propranolol and sotalol pharmacokinetics in obese subjects. *J Pharm Pharmacol.* 1990;42:344–348.

Quetiapine Fumarate

Product Availability

Solid	• Tablet:
	   ○ Immediate-release: 25 mg, 50 mg, 100 mg, 200 mg, 300 mg, 400 mg (base) (Seroquel® [AstraZeneca]; others)
	   ○ Extended-release: 50 mg, 150 mg, 200 mg, 300 mg, 400 mg (base) (Seroquel® XR [AstraZeneca]; others)

Physicochemical (drug)

Molecular weight: • 383.51 (salt 883.09)	Permeability: • LogP 2.94 • LogD 2.85 (pH 7.4)	Water solubility: • 0.038 mg/mL
pKa: • 6.87	Classification: • BCS Class 2; BDDCS Class n/a	

Pharmaceutical (product)

Solid	• Immediate-release tablet products may be film-coated and may disperse after crushing. • Do not crush or chew extended-release tablet

Pharmacokinetic (patient)

Absorption	• Specific site not known; t_{max} ~1.5 hours after an oral dose (immediate-release) • Bioavailability ~9%
Transport	• Substrate for P-glycoprotein efflux • Plasma protein binding ~83% • V_d ~10 L/kg
Metabolism	• Extensive hepatic metabolism via CYP3A4 (sulfoxidation, dealkylation, and hydroxylation) to >12 metabolites (including norquetiapine) excreted in urine and feces • Cl ~80–100 L/h

Enteral Administration and Nutrition Considerations

Compatibility, Stability, and Bioavailability Considerations
- Drug administration via enteral access device was successful in managing critically ill patients with delirium receiving EN; the tablet was crushed and dispersed in 10 mL water, the feeding tube was flushed with 25 mL sterile water before and 50 mL sterile water after each dose, and the feeding was stopped 30 minutes prior to drug administration and restarted immediately afterward.[1]
- Incorporating quetiapine into solid lipid nanoparticle formulations under study revealed good stability and improved oral bioavailability (3.7-fold) in an animal model.[2]

Drug-Nutrition Interactions
- Drug may influence nutrition status directly or indirectly:
  - o Increased appetite, weight gain
  - o CNS: movement disorders (eg, akathisia, dystonia), dizziness, sedation, blurred vision
  - o GI: cheilitis, dry mouth, nausea, vomiting, dyspepsia, abdominal pain, constipation or diarrhea, fecal incontinence
  - o Metabolic: hyperglycemia, dyslipidemia, polydipsia
  - o Other: elevated CK, arthralgia
- No data on the influence of malnutrition or obesity on drug disposition.
- No known influence of food on oral absorption or bioavailability.

Recommendations

Gastric	• Crush and disperse immediate-release tablet in water prior to administration. • No need to hold EN beyond the time required to flush-administer-flush feed.
Postpyloric	• As above. • Monitor for any unexpected change in effect.

References

1. Devlin JW, Roberts RJ, Fong JJ, et al. Efficacy and safety of quetiapine in critically ill patients with delirium: a prospective, multicenter, randomized, double-blind, placebo-controlled pilot study. *Crit Care Med.* 2010;38:419–427.
2. Narala A, Veerabrahma K. Preparation, characterization and evaluation of quetiapine fumarate solid lipid nanoparticles to improve the oral bioavailability. *J Pharmaceut.* 2013;ID 265741 (7 pages). doi:10.1155/2013/265741.

Quinapril Hydrochloride

Product Availability

Solid	• Tablet: 5 mg, 10 mg, 20 mg, 40 mg (base) (Accupril® [Pfizer]; others)

Physicochemical (drug)

Molecular weight: • 438.53 (salt 474.98)	Permeability: • LogP 3.2 • LogD 2.26 (pH 7.4)	Water solubility: • 0.1 mg/mL
pKa: • 5.2	Classification: • BCS Class 1; BDDCS Class 2	

Pharmaceutical (product)

Solid	• Non-film-coated tablets may disperse in water after crushing.

Pharmacokinetic (patient)

Absorption	• Specific site not known; t_{max} ~1 hour after an oral dose • Bioavailability ~50%–60%
Transport	• Plasma protein binding ~97% • V_d ~0.2 L/kg
Metabolism	• Hepatic esterases convert quinapril to quinaprilat, and the drug is eliminated by renal excretion. • Cl ~1 mL/min/kg

Enteral Administration and Nutrition Considerations

Compatibility, Stability, and Bioavailability Considerations

- Although water-soluble, the drug is unstable in an aqueous solution with a pH-dependent rate of decomposition and formation of degradation products, with best stability for up to 24 hours at pH 5.5–5.7.[1,2]
- One tablet excipient (magnesium carbonate) released into the aqueous environment raises the pH to unstable levels.[2]
- An oral preparation made from crushed tablets placed in a buffer solution (K-Phos Neutral/Bicitra [1:1] in sterile water) was diluted in OraSweet, OraSweet SF, or simple syrup; when stored in polyethylene terephthalate bottles, this preparation remained stable (HPLC analysis) for 24 hours at 25°C with 65% relative humidity and for up to 6 weeks at 5°C.[2]

Drug-Nutrition Interactions

- Drug may influence nutrition status directly or indirectly:
  - CNS: dizziness, headache, fatigue
  - GI: dysgeusia, stomatitis, nausea, abdominal pain, diarrhea
  - Metabolic: hyperkalemia, anemia, hypoglycemia

- No data on the influence of malnutrition or obesity on drug disposition.
- Influence of food on oral absorption or bioavailability:
  - Food may reduce rate of absorption but without usually an effect on oral bioavailability.
  - High-fat meal may reduce oral bioavailability by up to 25%–30%.

Recommendations

Gastric	• Crush and disperse tablet in water prior to administration. • No need to hold EN beyond the time required to flush-administer-flush.
Postpyloric	• As above. • Monitor for any unexpected change in effect.

References

1. Freed AL, Kolodsick K, Silbering S, et al. The development and stability assessment of extemporaneously pediatric formulations of Accupril. American Association of Pharmaceutical Scientists Annual Meeting and Expo; 2003.
2. Freed AL, Silbering SB, Kolodsick KJ, et al. The development and stability assessment of extemporaneous pediatric formulations of Accupril. *Int J Pharm.* 2005;304:135–144.

Rabeprazole Sodium

Product Availability

Solid	• Tablet: 20 mg (Aciphex® [Eisai]; others) • Capsule: 5 mg, 10 mg (Aciphex® Sprinkle™ [Avadel Pharm])

Physicochemical (drug)

Molecular weight: • 359.45 (salt 381.43)	Permeability: • LogP 2.08 (calc) • LogD n/a	Water solubility: • 0.34 mg/mL
pKa: • 1.9, 3.2, 4.2	Classification: • BCS Class 3; BDDCS Class 1	

Pharmaceutical (product)

Solid	• Do not crush or chew the tablet or capsule contents; they are modified-release.

Pharmacokinetic (patient)

Absorption	• Specific site not known; t_{max} ~3.5 hours after an oral dose • Bioavailability ~52%
Transport	• Plasma protein binding ~96% • V_d ~0.34–0.98 L/kg
Metabolism	• Extensive metabolism via CYP3A4 and CYP2C19, with most metabolites eliminated renally • Cl ~280 mL/min

Enteral Administration and Nutrition Considerations

Compatibility, Stability, and Bioavailability Considerations
- In healthy adults under fasted conditions, mixtures of the capsule granules combined with small amounts of yogurt (1 Tbsp), applesauce (1 Tbsp), infant formula (5 mL), or a suspension vehicle resulted in equivalent oral bioavailability; the vehicles had pH values between 3.6 and 7.2, in which the granules remained stable for up to 30 minutes.[1]

Drug-Nutrition Interactions
- Drug may influence nutrition status directly or indirectly:
  - CNS: headache, dizziness
  - GI: vomiting, abdominal pain, atrophic gastritis with long-term use, diarrhea including an association with *Clostridium difficile*
  - Metabolic: osteoporosis, hypomagnesemia, vitamin B_{12} malabsorption
  - Other: arthralgia
- No data on the influence of malnutrition or obesity on drug disposition.
- Influence of food on oral absorption or bioavailability:
  - Although food slows the rate of absorption, there is no difference in oral bioavailability.[2]

Recommendations

Gastric	• If there is no therapeutic alternative (eg, esomeprazole, lansoprazole), prepare a dispersion of tablets in sodium bicarbonate solution prior to administration. • No need to hold EN beyond the time required to flush-administer-flush.
Postpyloric	• As above. • Monitor for any unexpected change in effect.

References

1. Thyssen A, Solanki B, Treem W. Randomized, open-label, single-dose, crossover, relative bioavailability study in healthy adults, comparing the pharmacokinetics of rabeprazole granules, administered using soft food or infant formula as dosing vehicle versus suspension. *Clin Ther*. 2012;34:1636–1645.
2. Yasuda S, Ohnishi A, Ogawa T, et al. Pharmacokinetic properties of E3810, a new proton pump inhibitor, in healthy male volunteers. *Int J Clin Pharmacol Ther*. 1994;32:466–473.

Raloxifene Hydrochloride

Product Availability

Solid	• Tablet: 60 mg (Evista* [Lilly]; others)

Physicochemical (drug)

Molecular weight: • 473.60 (salt 510.05)	Permeability: • LogP 5.20 • LogD n/a	Water solubility: • 0.3 mg/mL (25°C)
pKa: • ~8–9	Classification: • BCS Class 2; BDDCS Class 2	

Pharmaceutical (product)

Solid	• Tablets are film-coated. • Do not crush (unacceptable taste; teratogenic potential; avoid direct contact).

Pharmacokinetic (patient)

Absorption	• Specific site not known; t_{max} ~3.5 hours after an oral dose • Bioavailability <5%
Transport	• Substrate for P-glycoprotein efflux and possibly MRP efflux • Plasma protein binding ≥95% to albumin and α_1-acid glycoprotein • V_d ~2348 L/kg
Metabolism	• Extensive first-pass metabolism (intestine and liver) to 3 glucuronic acid conjugates via UGT (including UGT1A8, UGT1A10), then excreted through bile with some enterohepatic circulation possible • Cl ~44 L/h

Enteral Administration and Nutrition Considerations

Compatibility, Stability, and Bioavailability Considerations
- A saturated aqueous solution has pH ~4.5 at 25°C.
- Several novel formulations being investigated may improve drug dissolution and oral bioavailability:
  - A mixed-micelle formulation increased oral bioavailability (1.5-fold) in an animal model.[1]
  - A nanoparticle formulation increased oral bioavailability (7.5-fold) in an animal model compared with pure drug.[2]
  - Formulation as a microemulsion increased oral bioavailability (4.3-fold) in an animal model compared with plain drug suspension.[3]

- o A nanostructured lipid carrier enhanced dissolution and oral bioavailability (3.75-fold) compared with a simple susupension.[4]
- o Another solid lipid nanoparticle formulation increased oral bioavailability (2.7-fold) compared with free drug.[5]

Drug-Nutrition Interactions
- Drug may influence nutrition status directly or indirectly:
  - o Weight gain
  - o CNS: headache, depression, insomnia, vertigo
  - o GI: nausea, vomiting, dyspepsia, diarrhea
  - o Other: leg cramps, myalgia, arthralgia
- No data on the influence of malnutrition or obesity on drug disposition.
- No known influence of food on oral absorption or bioavailability.

Recommendations

Gastric	• Not recommended for administration by enteral access devices.
Postpyloric	• As above.

References

1. Kanade R, Boche M, Pokharkar V. Self-assembling raloxifene loaded mixed micelles: formulation optimization, in vitro cytotoxicity and in vivo pharmacokinetics. *AAPS Pharmscitech*. 2018;19(3):1105–1115. Epub 2017 Nov 27. doi:10.1208/s12249-017-0919-6.
2. Varshosaz J, Minaiyan M, Dayyani L. Poly(methyl vinyl ether-co-maleic acid) for enhancement of solubility, oral bioavailability and anti-osteoporotic effects of raloxifene hydrochloride. *Eur J Pharm Sci*. 2018;112:195–206.
3. Shah N, Seth A, Balaraman R, et al. Oral bioavailability enhancement of raloxifene by developing microemulsion using d-optimal mixture design: optimization and in-vivo pharmacokinetic study. *Drug Dev Ind Pharm*. 2017;4:1–10.
4. Shah NV, Seth AK, Balaraman R, et al. Nanostructured lipid carriers for oral bioavailability enhancement of raloxifene: design and in vivo study. *J Adv Res*. 2016;7:423–434.
5. Tran TH, Ramasamy T, Cho HJ, et al. Formulation and optimization of raloxifene-loaded solid lipid nanoparticles to enhance oral bioavailability. *J Nanosci Nanotechnol*. 2014;14:4820–4831.

Ramipril

Product Availability

Solid	• Tablet: 1.25 mg, 2.5 mg, 5 mg, 10 mg (various) • Capsule: 1.25 mg, 2.5 mg, 5 mg, 10 mg (Altace® [King Pharms]; others)

Physicochemical (drug)

Molecular weight: • 416.52	Permeability: • LogP 2.90 • LogD 1.76 (pH 7.4)	Water solubility: • 0.004 mg/mL
pKa: • 3.2	Classification: • BCS Class 1; BDDCS Class 1	

Pharmaceutical (product)

Solid	• Non-film-coated tablets disperse in water. • Capsule contents may disperse in water.

Pharmacokinetic (patient)

Absorption	• Specific site not known; t_{max} ~2 hours after an oral dose • Bioavailability ~28%
Transport	• Plasma protein binding ~73% (ramiprilat ~56%) • V_d ~1.2 L/kg
Metabolism	• Ester group cleavage converts most of the drug to its active metabolite, ramiprilat, which then undergoes glucuronidation before renal and biliary excretion. • Cl ~23 mL/min/kg

Enteral Administration and Nutrition Considerations

Compatibility, Stability, and Bioavailability Considerations

- Aqueous solution of ramipril remained stable (HPLC analysis) at pH 3 and pH 5, and stable to oxidation; however, at a pH of 8, the aqueous solution results in rapid and extensive drug loss.[1]
- Three different preparation methods were compared (open crushing with mortar and pestle followed by suspension in water; closed crushing in a commercial tablet crusher and then open suspension in water; or closed crushing and confined suspension in water in a different commercial device); although the methods were similar in the efficiency of preparation, the fully closed method prevented particle aerosolization.[2]
- An extemporaneously compounded oral solution prepared from capsule contents (1.25 mg, 2.5 mg, 5 mg) dispersed in 120 mL of deionized water, stored in polyethylene terephthalate containers, remained stable (HPLC analysis) for 24 hours at 23°C and for 48 hours at 3°C; the drug was also similarly stable when dispersed in 120 mL apple juice.[3]

- An extemporaneously compounded oral microemulsion prepared from drug dissolved in clove oil with polysorbate-20 and water (5:30:65) appeared stable without phase separation or creaming; however, it was not tested any further.[4]
- A nanoemulsion formulation under study enhanced drug dissolution and improved oral bioavailability (2.3- to 5.4-fold) compared with the marketed conventional products.[5]

Drug-Nutrition Interactions
- Drug may influence nutrition status directly or indirectly:
  o CNS: fatigue, headache, dizziness
  o GI: nausea, vomiting, abdominal pain, diarrhea
  o Metabolic: hyperkalemia, angioedema (including of intestine, manifest as abdominal pain)
- No data on the influence of malnutrition or obesity on drug disposition.
- Influence of food on oral absorption or bioavailability:
  o Slight influence of food on rate of absorption, but no influence on oral bioavailability.

Recommendations

Gastric	• Disperse tablet (or capsule contents) in water just prior to administration. • No need to hold EN beyond the time required to flush-administer-flush.
Postpyloric	• As above. • Monitor for any unexpected change in effect.

References
1. Hanysova L, Vaclavkova M, Dohnal J, et al. Stability of ramipril in solvents of different pH. *J Pharm Biomed Anal.* 2005;37:1179–1183.
2. Salmon D, Pont E, Chevallard H, et al. Pharmaceutical and safety considerations of tablet crushing in patients undergoing enteral intubation. *Int J Pharm.* 2013;443:146–153.
3. Allen LV, Stiles ML, Prince SJ, et al. Stability of ramipril in water, apple juice, and applesauce. *Am J Health-Syst Pharm.* 1995;52:2433–2436.
4. Nirmala MJ, Chandrasekaran N, Mukherjee A. Enhanced solubilization of aqueous insoluble anti-hypertensive drug. *Int J Pharm Pharmaceut Sci.* 2012;4:366–368.
5. Shafiq S, Shakeel F, Talegaonkar S, et al. Development and bioavailability assessment of ramipril nanoemulsion formulation. *Eur J Pharm Biopharm.* 2007;66:227–243.

Ranitidine Hydrochloride

Product Availability

Solid	• Tablet: 75 mg, 150 mg, 300 mg (base) (Zantac® [GSK]; others)
Liquid	• Oral solution: 15 mg/mL (base) (Zantac® [GSK]; others)

Physicochemical (drug)

Molecular weight: • 314.41 (salt 350.86)	Permeability: • LogP 0.27 • LogD 0.54 (pH 7.4), −1.28 (pH 6.5, calc)	Water solubility: • 555–660 mg/mL
pKa: • 2.7, 8.2	Classification: • BCS Class 3; BDDCS Class 3	

Pharmaceutical (product)

Solid	• Film-coated tablets do not disperse in water.

Liquid	• Oral solution:
	  ○ pH 6.88[1]
	  ○ Osmolality 637 mOsm/kg[1]
	  ○ Viscosity n/a
	  ○ May contain ethanol, saccharin, and sorbitol; peppermint-flavored
	  ○ Store at <25°C but avoid freezing.

Note	• Tablet, oral solution, and previously available effervescent tablet are considered bioequivalent.

Pharmacokinetic (patient)

Absorption	• Proximal small intestine (duodenum, jejunum); t_{max} ~2–3 hours after an oral dose • Bioavailability ~50%
Transport	• Substrate for P-glycoprotein efflux • Plasma protein binding ~10%–19% • V_d ~1.2–1.9 L/kg
Metabolism	• Extensive first-pass effect, with hepatic metabolism to desmethylranitidine, ranitidine N-oxide, and S-oxide, all of which are excreted mostly in bile, with some excretion of metabolites or unchanged drug in urine • Cl ~35 L/h

Enteral Administration and Nutrition Considerations

Compatibility, Stability, and Bioavailability Considerations
- Ranitidine is hygroscopic.[2]
- A 1% aqueous solution has a pH of 4.5–6.0, and aqueous solutions remain stable in the pH range 5.0–6.6.[3]

- A pharmacy-prepared ranitidine solution (50 mg/mL) had an osmolality of 2911 mOsm/kg, which decreased to 580 mOsm/kg when diluted 4:1 with water.[4]
- An extemporaneously compounded suspension (150 mg/10 mL) prepared from tablets (150 mg) suspended in distilled water/simple syrup (1:1), stored in amber glass bottles at 25°C, resulted in ≤9% drug loss (HPLC analysis) in 7 days; however, the suspension needs to be shaken well before measuring out dose based on rapid sedimentation.[5]
- An extemporaneously compounded oral suspension using OraPlus as the suspending vehicle and stored in plastic containers at room temperature resulted in 16% drug loss (HPLC analysis) at 6 weeks, but no loss when stored under refrigeration.[6]
- An extemporaneously compounded oral solution (5 mg/mL) prepared from pure powder, effervescent tablets, or effervescent granules in sterile water and stored in glass at 4°C remained stable (HPLC analysis) for 28 days, 54 days, or 6 days, respectively.[7]
- An extemporaneously compounded oral suspension (15 mg/mL) prepared from drug powder in SyrSpend SF PH4, stored in low-actinic plastic containers at 2°C–8°C or at room temperature, remained stable (HPLC analysis) for 58 days (refrigeration) or 36 days (room temperature).[8]
- Compatibility of ranitidine admixed with EN formulations varies by drug form and feeding product:
  - Under simulated clinical conditions, the commercial oral solution combined (1:1) with Osmolite 1.2 would result in no clogging of an 8 Fr or a 20 Fr feeding tube.[1]
  - A 10 mg dose of oral solution (commercial syrup, or 300 mg tablet crushed and dispersed in 20 mL deionized water) added to 50 mL of each EN formula (Ensure, Ensure Plus, Jevity, Nutren 1.0, Nutren 1.0 with Fiber, Nutren 2.0, Peptamen, Sustacal), stored at 22°C–25°C under fluorescent light for 9 hours followed by 15 hours of dark, appeared physically compatible (no flocculation or phase separation); however, significant drug loss (HPLC analysis) occurred in both Ensure Plus and in Nutren 2.0.[9]
- Administration via jejunostomy is expected to yield serum concentrations similar to nasogastric administration.[10]

Drug-Nutrition Interactions
- Drug may influence nutrition status directly or indirectly:
  - CNS: headache, dizziness, vertigo
  - GI: nausea, vomiting, abdominal discomfort, constipation, rare pancreatitis and hepatitis
  - Other: arthralgia, myalgia

- Influence of malnutrition or obesity on drug disposition:
  - Body weight–normalized volume of distribution is decreased in obesity, although total clearance remained unchanged; this suggests use of a lean body weight if using weight-based dosing.[11]
- No known influence of food on oral absorption or bioavailability.

Recommendations

Gastric	• Use oral solution, with or without dilution prior to administration. • No need to hold EN beyond the time required to flush-administer-flush.
Postpyloric	• Consider diluting oral solution (1:1) prior to administration. • Monitor for any unexpected change in effect.

References

1. Klang M, McLymont V, Ng N. Osmolality, pH, and compatibility of selected oral liquid medications with an enteral nutrition product. *JPEN J Parenter Enteral Nutr.* 2013;37: 689–694.
2. Church C, Smith J. How stable are medicines moved from original packs into compliance aids? *Pharm J.* 2006;276:75–81.
3. Ferreira MO, Bahia MF, Costa P. Stability of ranitidine hydrochloride in different aqueous solutions. *Eur J Hosp Pharm Sci.* 2004;10:60–63.
4. Fernández Polo A, Cabañas Poy MJ, Clemente Bautista S, et al. Osmolality of oral liquid dosage forms to be administered to newborns in a hospital. *Farm Hosp.* 2007;31: 311–314.
5. Karnes HT, Harris SR, Garnett WR, et al. Concentration uniformity of extemporaneously prepared ranitidine suspension. *Am J Hosp Pharm.* 1989;46:304–307.
6. Lifshin LS, Fox JL. Stability of extemporaneously prepared ranitidine hydrochloride suspension. Paper presented at American Society of Health-System Pharmacists Annual Meeting; 1992.
7. Schlatter J, Saulnier J-L. Stability of ranitidine oral solutions prepared from commercial forms. *Eur Hosp Pharm.* 1998;4:23–25.
8. Geiger CM, Sorenson B, Whaley P. Stability assessment of 10 active pharmaceutical ingredients compounded in SyrSpend SF. *Int J Pharm Compd.* 2015;19:420–427.
9. Crowther RS, Bellanger R, Szauter KEM. In vitro stability of ranitidine hydrochloride in enteral nutrient formulas. *Ann Pharmacother.* 1995;29:859–862.
10. Adams D. Administration of drugs through a jejunostomy tube. *Br J Intens Care.* 1994;4: 10–17.
11. Davis RL, Quenzer RW, Bozigian HP, Warner CW. Pharmacokinetics of ranitidine in morbidly obese woman. *DICP Ann Pharmacother.* 1990;24:1040–1043.

Risedronate Sodium

Product Availability

Solid	• Tablet:
	   ○ Immediate-release: 5 mg, 30 mg, 35 mg, 150 mg (Actonel®
	     [Apil]; others)
	   ○ Delayed-release: 35 mg (Atelvia® [Apil])

Physicochemical (drug)

Molecular weight: • 283.12 (salt 305.1)	Permeability: • LogP −3.60 • LogD n/a	Water solubility: • 52.7 mg/mL
pKa: • 1.6, 2.2, 5.9, 7.1, 11.7	Classification: • BCS Class 3; BDDCS Class 3	

Pharmaceutical (product)

Solid	• Many tablet products are film-coated. • The non-film-coated immediate-release tablet disperses rapidly (within 3 minutes) in water without crushing. • Do not crush products (oropharyngeal mucosal irritant), especially not the delayed-release product.

Pharmacokinetic (patient)

Absorption	• Throughout the small intestine; t_{max} ~1 hour after an oral dose (immediate-release) • Bioavailability ~1%
Transport	• Plasma protein binding ~24% • V_d ~6.3–13.8 L/kg
Metabolism	• No known metabolism • Cl ~122 mL/min

Enteral Administration and Nutrition Considerations

Compatibility, Stability, and Bioavailability Considerations
- Bisphosphonates remained clinically effective when administered via enteral feeding tube.[1]
- Aqueous risedronate solutions made from the 5 mg tablet or the 35 mg tablet in 60 mL of sterile water had a pH of 6.2 or 5.5, respectively, and remained stable (HPLC analysis) when drawn up and stored in polypropylene syringes for 4 hours.[2]
- The aqueous dispersions described above were successfully delivered through enteral access devices (12 Fr polyurethane nasoenteric tube, 18 Fr and 22 Fr gastrostomy tubes of polyurethane and silicone) with a 30 mL flush before and after drug administration.[2]
- Risedronate dissolved in 180 mL of water before the addition of thickening agents (NutraThik, Thick&Easy, Thick-It, ThickenUp, or

Thik&Clear), and then stored at room temperature, resulted in no significant drug loss (HPLC analysis) in 24 hours; viscosity was not reported.[3]

- A risedronate adduct formulation with titanium dioxide being studied resulted in a near doubling of oral bioavailability in an animal model compared with the free drug.[4]

Drug-Nutrition Interactions
- Drug may influence nutrition status directly or indirectly:
  o CNS: headache, dizziness
  o GI: esophageal ulceration/perforation, nausea, dyspepsia, abdominal pain, diarrhea or constipation
  o Metabolic: peripheral edema, hypocalcemia
  o Other: back pain, arthralgia, myalgia, osteonecrosis/myelitis (jaw)
- No data on the influence of malnutrition or obesity on drug disposition.
- Influence of food on oral absorption or bioavailability:
  o Food decreases oral bioavailability; drug should be administered on an empty stomach.
  o High concentrations of metal cations, as found in food, supplements, or mineral water, decrease oral bioavailability.

Recommendations

Gastric	• If there is no therapeutic alternative (injectable), disperse the once-weekly (35 mg) tablet in water (60 mL) prior to administration. • Flush enteral access device well and, if practical, maintain patient in an upright position for 30 minutes. • Hold EN by at least 2 hours before and after drug administration.
Postpyloric	• As above. • Monitor for any unexpected change in effect.
Other	• Correct patient hypocalcemia or vitamin D deficiency prior to therapy with risedronate; maintain adequate calcium and vitamin D status.

References

1. Tanner S, Taylor HM. Feeding tube administration of bisphosphonates for treating osteoporosis in institutionalized patients with developmental disabilities. *Bone.* 2004;34:(Suppl 1):S97–S98.
2. Dansereau RJ, Crail DJ. Extemporaneous procedures for dissolving risedronate tablets for oral administration and for feeding tubes. *Ann Pharmacother.* 2005;39:63–67.
3. Dansereau RJ, Crail DJ. Compatibility of risedronate sodium tablets with food thickeners. *Am J Health-Syst Pharm.* 2008;65:2133–2136.
4. Dissette V, Bozzi P, Bignozzi CA, et al. Particulate adducts based on sodium risedronate and titanium dioxide for the bioavailability enhancement of oral administered bisphosphonates. *Eur J Pharm Sci.* 2010;41:328–336.

Risperidone

Product Availability

Solid	• Tablet:
	  o Immediate-release: 0.25 mg, 0.5 mg, 1 mg, 2 mg, 3 mg, 4 mg (Risperdal® [Janssen]; others)
	  o Orally disintegrating: 0.5 mg, 1 mg, 2 mg, 3 mg, 4 mg (Risperdal® M-Tab [Janssen]; others)

Liquid	• Oral solution: 1 mg/mL (Risperdal® [Janssen]; others)

Physicochemical (drug)

Molecular weight: • 410.49	Permeability: • LogP 3.04 • LogD 2.52 (pH 7.4)	Water solubility: • ~2 mg/mL
pKa: • 1.2, 8.8	Classification: • BCS Class 1 or 2; BDDCS Class 1	

Pharmaceutical (product)

Solid	• Tablet products may disperse in water. • Orally disintegrating tablets disperse in water; depending on product, they may contain aspartame (phenylalanine caution), mannitol, sorbitol, or maltitol.

Liquid	• Oral solution:
	  o pH n/a
	  o Osmolality n/a
	  o Viscosity n/a
	  o May or may not contain sweeteners
	  o Store at controlled room temperature and protect from light.

Note	• The orally disintegrating tablet and immediate-release tablet are considered bioequivalent.

Pharmacokinetic (patient)

Absorption	• Specific site not known; t_{max} ~1–2 hours after an oral dose • Bioavailability ~70% (solution has slightly higher relative bioavailability than tablet)
Transport	• Substrate for P-glycoprotein efflux • Plasma protein binding ~88% to albumin and α_1-acid glycoprotein • V_d ~1–2 L/kg
Metabolism	• Undergoes metabolism via CYP2D6 to an active metabolite, 9-OH-risperidone (the latter is also marketed as paliperidone), with excretion predominantly through the urine • Cl ~5.4 mL/min/kg; varies depending on CYP2D6 metabolizer phenotype

Enteral Administration and Nutrition Considerations

Compatibility, Stability, and Bioavailability Considerations
- The commercial oral solution is physically compatible in water, orange juice, low-fat milk, and coffee, but it is not compatible in cola or tea.
- Risperidone oral solution (3 mL) diluted with bottled water, green tea, black tea, or oolong tea to 100 mL, stored at room temperature for 24 hours, resulted in cloudiness with a white precipitate in all the tea solutions; the precipitate was identified (isothermal microcalorimetry) to be a 1:1 molar ratio of the drug complexed with tannins, which complexes ~30%–80% of the drug.[1,2]
- An oral solution formulation was considered not bioequivalent with the tablet formulation in a group of healthy volunteers under fasted conditions.[3]
- Despite slight differences in the rate and extent of absorption between the conventional tablet and oral solution, the clinical effectiveness as studied in acutely ill patients with schizophrenia was no different between formulations.[4]
- A self-emulsifying formulation under study improved dissolution and intestinal permeability compared with pure drug and marketed formulation.[5]
- An emulsion formulation enriched with ω-3/ω-6 fatty acids under investigation remained stable over time.[6]
- Oral solution administered via a nasogastric enteral access device (12 Fr, 91 cm long, polyurethane tube) 30 minutes prior to intermittent feeding (400 mL of Nutrison Protein Plus Multifibre at 200 mL/h), with 10 mL flush before and after drug administration (type of fluid not reported), resulted in lower serum concentrations and clinical effects in a patient with paranoid schizophrenia compared with administration of oral doses.[7]

Drug-Nutrition Interactions
- Drug may influence nutrition status directly or indirectly:
  - Increased appetite, weight gain
  - CNS: movement disorders (eg, akathisia, dystonia), dizziness, sedation, blurred vision
  - GI: cheilitis, dry mouth, nausea, vomiting, dyspepsia, abdominal pain, constipation or diarrhea, fecal incontinence
  - Metabolic: hyperglycemia, dyslipidemia, polydipsia
  - Other: elevated CK, arthralgia
- No data on the influence of malnutrition or obesity on drug disposition.
- Influence of food on oral absorption or bioavailability:
  - Food has no significant influence on rate or extent of oral drug absorption.

Recommendations

Gastric	• Use oral solution with dilution in water prior to administration. • Alternative: Disperse tablet (immediate- or orally disintegrating) in water prior to administration. • No need to hold EN beyond the time required to flush-administer-flush.
Postpyloric	• As above. • Monitor for any unexpected change in effect.

References

1. Aki H, Ohta M, Fukusumi K, et al. Evaluation of compatibility of risperidone with soft drinks and interactions of risperidone with tea tannin using isothermal titration microcalorimetry. *Iryo Yakugaku (Jpn J Health Care Sci)*. 2006;32:190–198.
2. Aki H, Okamoto Y, Kimura T. Compatibility and stability tests of risperidone with soft-drinks by isothermal titration microcalorimetry. *J Therm Anal Calorim*. 2006;85: 681–684.
3. van Os S, Relleke M, Piniella PM. Lack of bioequivalence between generic risperidone oral solution and originator risperidone tablets. *Int J Clin Pharmacol Ther*. 2007;45: 293–299.
4. Kusumi I, Honda M, Ito K, et al. Risperidone oral solution versus standard tablets for the acute treatment of patients with schizophrenia. *Progr Neuro-Psychopharmacol Biol Psych*. 2011;35:537–540.
5. Bandi S, Sanka K, Bakshi V. Enhanced oral delivery of risperidone through a novel self-nanoemulsifying powder (SNEP) formulations: in-vitro and ex-vivo assessment. *J Microencapsul*. 2016;33:544–553.
6. Igartúa DE, Calienni MN, Feas DA, et al. Development of nutraceutical emulsions as risperidone delivery systems: characterization and toxicological studies. *J Pharm Sci*. 2015;104:4142–4152.
7. Oriolo G, Barbosa L, Imaz ML, et al. Plasma levels of oral risperidone during enteral nutrition in a pregnant schizophrenic patient. *Ther Adv Psychopharmacol*. 2015;5:133–137.

Ropinirole Hydrochloride

Product Availability

Solid	• Tablet:
	  ○ Immediate-release: 0.25 mg, 0.5 mg, 1 mg, 2 mg, 3 mg, 4 mg, 5 mg (base) (Requip® [GSK]; others)
	  ○ Extended-release: 2 mg, 4 mg, 6 mg, 8 mg, 12 mg (Requip® XL [GSK]; others)

Physicochemical (drug)

Molecular weight: • 260.38 (salt 296.84)	Permeability: • LogP 2.70 • LogD n/a	Water solubility: • 133 mg/mL
pKa: • 10.2	Classification: • BCS Class n/a; BDDCS Class 1	

Pharmaceutical (product)

Solid	• Many tablet products are film-coated. • The non-film-coated immediate-release tablets may disperse in water. • Do not crush extended-release tablet product.

Pharmacokinetic (patient)

Absorption	• Specific site not known; t_{max} ~1.5 hours after an oral dose. • Bioavailability ~45%–55%
Transport	• Plasma protein binding ~40% • V_d ~7.5 L/kg
Metabolism	• Extensive metabolism via CYP1A2 to the N-despropyl and hydroxyl metabolites, which may undergo glucuronidation prior to renal excretion • Cl ~47 L/h

Enteral Administration and Nutrition Considerations

Compatibility, Stability, and Bioavailability Considerations
• No data are available.

Drug-Nutrition Interactions
• Drug may influence nutrition status directly or indirectly:
  ○ CNS: somnolence, fatigue, syncope, dyskinesia, visual abnormalities
  ○ GI: anorexia, nausea, vomiting, abdominal pain
  ○ Metabolic: dependent edema
• No data on the influence of malnutrition or obesity on drug disposition.
• Influence of food on oral absorption or bioavailability:
  ○ Food, including a high-fat meal, may reduce the rate of absorption but without an influence on oral bioavailability.

Recommendations

Gastric	• Disperse immediate-release tablet in water just prior to administration. • No need to hold EN beyond the time required to flush-administer-flush. • Consider administration in close proximity to intermittent feeds to alleviate GI complaints.
Postpyloric	• As above. • Monitor for any unexpected change in effect.

Rosuvastatin Calcium

Product Availability

Solid	• Tablet: 5 mg, 10 mg, 20 mg, 40 mg (base) (Crestor® [IPR Pharma]; others)

Physicochemical (drug)

Molecular weight: • 481.55 (salt 1001.14)	Permeability: • LogP 1.90 (calc) • LogD –0.89 (pH 7.4)	Water solubility: • 0.02 mg/mL
pKa: • 4.0	Classification: • BCS Class 2; BDDCS Class 3	

Pharmaceutical (product)

Solid	• Many tablet products are film-coated, but some generic products may disperse in water.

Pharmacokinetic (patient)

Absorption	• Specific site not known; t_{max} ~5 hours after an oral dose • Bioavailability ~20%
Transport	• Plasma protein binding ~90%, mostly to albumin • V_d ~1.7 L/kg
Metabolism	• Approximately 10% metabolized via CYP2C9 to N-desmethyl-rosuvastatin, which is pharmacologically active; eliminated primarily in feces, with minimal renal excretion • Cl ~11 mL/min/kg

Enteral Administration and Nutrition Considerations

Compatibility, Stability, and Bioavailability Considerations
- A nanoparticle formulation under study remained stable for 3 months and improved oral bioavailability in an animal model compared with the marketed tablet formulation.[1]
- A nanodispersion formulation that incorporated oleic acid enhanced intestinal permeability and oral bioavailability in an animal model compared with an aqueous suspension or tablet formulation.[2]
- Another solid lipid nanoparticle formulation also increased oral bioavailability and improved antilipidemic effects in an animal model compared with an aqueous suspension.[3]

Drug-Nutrition Interactions
- Drug may influence nutrition status directly or indirectly:
  - CNS: cognitive impairment, confusion, headache
  - GI: nausea, dyspepsia, abdominal pain, constipation or diarrhea, elevated aminotransferases (AST, ALT), rare hepatic failure

- o Metabolic: glucose intolerance, proteinuria
- o Other: myopathy (pain, tenderness, weakness) including immune-mediated and necrotizing, rhabdomyolysis
- No data on the influence of malnutrition or obesity on drug disposition.
- No known influence of food on oral absorption or bioavailability.

Recommendations

Gastric	• If there is no therapeutic alternative (eg, atorvastatin), crush and/or disperse tablet in water just prior to administration. • No need to hold EN beyond the time required to flush-administer-flush.
Postpyloric	• As above. • Monitor for any unexpected change in effect.

References

1. Gabr MM, Mortada SM, Sallam MA. Carboxylate cross-linked cyclodextrin: a nanoporous scaffold for enhancement of rosuvastatin oral bioavailability. *Eur J Pharm Sci.* 2018;111:1–12.
2. Gabr MM, Mortada SM, Sallam MA. Hexagonal liquid crystalline nanodispersions proven superiority for enhanced oral delivery of rosuvastatin: in vitro characterization and in vivo pharmacokinetic study. *J Pharm Sci.* 2017;106:3103–3112.
3. Dudhipala N, Veerabrahma K. Improved anti-hyperlipidemic activity of rosuvastatin calcium via lipid nanoparticles: pharmacokinetic and pharmacodynamics evaluation. *Eur J Pharm Biopharm.* 2017;110:47–57.

Sertraline Hydrochloride

Product Availability

Solid	• Tablet: 25 mg, 50 mg, 100 mg (base) (Zoloft® [Pfizer]; others)
Liquid	• Oral solution: 20 mg/mL (base) (Zoloft® [Pfizer]; others)

Physicochemical (drug)

Molecular weight: • 306.24 (salt 342.69)	Permeability: • LogP 2.90 • LogD 2.74 (pH 7.4)	Water solubility: • 3.8 mg/mL
pKa: • 9.16	Classification: • BCS Class 1; BDDCS Class 1	

Pharmaceutical (product)

Solid	• Many tablet products are film-coated. • Tablets can be crushed to disperse in water.

Liquid	• Oral solution:
	  ○ pH n/a
	  ○ Osmolality n/a
	  ○ Viscosity n/a
	  ○ May contain alcohol and glycerin; menthol-flavored
	  ○ A dose of this concentrated solution is intended to be diluted with water (120 mL) immediately before administration.
	  ○ Store at controlled room temperature.

Note	• Tablet and oral solution considered to be bioequivalent.

Pharmacokinetic (patient)

Absorption	• Specific site not known; t_{max} ~4–8 hours after an oral dose • Absorption is more complete and quicker from the duodenum (~100%) compared with the ileum (~66%) • Bioavailability ~20%–40%
Transport	• Plasma protein binding ~98% to albumin and α_1-acid glycoprotein • V_d at least ~20 L/kg
Metabolism	• Extensive first-pass metabolism; demethylated by CYP3A (more than by CYP2D6 or CYP2C19) to N-desmethyl-sertraline, which undergoes further reaction to glucuronic acid metabolites excreted in urine and feces • Cl ~1.3 L/h/kg

Enteral Administration and Nutrition Considerations

Compatibility, Stability, and Bioavailability Considerations
- An extemporaneously compounded oral suspension (10 mg/mL) prepared from drug powder in SyrSpend SF PH4, stored in low-actinic containers at 2°C–8°C or 20°C–25°C, remained stable (HPLC analysis) for 90 days at both temperatures.[1]
- A self-nanoemulsifying formulation under study increased drug dissolution and oral bioavailability in an animal model compared with a simple aqueous suspension.[2]
- Oral bioavailability was significantly reduced (~60%) at 9–15 months following gastric bypass (CYP2D6/C19 poor and ultra-rapid metabolizers excluded) compared with matched controls, with risk for clinical exacerbation of underlying disorder.[3,4]
- The drug solution may better maintain therapeutic effects following gastric bypass than the tablet.[4]

Drug-Nutrition Interactions
- Drug may influence nutrition status directly or indirectly:
  - Weight loss (minimal)
  - CNS: headache, dizziness, tremor
  - GI: anorexia, dry mouth, nausea, diarrhea
  - Metabolic: hyponatremia
  - Other: back pain, myalgia
- No data on the influence of malnutrition or obesity on drug disposition.
- Influence of food on oral absorption or bioavailability:
  - Food may delay rate of absorption with a slight increase in oral bioavailability.
  - Grapefruit juice (240 mL) administered along with a daily dose of drug for 7 days resulted in elevated trough concentrations associated with decreased drug metabolism.[5]

Recommendations

Gastric	• Crush and disperse tablet in water just prior to administration. • No need to hold EN beyond the time required to flush-administer-flush.
Postpyloric	• As above. • Monitor for any unexpected change in effect.

References
1. Polonini HC, Loures S, de Araujo EP, et al. Stability of allopurinol, amitriptyline hydrochloride, carbamazepine, domperidone, isoniazid, ketoconazole, lisinopril, naproxen, paracetamol (acetaminophen), and sertraline hydrochloride in SyrSpend SF PH4 oral suspensions. *Int J Pharm Compd.* 2016;20:426–434.

2. Rahman MA, Mujahid M, Hussain A. Self-emulsifying pellets prepared by extrusion/ spheronization: in vitro/in vivo evaluation. *Recent Pat Drug Deliv Formul.* 2016;10: 245–252.
3. Roerig JL, Steffen K, Zimmerman C, et al. Preliminary comparison of sertraline levels in postbariatric surgery patients versus matched nonsurgical cohort. *Surg Obes Relat Dis.* 2012;8:62–66.
4. Hamad GG, Helsel JC, Perel JM, et al. The effect of gastric bypass on the pharmacokinetics of serotonin reuptake inhibitors. *Am J Psychiatry.* 2012;169:256–263.
5. Lee AJ, Chan WK, Harralson AF, et al. The effects of grapefruit juice on sertraline metabolism: an in vitro and in vivo study. *Clin Ther.* 1999;21:1890–1899.

Sildenafil Citrate
Product Availability

Solid	• Tablet: 20 mg, 25 mg, 50 mg, 100 mg (base) (Viagra® [Pfizer]; others)
Liquid	• Powder for oral suspension: 10 mg/mL (base) (Revatio® [Pfizer]; others)

Physicochemical (drug)

Molecular weight:	Permeability:	Water solubility:
• 474.59	• LogP 1.98 (calc)	• 3.5 mg/mL
	• LogD n/a	
pKa:	**Classification:**	
• 6.5, 9.2	• BCS Class 1; BDDCS Class 1	

Pharmaceutical (product)

Solid	• Many tablet products are film-coated. • Non-film-coated tablets can be crushed to disperse in water.
Liquid	• Oral suspension (reconstituted): o pH 3.5–4 o Osmolality n/a o Viscosity n/a o May contain sorbitol and sucralose; grape-flavored o Store at room temperature or refrigerated for up to 60 days from initial reconstitution.
Note	• Tablet and powder for oral suspension are considered bioequivalent.

Pharmacokinetic (patient)

Absorption	• Specific site not known; t_{max} ~1 hour after an oral dose • Bioavailability ~40%
Transport	• Substrate for P-glycoprotein and BCRP efflux • Plasma protein binding ~96% • V_d ~105 liters
Metabolism	• Extensive first-pass metabolism; metabolized by CYP3A4 much more than by CYP2C9; of the ~16 metabolites that are predominantly excreted in feces over urine, the major and active metabolite formed is N-desmethyl sildenafil • Cl ~41 L/h

Enteral Administration and Nutrition Considerations

Compatibility, Stability, and Bioavailability Considerations

- The official USP oral suspension formulation (2.5 mg/mL) prepared from tablets in OraSweet/OraPlus (1:1) is expected to have a pH of 3.9–4.9 and is assigned a BUD of 90 days.
- An oral sildenafil liquid (0.9 mg/mL) prepared from tablets crushed and diluted with lactose and dissolved in sterile water was used to manage pulmonary arterial hypertension in an infant.[1]
- An extemporaneous preparation (2 mg/mL) made from tablets (50 mg) in Orabase was successfully administered to infants with persistent pulmonary hypertension of the newborn through an orogastric tube, resulting in improved oxygenation compared with those receiving placebo.[2]
- An extemporaneously compounded oral suspension (2 mg/mL) prepared from drug powder in citrate buffer, syrup, and distilled water, stored at 4°C or 25°C, remained stable (ultraviolet spectrophotometric analysis) for 90 days.[3]
- Extemporaneously compounded oral suspensions (2.5 mg/mL) were prepared from Viagra or Revatio tablets (which have differing formulations), using 1% methylcellulose/simple syrup (1:1), methylcellulose/simple syrup (1:7), or OraSweet/OraPlus (1:1) as suspension vehicles, and stored in amber plastic bottles at 4°C or 25°C for 91 days. There were no changes in pH, color, odor, or turbidity, and the drug from either tablet formulation remained stable (HPLC analysis) the entire duration in each vehicle.[4-6]
- An extemporaneously compounded suspension (10 mg/mL) was prepared from tablets (20 mg) in OraSweet/OraPlus (3:1) and stored in enteral syringes prior to administration in healthy adult volunteers in a randomized crossover study. The oral bioavailability of the suspension was comparable with that of the intact tablet despite having a lower peak serum concentration.[7]
- Orally disintegrating formulations (tablet or film) under development were bioequivalent to the conventional tablets in healthy men under fasted conditions.[8,9]

Drug-Nutrition Interactions

- Drug may influence nutrition status directly or indirectly:
  - CNS: headache, visual disturbances, tremor
  - GI: glossitis, nausea, dyspepsia, diarrhea
  - Metabolic: dysglycemia
  - Other: myalgia
- No data on the influence of malnutrition or obesity on drug disposition.

- Influence of food on oral absorption or bioavailability:
  - ○ Food, especially a high-fat meal (980 kcal, 68 g fat), may delay rate of absorption with a clinically minor decrease (~11%) in oral bioavailability compared with the fasted state.[10]
  - ○ Grapefruit juice (250 mL) administered with or 1 hour before drug administration increased oral bioavailability (0.8- to 2.6-fold increase) compared with water.[11]
  - ○ Pummelo juice (250 mL) reduced oral bioavailability by ~40% in healthy volunteers compared with water.[12]
  - ○ Seville orange juice (250 mL/d for 3 days), but not lemon juice, increased oral bioavailability of the drug by 44% in healthy subjects compared with the same volume of water.[13]

Recommendations

Gastric	• Use reconstituted oral suspension and further dilute (at least 1:1) in water prior to administration. • No need to hold EN beyond the time required to flush-administer-flush.
Postpyloric	• As above. • Monitor for any unexpected change in effect.

References

1. Hon KL, Cheng KL, Siu KL, et al. Oral sildenafil for treatment of severe pulmonary hypertension in an infant. *Biol Neonate.* 2005;88:109–112.
2. Baquero H, Soliz A, Neira F, et al. Oral sildenafil in infants with persistent pulmonary hypertension of the newborn: a pilot randomized blinded study. *Pediatrics.* 2006;117: 1077–1083.
3. Provenza N, Calpena AC, Mallandrich M, et al. Design and physicochemical stability studies of paediatric oral formulations of sildenafil. *Int J Pharm.* 2014;460:234–239.
4. Nahata MC, Morosco RS, Brady MT. Extemporaneous sildenafil citrate oral suspensions for the treatment of pulmonary hypertension in children. *Am J Health-Syst Pharm.* 2006; 63:254–257.
5. Nahata MC, Morosco RS, Zuacha J. Stability of sildenafil citrate in two extemporaneously prepared oral dosage forms stored under refrigeration and at room temperature. Presentation at American Society of Health-System Pharmacists Midyear Clinical Meeting; 2007.
6. Nahata MC. Extended stability of morphine and sildenafil for oral use in infants and young children. *Int J Pharm Compd.* 2016;20:247–249.
7. Gao X, Ndongo M-N, Checchio TM, et al. A randomized, open-label 3-way crossover study to investigate the relative bioavailability and bioequivalence of crushed sildenafil 20 mg tablets mixed with apple sauce, extemporaneously prepared suspension (EP), and intact sildenafil 20 mg tablets in healthy volunteers under fasting conditions. *Clin Pharmacol Drug Dev.* 2015;4:74–80.
8. Damle B, Duczynski G, Jeffers BW, et al. Pharmacokinetics of a novel orodispersible tablet of sildenafil in healthy subjects. *Clin Ther.* 2014;36:236–244.
9. Radicioni M, Castiglioni C, Giori A, et al. Bioequivalence study of a new sildenafil 100 mg orodispersible film compared to the conventional film-coated 100 mg tablet administered to healthy male volunteers. *Drug Des Dev Ther.* 2017;11:1183–1192.

10. Nichols DJ, Muirhead GJ, Harness JA. Pharmacokinetics of sildenafil citrate after single oral doses in healthy male subjects: absolute bioavailability, food effects and dose proportionality. *Br J Clin Pharmacol.* 2002;53(Suppl 1):5S–12S.

11. Jetter A, Kinzig-Schippers M, Walchner-Bonjean M, et al. Effects of grapefruit juice on the pharmacokinetics of sildenafil. *Clin Pharmacol Ther.* 2002;71:21–29.

12. Al-Ghazawi MA, Tutunji MS, AbuRuz SM. The effects of pummelo juice on pharmacokinetics of sildenafil in healthy adult male Jordanian volunteers. *Eur J Clin Pharmacol.* 2010;66:159–163.

13. Abdelkawy KS, Donia AM, Turner RB, Elbarbry F. Effects of lemon and Seville orange juices on the pharmacokinetic properties of sildenafil in healthy subjects. *Drugs R D.* 2016;16:271–278.

Simvastatin

Product Availability

Solid	• Tablet: 5 mg, 10 mg, 20 mg, 40 mg, 80 mg (Zocor® [Merck]; others)
Liquid	• Oral suspension: 20 mg/5 mL, 40 mg/5 mL (FloLipid® [TCG Fluent Pharm])

Physicochemical (drug)

Molecular weight: • 418.58	Permeability: • LogP 4.68 • LogD 4.68 (pH 7.4)	Water solubility: • ≤0.03 mg/mL
pKa: • n/a	Classification: • BCS Class 2; BDDCS Class 2	

Pharmaceutical (product)

Solid	• Many tablet products are film-coated. • Non-film-coated tablets may be crushed and then dispersed in water.
Liquid	• Oral suspension: o pH n/a o Osmolality n/a o Viscosity n/a o May contain acesulfame potassium and propylene glycol; strawberry-flavored o Store at controlled room temperature; use within 1 month of first opening.

Pharmacokinetic (patient)

Absorption	• Specific site not known; t_{max} ~1–2 hours after an oral dose • Bioavailability <5%
Transport	• Substrate for OATP uptake • Plasma protein binding ≥90% • V_d ~230 liters
Metabolism	• Simvastatin is a prodrug requiring hydrolysis (CYP3A4) to the active mevinolinic acid • Cl ~7.6 mL/min/kg

Enteral Administration and Nutrition Considerations

Compatibility, Stability, and Bioavailability Considerations
- An extemporaneously compounded oral suspension (1 mg/mL) prepared from drug powder in SyrSpend SF PH4, stored in low-actinic plastic containers at 2°C–8°C, remained stable (HPLC analysis) for 90 days.[1]

- A nanocrystal formulation under study enhanced dissolution and improved oral bioavailability compared with plain simvastatin.[2]
- Using a nanostructured lipid formulation resulted in significant improvement in oral bioavailability (~4-fold) and hypolipidemic effect in an animal model.[3]
- Coamorphous simvastatin–amino acid formulations being evaluated suggest they have a stability and dissolution advantage compared with the crystalline formulation (or even the amorphous form alone) in aqueous and simulated intestinal fluids.[4]
- Compared with pure drug, a solid dispersion formulation that used nonfat milk as a carrier enhanced drug solubility (~30-fold) with conversion to the amorphous form.[5]
- Based on data modeling, oral bioavailability is expected to remain relatively unchanged following gastric bypass surgery.[6]

Drug-Nutrition Interactions
- Drug may influence nutrition status directly or indirectly:
  o CNS: cognitive impairment, confusion, headache
  o GI: nausea, dyspepsia, abdominal pain, constipation or diarrhea, elevated aminotransferases (AST, ALT), rare hepatic failure
  o Metabolic: glucose intolerance, proteinuria
  o Other: myopathy (pain, tenderness, weakness) including immune-mediated and necrotizing, rhabdomyolysis
- No data on the influence of malnutrition or obesity on drug disposition.
- Influence of food on oral absorption or bioavailability:
  o A high-fat meal (954 kcal, 57% fat) reduced peak drug concentrations and oral bioavailability (~20%) of the drug from the suspension.
  o Grapefruit juice (200 mL daily to 400 mL three times daily) before or with drug administration significantly increased oral bioavailability (3.3- to 7-fold) compared with water.[7-9]

Recommendations

Gastric	• Crush and disperse non-film-coated tablet in water prior to administration.
	• Alternative: Dilute oral suspension in water (at least 1:1) prior to administration.
	• No need to hold EN beyond the time required to flush-administer-flush.
Postpyloric	• As above.
	• Monitor for any unexpected change in effect.

References

1. Geiger CM, Sorenson B, Whaley P. Stability assessment of 10 active pharmaceutical ingredients compounded in SyrSpend SF. *Int J Pharm Compd.* 2015;19:420–427.

2. Jiang T, Han N, Zhao B, Xie Y, Wang S. Enhanced dissolution rate and oral bioavailability of simvastatin nanocrystal prepared by sonoprecipitation. *Drug Dev Ind Pharm.* 2012;38: 1230–1239.
3. Fathi HA, Allam A, Elsabahy M, Fetih G, El-Badry M. Nanostructured lipid carriers for improved oral delivery and prolonged antihyperlipidemic effect of simvastatin. *Colloids Surf B Biointerfaces.* 2018;162:236–245.
4. Heikkinen AT, DeClerck L, Löbmann K, et al. Dissolution properties of co-amorphous drug-amino acid formulations in buffer and biorelevant media. *Pharmazie.* 2015;70: 452–457.
5. Sonar PA, Behera AL, Banerjee SK, Gaikwad DD, Harer SL. Preparation and characterization of simvastatin solid dispersion using skimmed milk. *Drug Dev Ind Pharm.* 2015;41:22–27.
6. Darwich AS, Pade D, Ammori BJ, et al. A mechanistic pharmacokinetic model to assess modified oral drug bioavailability post bariatric surgery in morbidly obese patients: interplay between CYP3A gut wall metabolism, permeability and dissolution. *J Pharm Pharmacol.* 2012;64:1008–1024.
7. Lilja JJ, Kivisto KT, Neuvonen PJ. Grapefruit juice-simvastatin interaction: effect on serum concentrations of simvastatin, simvastatin acid, and HMG-CoA reductase inhibitors. *Clin Pharmacol Ther.* 1998;64:477–483.
8. Lilja JJ, Kivisto KT, Neuvonen PJ. Duration of effect of grapefruit juice on the pharmacokinetics of the CYP3A4 substrate simvastatin. *Clin Pharmacol Ther.* 2000;68: 384–390.
9. Lilja JJ, Neuvonen M, Neuvonen PJ. Effects of regular consumption of grapefruit juice on the pharmacokinetics of simvastatin. *Br J Clin Pharmacol.* 2004;58:56–60.

Sitagliptin Phosphate

Product Availability

Solid	• Tablet: 25 mg, 50 mg, 100 mg (base) (Januvia® [Merck]; others)

Physicochemical (drug)

Molecular weight: • 407.32 (salt 505.31)	Permeability: • LogP 1.5 • LogD n/a	Water solubility: • 0.18 mg/mL
pKa: • 8.8	Classification: • BCS Class n/a; BDDCS Class 3	

Pharmaceutical (product)

Solid	• Many tablet products are film-coated and may be difficult to crush before dispersing in water.

Pharmacokinetic (patient)

Absorption	• Specific site not known; t_{max} within ~2–4 hours after an oral dose • Bioavailability ~87%
Transport	• Substrate for P-glycoprotein efflux • Substrate for organic anion transporter (OAT3) uptake • Plasma protein binding ~38% • V_d ~198 liters
Metabolism	• Some metabolism by CYP3A4 and CYP2C8 to inactives, but most of the dose is excreted unchanged mainly in urine. • Cl ~350–420 mL/min

Enteral Administration and Nutrition Considerations

Compatibility, Stability, and Bioavailability Considerations
• No data are available.

Drug-Nutrition Interactions
• Drug may influence nutrition status directly or indirectly:
  o CNS: headache
  o GI: stomatitis, pancreatitis
  o Metabolic: angioedema, peripheral edema, rare hypoglycemia
  o Other: severe arthralgia, myalgia
• No data on the influence of malnutrition or obesity on drug disposition.
• Influence of food on oral absorption or bioavailability:
  o Food, including a high-fat meal (~900 kcal, 57% fat), has no influence on oral absorption or bioavailability relative to administration in the fasted state.[1]

Recommendations

Gastric	• Crush and/or disperse tablet in water prior to administration. • No need to hold EN beyond the time required to flush-administer-flush.
Postpyloric	• As above. • Monitor for any unexpected change in effect.

Reference

1. Bergman A, Ebel D, Liu F, et al. Absolute bioavailability of sitagliptin, an oral dipeptidyl peptidase-4 inhibitor, in healthy volunteers. *Biopharm Drug Disp.* 2007;28:315–322.

Spironolactone

Product Availability

Solid	• Tablet: 25 mg, 50 mg, 100 mg (Aldactone® [GD Searle]; others)
Liquid	• Oral suspension: 25 mg/5 mL (CaroSpir® [CMP Pharma])

Physicochemical (drug)

Molecular weight: • 416.58	Permeability: • LogP 2.26 • LogD 2.26 (pH 7.4)	Water solubility: • ~0.03 mg/mL
pKa: • n/a	Classification: • BCS Class 2; BDDCS Class 2	

Pharmaceutical (product)

Solid	• Some tablet products are film-coated. • Non-film-coated tablets can be dispersed in water.
Liquid	• Oral suspension (reconstituted): o pH ~4.5 o Osmolality n/a o Viscosity: viscous o May contain saccharin and glycerin; banana-flavored o Store at controlled room temperature and use within 30 days. o Shake product very well before measuring out the dose.
Note	• Tablet and suspension formulations are not necessarily bioequivalent.

Pharmacokinetic (patient)

Absorption	• Specific site not known; t_{max} ~1–4 hours after an oral dose (tablet) • Bioavailability ~90%
Transport	• Plasma protein binding >90% • V_d ~10 L/kg
Metabolism	• Extensive metabolism by deacetylation (and possibly other mechanisms) prior to dethiolation to form canrenone (major metabolite) and others, all of which are excreted primarily in urine • Cl ~93 mL/min/kg

Enteral Administration and Nutrition Considerations

Compatibility, Stability, and Bioavailability Considerations

- Optimal stability for spironolactone is seen at pH ~4.5.[1,2]
- The official USP formulation for oral suspension (5 mg/mL) prepared from tablets in OraBlend is expected to have pH of 3.6–4.6 and provided a BUD of 90 days when refrigerated.

- An extemporaneously compounded suspension (1 mg/mL) prepared from tablets in ethanol, carboxymethylcellulose 1.5%, syrup NF, and purified water, stored in amber glass bottles at 4°C or 22°C, remained stable (HPLC analysis) for 91 days.[3]
- An extemporaneously compounded suspension (2 mg/mL) prepared from powder in ethanol, simple syrup, and a preservative, stored in amber bottles at 24°C, remained stable (HPLC analysis) for 160 days.[4]
- An oral liquid (2 mg/mL) prepared from tablets using multiple solvents (ethanol PEG 400, propylene glycol, and glycerin), stored in amber glass bottles at 40°C, remained stable (HPLC analysis) for 93 days.[5]
- A liquid preparation (2.5 mg/mL) using a nonaqueous vehicle (ethanol, propylene glycol, and glycerol) remained stable for 4 months when stored in amber glass at 19°C.[6]
- An oral suspension (2.5 mg/mL) prepared from tablets (25 mg) in simple syrup, stored in amber glass bottles at 5°C or 22°C, remained stable (HPLC analysis) for up to 60 days when also preserved with 0.2% potassium sorbate.[7]
- Extemporaneously compounded suspensions (2.5, 5, and 10 mg/mL) prepared from tablets in water or cherry syrup, stored in glass prescription bottles at 5°C or 30°C, remained stable (HPLC analysis) for 4 weeks.[8]
- An extemporaneously compounded oral liquid (10 mg/mL) had a pH of 4.28.
- An extemporaneously compounded oral suspension (5 mg/mL) prepared from tablets (25 mg) in a complex recipe and stored in amber glass bottles at 5°C–7°C or 21°C–25°C remained stable (HPLC analysis) for 21 days (room temperature) or 60 days (refrigerated).[9]
- Another extemporaneous suspension (5 mg/mL) prepared from tablets using a complex recipe including carboxymethylcellulose, Veegum, sorbitol, and distilled water, stored in amber bottles at 5°C or 30°C, remained stable (HPLC analysis) for 90 days.[10]
- An extemporaneously compounded oral suspension (5 mg/mL) prepared from drug powder in a vehicle that included carboxymethylcellulose, propylene glycol, saccharin, parabens, ethanol, and sterile water, stored in amber glass at 2°C–8°C or 23°C–27°C, remained stable (HPLC analysis) for 7 days; reported pH was 6.4.[11]
- Three extemporaneous suspensions (25 mg/mL) prepared from tablets but differing in suspending vehicle (OraSweet/OraPlus [1:1], OraSweet SF/OraPlus [1:1], or cherry syrup/simple syrup [1:4]), stored in polyethylene terephthalate plastic bottles at 5°C or 25°C, remained stable (HPLC analysis) for 60 days.[12]
- An extemporaneously compounded oral suspension (25 mg/mL) prepared from drug powder in SyrSpend SF PH4 and in SyrSpend SF PH4 Cherry, stored in low-actinic plastic at 2°C–8°C, remained stable (HPLC analysis) for 90 days.[13]

- A solid dispersion formulation under study exhibited a 2.5-fold increase in drug solubility compared with the pure drug.[14]
- A nanoparticle formulation being investigated revealed good stability with rapid and complete release in simulated gastric fluid; it is expected to improve oral bioavailability while requiring only small volumes for administration.[15]
- A nanosuspension formulation under development resulted in greater cell membrane permeability, compared with a saturated solution of micronized drug particles, and is expected to improve oral bioavailability.[16]

Drug-Nutrition Interactions

- Drug may influence nutrition status directly or indirectly:
  - CNS: headache, drowsiness, lethargy, ataxia
  - GI: anorexia, nausea, vomiting, gastric ulceration, abdominal cramping, diarrhea
  - Metabolic: hyperkalemia, hyponatremia, elevated BUN
- No data on the influence of malnutrition or obesity on drug disposition.
- Influence of food on oral absorption or bioavailability:
  - Food increases the oral bioavailability of the tablet and suspension by at least 90%.

Recommendations

Gastric	• Disperse non-film-coated tablet in water just prior to administration. • Alternative: Use an oral suspension diluted with water (at least 1:1) prior to administration. • No need to hold EN beyond the time required to flush-administer-flush.
Postpyloric	• As above. • Monitor for any unexpected change in effect.

References

1. Pramar Y, Gupta VD. Preformulation studies of spironolactone: effect of pH, two buffer species, ionic strength, and temperature on stability. *J Pharm Sci.* 1991;80:551–553.
2. Glass BD, Haywood A. Stability considerations in liquid dosage forms extemporaneously prepared from commercially available products. *J Pharm Pharmaceut Sci.* 2006;9:398–426.
3. Nahata MC, Morosco RS, Hipple TF. Stability of spironolactone in an extemporaneously prepared suspension at two temperatures. *Ann Pharmacother.* 1993;27:1198–1199.
4. Gupta VD, Gibbs CW, Ghanekar AG. Stability of pediatric liquid dosage forms of ethacrynic acid, indomethacin, methyldopate hydrochloride, prednisone, and spironolactone. *Am J Hosp Pharm.* 1978;35:1382–1385.
5. Pramar Y, Gupta VD, Bethea C. Development of a stable oral liquid dosage form of spironolactone. *J Clin Pharm Ther.* 1992;17:245–248.
6. McKnight DL. The formulation of spironolactone solution for paediatric use. *Aust J Hosp Pharm.* 1993;23:83.
7. Salgado AC, Rosa ML, Duarte MA, et al. Stability of spironolactone in an extemporaneously prepared aqueous suspension: the importance of microbiological quality of compounded paediatric formulations. *Eur J Hosp Pharm Sci.* 2005;11:68–73.

8. Mathur LK, Wickman A. Stability of extemporaneously compounded spironolactone suspensions. *Am J Hosp Pharm.* 1989;46:2040–2042.
9. Peterson GM, Meaney MF, Reid CA. Stability of extemporaneously prepared mixtures of metoprolol and spironolactone. *Aust J Hosp Pharm.* 1989;19:344–346.
10. Alexander KS, Vangala SSKS, White DB, et al. The formulation development and stability of spironolactone suspension. *Int J Pharm Compd.* 1997;1:195–199.
11. Mendes C, Costa AP, Oliviera PR, et al. Physicochemical and microbiological stability of extemporaneous anti-hypertensive pediatric suspensions for hospital use. *Pharm Dev Technol.* 2013;18:813–820.
12. Allen LV, Erickson MA. Stability of ketoconazole, metolazone, metronidazole, procainamide hydrochloride, and spironolactone in extemporaneously compounded oral liquids. *Am J Health-Syst Pharm.* 1996;53:2073–2078.
13. Geiger CM, Sorenson B, Whaley P. Stability assessment of 10 active pharmaceutical ingredients compounded in SyrSpend SF. *Int J Pharm Compd.* 2015;19:420–427.
14. Shamsuddin MF, Ansari SH, Ali J. Development and evaluation of solid dispersion of spironolactone using fusion method. *Int J Pharm Investig.* 2016;6:63–68.
15. Blouza IL, Charcosset C, Sfar S, Fessi H. Preparation and characterization of spironolactone-loaded nanocapsules for paediatric use. *Int J Pharm.* 2006;325:124–131.
16. Lenhardt T, Vergnault G, Grenier P, Scherer D, Langguth P. Evaluation of nanosuspensions for absorption enhancement of poorly soluble drugs: in vitro transport studies across intestinal epithelial monolayers. *AAPS J.* 2008;10:435–438.

Sumatriptan Succinate

Product Availability

Solid	• Tablet: 25 mg, 50 mg, 100 mg (base) (Imitrex® [GSK]; others)

Physicochemical (drug)

Molecular weight:	Permeability:	Water solubility:
• 295.41 (salt 413.49)	• LogP 0.93	• 21.4 mg/mL
	• LogD −1.17 (pH 7.4)	
pKa:	Classification:	
• 4.21, 5.67, 9.63, 12.00	• BCS Class 3; BDDCS Class 1	

Pharmaceutical (product)

Solid	• Some tablet products are film-coated.
	• Non-film-coated tablet may disperse in water.

Pharmacokinetic (patient)

Absorption	• Specific site not known; t_{max} <1 hour after an oral dose
	• Bioavailability ~15%
Transport	• Substrate for P-glycoprotein efflux
	• Plasma protein binding ~14%–21%
	• V_d ~2.4 L/kg
Metabolism	• Metabolized extensively by monoamine oxidase A and glucuronosyltransferase prior to excretion
	• Cl ~1.2 L/min

Enteral Administration and Nutrition Considerations

Compatibility, Stability, and Bioavailability Considerations

- The official USP formulation yields a 5 mg/mL oral suspension with a pH between 3.6 and 4.6 and is provided a BUD of 14 days when stored at 2°C–8°C.
- Using a variety of suspending vehicles (OraSweet/OraPlus, OraSweet SF/OraPlus, Syrpalta), sumatriptan suspension stored in amber glass bottles at 4°C remained stable (HPLC analysis) for 21 days regardless of vehicle, but losses exceeded 10% by 28 days.[1]
- Orally disintegrating tablets under development for buccal or sublingual use exhibit much more rapid disintegration with higher bioavailability (~1.3–1.4 fold) compared with the conventional oral tablet or aqueous solution.[2,3]

Drug-Nutrition Interactions

- Drug may influence nutrition status directly or indirectly:
  - CNS: fatigue, vertigo
  - GI: dysgeusia, nausea, vomiting, dysphagia, abdominal discomfort, obstruction

- o Metabolic: dysglycemia
- o Other: myalgia
- No data on the influence of malnutrition or obesity on drug disposition.
- Influence of food on oral absorption or bioavailability:
  - o A high-fat meal may increase the rate and the extent of absorption (~10%–15%)

Recommendations

Gastric	• If there is no therapeutic alternative (eg, transdermal, nasal, sublingual administration), disperse tablets in water prior to administration. • No need to hold EN beyond the time required to flush-administer-flush.
Postpyloric	• As above. • Monitor for any unexpected change in effect.

References

1. Fish DN, Beall HD, Goodwin SD, et al. Stability of sumatriptan succinate in extemporaneously prepared oral liquids. *Am J Health-Syst Pharm.* 1997;54:1619–1622.
2. Shivanand K, Raju SA, Nizamuddin S, Jayakar B. In vivo bioavailability studies of sumatriptan succinate buccal tablets. *DARU J Pharm Sci.* 2011;19:224–230.
3. Tayel SA, El Nabarawi MA, Amin MM, AbouGhaly MHH. Comparative study between different ready-made orally disintegrating platforms for the formulation of sumatriptan succinate sublingual tablets. *AAPS PharmSciTech.* 2017;18:410–423.

Tamsulosin Hydrochloride

Product Availability

Solid	• Capsule: 0.4 mg (Flomax® [Boehringer Ingelheim]; others)

Physicochemical (drug)

Molecular weight: • 408.52 (salt 444.97)	Permeability: • LogP 2.3 • LogD 0.89 (pH 7.4, calc)	Water solubility: • 10 mg/mL
pKa: • 9.3	Classification: • BCS Class 1; BDDCS Class 1	

Pharmaceutical (product)

Solid	• Do not crush, chew, or open capsule, which is a slow-release product.

Pharmacokinetic (patient)

Absorption	• Specific site not known; t_{max} ~4–5 hours after an oral dose (fasted) • Bioavailability ~90%
Transport	• Plasma protein binding ~94%–99% • V_d ~16 liters
Metabolism	• Extensively metabolized by CYP3A4 and CYP2D6, with subsequent conjugation with glucuronic acid and sulfate prior to excretion in urine • Cl ~2.9 L/h

Enteral Administration and Nutrition Considerations

Compatibility, Stability, and Bioavailability Considerations
• No data are available.

Drug-Nutrition Interactions
• Drug may influence nutrition status directly or indirectly:
  o CNS: headache, dizziness, blurred vision
  o GI: nausea, diarrhea
  o Other: back pain
• No data on the influence of malnutrition or obesity on drug disposition.
• Influence of food on oral absorption or bioavailability:
  o Food (light or high-fat meal) may reduce the rate of drug absorption and reduces oral bioavailability by ~30%.
  o Grapefruit juice is likely to increase oral bioavailability.

Recommendations

Gastric	• Do not administer via enteral access device; use therapeutic alternative.
Postpyloric	• As above.

Temazepam

Product Availability

Solid	• Capsule: 7.5 mg, 15 mg, 22.5 mg, 30 mg (Restoril® [Spec GX]; others)

Physicochemical (drug)

Molecular weight: • 300.75	Permeability: • LogP 2.19 • LogD 1.79 (pH 7.4)	Water solubility: • 0.6 mg/mL
pKa: • 1.5	Classification: • BCS Class n/a; BDDCS Class 1	

Pharmaceutical (product)

Solid	• Capsule contents may disperse in water. • Avoid manipulation or exposure if pregnant.

Pharmacokinetic (patient)

Absorption	• Specific site not known; t_{max} within ~1 hour after an oral dose • Bioavailability ~90%
Transport	• Plasma protein binding ~96% • V_d ~1.1 L/kg
Metabolism	• Metabolized to oxazepam (via CYP3A4/2C9) or to conjugates (via UGT2B7/15), which also conjugates oxazepam to glucuronic acid; all metabolites are predominantly excreted in urine • Cl ~0.87 mL/min/kg

Enteral Administration and Nutrition Considerations

Compatibility, Stability, and Bioavailability Considerations
• A fraction of the orally administered drug may be degraded by hydrolysis in acidic gastric fluid.[1]

Drug-Nutrition Interactions
• Drug may influence nutrition status directly or indirectly:
  o CNS: sedation, confusion, ataxia, altered behavior, amnesia
  o GI: vomiting, diarrhea
  o Other: back pain
• No data on the influence of malnutrition or obesity on drug disposition.
• No known influence of food on oral absorption or bioavailability.

Recommendations

Gastric	• Disperse capsule contents in water just prior to administration. • No need to hold EN beyond the time required to flush-administer-flush.
Postpyloric	• As above. • Monitor for any unexpected change in effect.

Reference

1. Yang TJ, Pu QL, Yang SK. Hydrolysis of temazepam in simulated gastric fluid and its pharmacological consequence. *J Pharm Sci.* 1994;83:1543–1547.

Terazosin Hydrochloride

Product Availability

Solid	• Capsule: 1 mg, 2 mg, 5 mg, 10 mg (various)

Physicochemical (drug)

Molecular weight:	Permeability:	Water solubility:
• 387.44 (salt 423.90)	• LogP 2.18 (calc)	• 24.2 mg/mL
	• LogD –4.64 (pH 7.4)	
pKa:	Classification:	
• 7.2	• BCS Class 3; BDDCS Class 1	

Pharmaceutical (product)

Solid	• Capsule contents may disperse in water.

Pharmacokinetic (patient)

Absorption	• Specific site not known; t_{max} ~1 hour after an oral dose
	• Bioavailability ≥90%
Transport	• Plasma protein binding ~90%–94%
	• V_d ~1.1 L/kg
Metabolism	• Minimal first-pass metabolism with excretion of parent and metabolites in feces and urine
	• Cl ~1.2 mL/min/kg

Enteral Administration and Nutrition Considerations

Compatibility, Stability, and Bioavailability Considerations
- A previously available liquid-filled soft gelatin capsule was prepared for enteral access device administration by dissolving the entire dosage form in 60 mL warm (100°F–110°F) water while stirring for 10–15 minutes.[1]

Drug-Nutrition Interactions
- Drug may influence nutrition status directly or indirectly:
  o Rare weight gain
  o CNS: headache, dizziness
  o GI: nausea
  o Metabolic: peripheral edema
  o Other: flu-like aches
- No data on the influence of malnutrition or obesity on drug disposition.
- Influence of food on oral absorption or bioavailability:
  o Food will delay drug absorption but without an influence on oral bioavailability.[2]

Recommendations

Gastric	• Disperse capsule contents in water just prior to administration. • No need to hold EN beyond the time required to flush-administer-flush.
Postpyloric	• As above. • Monitor for any unexpected change in effect.

References

1. Cheng L. Administration of terazosin capsules through feeding tubes. *Am J Health-Syst Pharm.* 1995;52:2031.
2. McNeil JJ, Drummer OH, Raymond K, Conway EL, Louis WJ. The influence of food on the oral bioavailability of terazosin. *Br J Clin Pharmacol.* 1991;32:775–776.

Ticagrelor

Product Availability

Solid	• Tablet: 60 mg, 90 mg (Brilinta® [AstraZeneca])

Physicochemical (drug)

Molecular weight: • 522.57	Permeability: • LogP 1.98 • LogD n/a	Water solubility: • 0.01 mg/mL
pKa: • 2.28, 13.48	Classification: • BCS Class 4; BDDCS Class 2	

Pharmaceutical (product)

Solid	• Tablet is film-coated and does not easily disperse in water. • Tablet may be crushed and dispersed in water (50 mL).

Pharmacokinetic (patient)

Absorption	• Specific site not known; t_{max} ~1–2 hours after an oral dose • Bioavailability ~30%–42%
Transport	• Substrate for P-glycoprotein efflux • Plasma protein binding ~99% • V_d ~88 liters
Metabolism	• Metabolized by CYP3A4/5 to an active metabolite with several other metabolites; excreted primarily through the biliary route • Cl n/a

Enteral Administration and Nutrition Considerations

Compatibility, Stability, and Bioavailability Considerations
- In 36 healthy volunteers, a crushed tablet (90 mg) dispersed in water (200 mL) and administered orally or through a nasogastric tube (size and material not reported) resulted in much more rapid absorption than a whole tablet taken with 200 mL water in a fasted state; both forms of the drug (crushed or whole) and both routes (oral or enteral) had similar bioavailability.[1]
- An extemporaneous suspension formulation delivered directly into the proximal small intestine under fasting conditions resulted in lower bioavailability (~11%) than the same formulation administered orally in a group of healthy volunteers.[2]
- When patients requiring primary percutaneous coronary intervention following ST-elevated myocardial infarction were administered crushed tablets (2 × 90 mg) dispersed in purified water (50 mL) by mouth, the patients experienced quicker drug exposure and more rapid clinical effects compared with those receiving intact tablets.[3]

- An extemporaneously compounded liquid prepared from 1 or 2 crushed tablets (90 mg) dispersed in purified water was evaluated for administration through 3 nasogastric tubes (1 polyvinyl chloride, 1 silicone, 1 polyurethane); the compound demonstrated stability (HPLC analysis) and delivery of at least 97% of drug.[4]
- Following cardiac arrest, 38 patients (71% of whom underwent therapeutic hypothermia) were administered crushed tablets (2 × 90 mg, then 90 mg twice daily) dispersed in water (20 mL) through a nasogastric tube (15 Fr, polyurethane) followed by 10 mL water flush; adequate platelet inhibition was achieved in 97% of these patients.[5]
- In 44 patients undergoing primary percutaneous coronary intervention following cardiac arrest, the administration of crushed tablets (2 × 90 mg, then 90 mg twice daily) dispersed in purified water (50 mL) through a nasogastric tube resulted in sufficient platelet inhibition at 12 hours in ≥88% of patients.[6]

Drug-Nutrition Interactions
- Drug may influence nutrition status directly or indirectly:
  - CNS: headache, dizziness, fatigue
  - GI: nausea, diarrhea
  - Other: back pain
- Influence of malnutrition or obesity on drug disposition:
  - In a study evaluating BMI on platelet response to ticagrelor following percutaneous coronary intervention for acute coronary syndrome, no differences in platelet reactivity was noted between obese and nonobese patients.[7]
- Influence of food on oral absorption or bioavailability:
  - A high-fat meal increases oral bioavailability by ~21%.
  - Grapefruit juice (200 mL 3 times daily for 4 days) increased oral bioavailability (2.2-fold) of the parent drug (but not the active metabolite) compared with the same regimen of water in healthy volunteers, with a significant increase in antiplatelet effect.[8]

Recommendations

Gastric	• If there is no therapeutic alternative, crush and disperse tablet in water just prior to administration. • No need to hold EN beyond the time required to flush-administer-flush.
Postpyloric	• As above. • Monitor for any unexpected change in effect.

References

1. Teng R, Carlson G, Hsia J. An open-label, randomized bioavailability study with alternative methods of administration of crushed ticagrelor tablets in healthy volunteers. *Int J Clin Pharmacol Ther.* 2015;53:182–189.

2. Teng R, Mya J. Absolute bioavailability and regional absorption of ticagrelor in healthy volunteers. *J Drug Assess*. 2014;3:43–50.
3. Alexopoulos D, Barampoutis N, Gkizas V, et al. Crushed versus integral tablets of ticagrelor in ST-segment elevation myocardial infarction patients: a randomized pharmacokinetic/pharmacodynamics study. *Clin Pharmacokinet*. 2016;55:359–367.
4. Crean B, Finnie C, Crosby A. Evaluation of crushing and naso-gastric tube passage ex vivo. *Drugs R D*. 2013;13:153–157.
5. Tilemann LM, Stiepak J, Zelniker T, et al. Efficacy of enteral ticagrelor in hypothermic patients after out-of-hospital cardiac arrest. *Clin Res Cardiol*. 2016;105:332–340.
6. Ratcovich H, Sadjadieh G, Andersson HB, et al. The effect of TIcagrelor administered through a nasogastric tube to COMAtose patients undergoing acute percutaneous coronary intervention: the TICOMA study. *EuroIntervention*. 2017;12:1782–1788.
7. Deharo P, Pankert M, Bonnet G, et al. Body mass index has no impact on platelet inhibition induced by ticagrelor after acute coronary syndrome, conversely to prasugrel. *Int J Cardiol*. 2014;176:1200–1202.
8. Holmberg MT, Tornio A, Joutsi-Korhonen L, et al. Grapefruit juice markedly increases the plasma concentrations and antiplatelet effects of ticagrelor in healthy subjects. *Br J Clin Pharmacol*. 2012;75:1488–1496.

Tizanidine Hydrochloride

Product Availability

Solid	• Tablet: 4 mg (base) (Zanaflex® [Covis Pharma]; others) • Capsule: 2 mg, 4 mg, 6 mg (base) (Zanaflex® [Covis Pharma]; others)

Physicochemical (drug)

Molecular weight: • 253.71 (salt 290.17)	Permeability: • LogP 1.4 • LogD n/a	Water solubility: • 0.133 mg/mL • 0.044 mg/mL (salt)
pKa: • 7.4	Classification: • BCS Class n/a; BDDCS Class 2	

Pharmaceutical (product)

Solid	• Tablet is not coated and may be crushed and dispersed in water. • Capsule contents may disperse in water. • Tablet and capsule are not necessarily bioequivalent, especially during the fed state.

Pharmacokinetic (patient)

Absorption	• Specific site not known; t_{max} ~1 hour after an oral dose • Bioavailability ~40%
Transport	• Plasma protein binding ~30% • V_d ~2.4 L/kg
Metabolism	• Extensive first-pass metabolism (via CYP1A2) to inactive metabolites, excreted mostly in the urine • Cl ~74 mL/min

Enteral Administration and Nutrition Considerations

Compatibility, Stability, and Bioavailability Considerations
  • Aqueous solubility decreases as pH of solution increases.
  • In healthy volunteers in the fasted state, administration of capsule contents (6 mg) sprinkled in apple sauce (30 mL) resulted in higher bioavailability (1.2-fold) than administration of the intact capsule by mouth.[1]

Drug-Nutrition Interactions
  • Drug may influence nutrition status directly or indirectly:
    o CNS: sedation, dizziness, dyskinesia
    o GI: dry mouth, vomiting, constipation, transaminitis
  • No data on the influence of malnutrition or obesity on drug disposition.

- Influence of food on oral absorption or bioavailability:
  - Food increases the drug's oral bioavailability by 10% (capsule) to 30% (tablet).
  - A high-fat meal (900–1000 kcal, 55%–60% fat) reduces the rate of absorption and oral bioavailability of the capsule relative to the tablet formulation.[2]

Recommendations

Gastric	• Disperse capsule contents in water just prior to administration. • No need to hold EN beyond the time required to flush-administer-flush.
Postpyloric	• As above. • Monitor for any unexpected change in effect.

References

1. Henney HR, Fitzpatrick A, Stewart J, Runyan JD. Relative bioavailability of tizanidine hydrochloride capsule formulation compared with capsule contents administered in applesauce: a single-dose, open-label, randomized, two-way, crossover study in fasted healthy adult subjects. *Clin Ther.* 2008;30:2263–2271.
2. Henney HR, Shah J. Relative bioavailability of tizanidine 4-mg capsule and tablet formulations after a standardized high-fat meal: a single-dose, randomized, open-label, crossover study in healthy subjects. *Clin Ther.* 2007;29:661–669.

Tolterodine Tartrate

Product Availability

Solid	• Tablet: 1 mg, 2 mg (Detrol® [Pharmacia & Upjohn]; others) • Capsule: Extended-release: 2 mg, 4 mg (Detrol® LA [Pharmacia & Upjohn]; others)

Physicochemical (drug)

Molecular weight: • 325.50 (salt 475.58)	Permeability: • LogP 5.24 (calc) • LogD 1.83 (pH 7.3)	Water solubility: • 12 mg/mL
pKa: • 9.87	Classification: • BCS Class 1; BDDCS Class 1	

Pharmaceutical (product)

Solid	• Tablet products may be film-coated. • Tablets may disperse in water. • Do not crush modified-release capsule or capsule contents.

Pharmacokinetic (patient)

Absorption	• Specific site not known; t_{max} ~1–2 hours after an oral dose (immediate-release) • Bioavailability varies between ~10%–74%; higher in individuals with poor-metabolizer CYP2D6 phenotype
Transport	• Plasma protein binding ~96%, especially to α_1-acid glycoprotein • V_d ~113 liters
Metabolism	• Metabolized by CYP2D6 and CYP3A4, with the latter predominant in forming an N-dealkylated metabolite in individuals with poor-metabolizer CYP2D6 phenotype; the major and active metabolite is 5-hydroxy-methyl tolterodine; excretion occurs through urine more than in feces • Cl ~7–9 L/min (extensive metabolizer), 0.2–0.3 L/min (poor metabolizer)

Enteral Administration and Nutrition Considerations

Compatibility, Stability, and Bioavailability Considerations
• No data are available.

Drug-Nutrition Interactions
• Drug may influence nutrition status directly or indirectly:
  ○ Rare weight gain
  ○ CNS: headache, dizziness, xerophthalmia

- o GI: dry mouth, abdominal pain, constipation
- o Other: flu-like symptoms
- No data on the influence of malnutrition or obesity on drug disposition.
- Influence of food on oral absorption or bioavailability:
  - o Food increases the oral bioavailability of the immediate-release tablet ~1.5-fold in extensive metabolizers but does not significantly influence the exposure to the active metabolite.[1]
  - o No meal effect was noted for the modified-release capsule.[2]

Recommendations

Gastric	• Disperse tablets in water just prior to administration. • No need to hold EN beyond the time required to flush-administer-flush.
Postpyloric	• As above. • Monitor for any unexpected change in effect.

References

1. Olsson B, Brynne N, Johansson C, Arnberg H. Food increases the bioavailability of tolterodine but not effective exposure. *J Clin Pharmacol.* 2001;41:298–304.
2. Olsson B, Szamosi J. Food does not influence the pharmacokinetics of a new extended release formulation of tolterodine for once daily treatment of patients with overactive bladder. *Clin Pharmacokinet.* 2001;40:135–143.

Topiramate

Product Availability

Solid	• Tablet: 25 mg, 50 mg, 100 mg, 200 mg, 300 mg, 400 mg (Topamax® [Janssen]; others)
	• Capsule:
	  o Granules:15 mg, 25 mg (Topamax® Sprinkle [Janssen]; others)
	  o Extended-release: 25 mg, 50 mg, 100 mg, 150 mg, 200 mg (Qudexy® XR [Upsher-Smith Labs]; other)

Physicochemical (drug)

Molecular weight: • 339.37	Permeability: • LogP 0.04 (calc) • LogD 2.25 (pH 7, calc)	Water solubility: • 9.8 mg/mL
pKa: • n/a	Classification: • BCS Class 1 or 3; BDDCS Class 3	

Pharmaceutical (product)

Solid	• Tablet products may be film-coated. • Tablet can be crushed and dispersed in water, but that is not recommended for oral administration (bitter taste is unacceptable). • Do not crush or chew capsule products (they contain coated granules or are extended-release). • Tablet and sprinkle capsule are considered to be bioequivalent.

Pharmacokinetic (patient)

Absorption	• Specific site not known; t_{max} ~2 hours after an oral dose (immediate-release) • Bioavailability approaches 100%.
Transport	• Plasma protein binding ~15%–41% • V_d ~0.9–1.1 L/kg
Metabolism	• Limited metabolism to at least 5 metabolites, but about 70% of drug dose is excreted unchanged renally • Cl ~1.2–1.3 L/h

Enteral Administration and Nutrition Considerations

Compatibility, Stability, and Bioavailability Considerations
- A saturated aqueous solution has a pH ~6.3.
- Topiramate has the greatest solubility in alkaline solution (pH ~9–10).
- The extended-release capsule (25 mg) granules were dispersed in 15 mL of deionized water and placed into an irrigation syringe for administration through gastrostomy tubes (14 Fr, 16 Fr, 18 Fr, 25 cm in length) and jejunostomy tubes (18 Fr, 75 cm in length); tubes were flushed with 15 mL deionized water before and with multiple portions

of deionized water after drug administration in this in vitro experiment; the use of water clogged the 14 Fr and 16 Fr tubes but was more successful in the 18 Fr gastrostomy and jejunostomy tubes.[1]

- Granules from the extended-release capsule (25 mg) were dispersed in 15 mL of sparkling water, apple juice, or Ketocal and placed into an irrigation syringe for administration through gastrostomy tubes (14 Fr, 25 cm in length); tubes were flushed with 15 mL deionized water before and with multiple portions of the diluent after drug administration in this in vitro experiment. Sparkling water allowed delivery of most of the granules but at the cost of 220 mL dosing volume; apple juice allowed most granules to be delivered at a dosing volume of 120 mL with minimal tube clogging; and Ketocal was successful at delivering all the granules without tube clogging.[1]
- Crushed tablets of topiramate doses (50–500 mg twice daily) dispersed in water (volume not reported) and administered by syringe through a nasogastric tube (size and type not reported) helped to control status epilepticus in a 12-year-old child who had been unresponsive to first- and second-line antiepileptic agents.[2]
- The administration of topiramate tablet crushed and delivered by nasogastric tube (details not reported) in 20 patients with refractory generalized convulsive status epilepticus was well tolerated and either successful or possibly successful in 16 (80%) of the patients.[3]

Drug-Nutrition Interactions
- Drug may influence nutrition status directly or indirectly:
  - Weight loss
  - CNS: cognitive dysfunction (eg, confusion, memory lapses), depression, fatigue, ataxia, visual disturbances (eg, diplopia, myopia)
  - GI: anorexia, altered taste, diarrhea
  - Metabolic: hyperchloremic (non-gap) metabolic acidosis, hypokalemia, hypophosphatemia, oligohydrosis with hyperthermia, hyperammonemia
- No data on the influence of malnutrition or obesity on drug disposition.
- No known influence of food on oral absorption or bioavailability.

Recommendations

Gastric	• Crush and/or disperse tablet in water just prior to administration. • No need to hold EN beyond the time required to flush-administer-flush.
Postpyloric	• As above. • Monitor for any unexpected change in effect.

References

1. Clark AM, Pellock JM, Holmay M, Anders B, Cloyd J. Clinical utility of topiramate extended-release capsules (USL255): bioequivalence of USL255 sprinkled and intact capsule in healthy adults and an in vitro evaluation of sprinkle delivery via enteral feeding tubes. *Epilepsy Behav*. 2016;57:105–110.
2. Shelton CM, Alford EL, Storgion S, Wheless J, Phelps SJ. Enteral topiramate in a pediatric patient with refractory status epilepticus: a case report and review of the literature. *J Pediatr Pharmacol Ther*. 2014;19:317–324.
3. Asadi-Pooya AA, Jahromi MJ, Izadi S, Emami Y. Treatment of refractory generalized convulsive status epilepticus with enteral topiramate in resource limited settings. *Seizure*. 2015;24:114–117.

Tramadol Hydrochloride

Product Availability

Solid	• Tablet:
	    o Immediate-release: 50 mg (Ultram® [Janssen]; others)
	    o Extended-release: 100 mg, 200 mg, 300 mg (various)
	 • Capsule (extended-release): 100 mg, 150 mg, 200 mg, 300 mg (ConZip® [Cipher Pharms]; others)

Physicochemical (drug)

Molecular weight: • 263.38 (salt 299.8)	Permeability: • LogP 2.63 • LogD 1.35 (pH 7)	Water solubility: • 0.8 mg/mL
pKa: • 9.41	Classification: • BCS Class 1; BDDCS Class 1	

Pharmaceutical (product)

Solid	• Immediate-release tablet may disperse in water. • Do not crush extended-release tablet or capsule products. • Capsule contains both extended-release and immediate-release constituents.

Pharmacokinetic (patient)

Absorption	• Specific site not known; t_{max} ~1.5–2 hours after an oral dose (immediate-release) • Bioavailability ~75%
Transport	• Plasma protein binding ~20% • V_d ~2.6–2.9 L/kg
Metabolism	• Extensively metabolized by CYP2D6 to an active O-desmethyl metabolite ("M1"), and by CYP3A4 to N-desmethyl tramadol ("M2"); excreted mostly via urine • Cl ~6–8 mL/min/kg

Enteral Administration and Nutrition Considerations

Compatibility, Stability, and Bioavailability Considerations
- The official USP oral suspension formulation (20 mg/mL) using OraBlend or OraSweet/OraPlus (1:1) is expected to have a pH of ~3.4–4.4 or 3.8–4.8, respectively, and has a BUD of 180 days or 90 days, respectively, at controlled room temperature.
- An extemporaneously compounded oral liquid (5 mg/mL) prepared from tablets (50 mg) in a vehicle of OraSweet NF/OraPlus (1:1) or strawberry syrup, stored in amber plastic bottles at 3°C–5°C and 23°C–25°C, remained stable (HPLC analysis) for 91 days.[1]

- An extemporaneously compounded oral suspension (10 mg/mL) prepared from drug powder in SyrSpend SF PH4, stored in low-actinic bottles at 2°C–8°C or 20°C–25°C, remained stable (HPLC analysis) for 90 days at both temperatures.[2]

Drug-Nutrition Interactions
- Drug may influence nutrition status directly or indirectly:
  - CNS: agitation and other mental status disturbances (as part of the serotonin syndrome), fatigue, confusion, visual disturbances
  - GI: anorexia, dysgeusia, nausea, vomiting, constipation more than diarrhea, abdominal pain, LFT abnormalities, and rare hyperamylasemia
  - Metabolic: proteinuria, rare hypoglycemia
  - Other: weakness
- No data on the influence of malnutrition or obesity on drug disposition.
- Influence of food on oral absorption or bioavailability:
  - No influence of food on oral bioavailability of immediate-release tablet.
  - Food may reduce the bioavailability of the extended-release tablet by ~16%.

Recommendations

Gastric	• Crush and/or disperse immediate-release tablet in water prior to administration. • No need to hold EN beyond the time required to flush-administer-flush.
Postpyloric	• As above. • Monitor for any unexpected change in effect.

References

1. Wagner DS, Johnson CE, Cichon-Hensley BK, et al. Stability of oral liquid preparations of tramadol in strawberry syrup and sugar-free vehicle. *Am J Health-Syst Pharm*. 2003;60: 1268–1270.
2. Polonini HC, Silva SL, Cunha CN, et al. Compatibility of cholecalciferol, haloperidol, imipramine hydrochloride, levodopa/carbidopa, lorazepam, minocycline hydrochloride, tacrolimus monohydrate, terbinafine, tramadol hydrochloride and valsartan in SyrSpend SF PH4 oral suspensions. *Pharmazie*. 2016;71:185–191.

Trazodone Hydrochloride

Product Availability

Solid	• Tablet: 50 mg, 100 mg, 150 mg, 300 mg (various)

Physicochemical (drug)

Molecular weight:	Permeability:	Water solubility:
• 371.87 (salt 408.32)	• LogP 3.80 • LogD 2.64 (pH 7.4)	• 0.2 mg/mL
pKa: • 6.7	Classification: • BCS Class n/a; BDDCS Class 2	

Pharmaceutical (product)

Solid	• Non-film-coated tablet products can be crushed and dispersed in water. • Sustained-release tablet product, which was discontinued, could not be crushed.

Pharmacokinetic (patient)

Absorption	• Specific site not known; t_{max} ~1 hour after an oral dose (immediate-release, fasted) • Bioavailability >50%
Transport	• Plasma protein binding ~89%–95% • V_d ~0.9–1.5 L/kg
Metabolism	• Extensively metabolized including hydroxylation and oxidation; CYP3A4 forms an active metabolite; metabolites subsequently undergo glucuronidation and are excreted mostly in urine with remainder excreted in bile • Cl ~2.3 mL/min/kg

Enteral Administration and Nutrition Considerations

Compatibility, Stability, and Bioavailability Considerations
- An extemporaneous oral suspension prepared from tablets in one of several vehicles (cherry syrup, simple syrup, Syrpalta, or Cologel), stored in a light-resistant container under refrigeration, remained stable for 30 days.[1]
- A trazodone liquid (10 mg/mL) prepared from tablets using Syrpalta as the vehicle, stored in amber glass bottles under refrigeration, remained stable for 30 days.[2]

Drug-Nutrition Interactions
- Drug may influence nutrition status directly or indirectly:
  - CNS: drowsiness, dizziness, confusion
  - GI: dry mouth, dysgeusia, nausea, vomiting, constipation
  - Metabolic: edema
  - Other: weakness, myalgia

- Influence of malnutrition or obesity on drug disposition:
  - Volume of distribution is increased in obesity both in absolute terms (162 vs 67 liters) and, more importantly, when indexed to body weight (1.43 vs 1.04 L/kg, P <0.001), while drug clearance remained unchanged (8.7 L/h), suggesting the use of total body weight for initial (loading) dose.[3]
- Influence of food on oral absorption or bioavailability:
  - Food may delay absorption but enhances oral bioavailability by ~20%.

Recommendations

Gastric	• Crush and disperse immediate-release tablet in water prior to administration. • No need to hold EN beyond the time required to flush-administer-flush.
Postpyloric	• As above. • Monitor for any unexpected change in effect.

References

1. Allen LV. Preparing a trazodone HCl suspension. *US Pharmacist.* 1990;15:54,57.
2. Pesko LJ. Compounding: trazodone oral liquid. *Am Druggist.* 1992;205:58.
3. Greenblatt DJ, Friedman H, Burstein ES, et al. Trazodone kinetics: effect of age, gender, and obesity. *Clin Pharmacol Ther.* 1987;42:193–200.

Valacyclovir Hydrochloride

Product Availability

Solid	• Tablet: 500 mg, 1000 mg (base) (Valtrex® [GSK]; others)

Physicochemical (drug)

Molecular weight:	Permeability:	Water solubility:
• 324.34 (salt 360.80)	• LogP −1.22 (calc) • LogD −1.22 (pH 7.4, calc)	• 174 mg/mL
pKa: • 1.90, 7.47, 9.43	Classification: • BCS Class 1; BDDCS Class 1	

Pharmaceutical (product)

Solid	• Tablet products may be film-coated and do not crush easily.

Pharmacokinetic (patient)

Absorption	• Specific site not known; t_{max} ~1 hour after an oral dose • Bioavailability ~54%
Transport	• Substrate for peptide uptake transporter(s) (eg, PepT1 and/or PhT1) • Plasma protein binding ~89%–95% • V_d ~7.4 liters
Metabolism	• Prodrug requires removal of valine by hydrolysis to form acyclovir and its active metabolite, acyclovir triphosphate; most is then excreted unchanged in urine • Cl ~3.5 L/h

Enteral Administration and Nutrition Considerations

Compatibility, Stability, and Bioavailability Considerations

- The official USP oral suspension (50 mg/mL) prepared from tablets in OraSweet/OraPlus (1:1) is expected to have pH 3.2–4.3 and provided a BUD of 14 days when refrigerated.
- The drug undergoes rapid hydrolysis in water or other aqueous media depending on pH; drug exhibits pH-dependent stability, optimal at pH ≤4, with hydrolysis increasing rapidly as pH increases.[1]
- The intestinal lumen pH may allow more degradation than gastric pH.[1]
- An extemporaneously compounded oral suspension (50 mg/mL) prepared from tablets (500 mg) suspended in OraPlus/OraSweet, OraPlus/OraSweet SF, or Syrpalta, stored in amber glass containers at 4°C for 60 days, exhibited over 10% drug loss (without decomposition products) (HPLC analysis) by 21 days (OraPlus) or 35 days (Syrpalta) without a change in pH.[2]

- An extemporaneous oral suspension (25 or 50 mg/mL) made from tablets (500 mg) in lots of 100 mL, each as described in the product information, and stored at refrigeration for no more than 28 days was well-tolerated after oral administration in young patients with bioavailability similar to that seen from intact tablets.[3]

Drug-Nutrition Interactions
- Drug may influence nutrition status directly or indirectly:
  o CNS: headache, confusion, encephalopathy
  o GI: nausea, vomiting, diarrhea, elevated transaminases
  o Metabolic: edema (facial)
- No data on the influence of malnutrition or obesity on drug disposition.
- Influence of food on oral absorption or bioavailability:
  o The rate and extent of absorption did not significantly change when administered with a high-fat meal (873 kcal, 51 g fat).

Recommendations

Gastric	• If there is no therapeutic alternative (eg, acyclovir), use a stable extemporaneously prepared suspension diluted with water (at least 1:1) just prior to administration. • No need to hold EN beyond the time required to flush-administer-flush.
Postpyloric	• Not recommended.
Other	• As with all antimicrobials, consider parenteral alternative for acutely ill patients to ensure therapeutic concentrations.

References
1. Granero GE, Amidon GL. Stability of valacyclovir: implications for its oral bioavailability. *Int J Pharm*. 2006;317:14–18.
2. Fish DN, Vidaurri VA, Deiter RG. Stability of valacyclovir hydrochloride in extemporaneously prepared oral liquids. *Am J Health-Syst Pharm*. 1999;56:1957–1960. .
3. Kimberlin DW, Jacobs RF, Weller S, et al. Pharmacokinetics and safety of extemporaneously compounded valacyclovir oral suspension in pediatric patients from 1 month through 11 years of age. *Clin Infect Dis*. 2010;50:221–228.

Valsartan

Product Availability

Solid	• Tablet: 40 mg, 80 mg, 160 mg, 320 mg (Diovan® [Novartis]; others)
Liquid	• Oral solution: 20 mg/5 mL (Prexxartan® [Carmel BioSci])

Physicochemical (drug)

Molecular weight:	Permeability:	Water solubility:
• 435.53	• LogP 5.8	• 0.02 mg/mL
	• Log D n/a	
pKa:	Classification:	
• 3.6	• BCS Class 2; BDDCS Class 4	

Pharmaceutical (product)

Solid	• Tablet products are often film-coated; they are unlikely to easily disperse in water without crushing.
Liquid	• Oral solution: o pH 5.7–6.2 o Osmolality n/a o Viscosity n/a o May contain propylene glycol and sucralose; grape-flavored o Store at room temperature.
Note	• Solution is not considered a therapeutic equivalent to tablet.

Pharmacokinetic (patient)

Absorption	• Specific site not known; t_{max} ~2 hours after an oral dose • Bioavailability ~10%–35%
Transport	• Substrate for OATP uptake and MRP2 efflux transporters • Plasma protein binding ~95%, mainly to albumin • V_d ~17 liters
Metabolism	• Unlike losartan, valsartan is not a prodrug. • Modest metabolism by CYP2C9 (~20%), eliminated primarily by biliary excretion mostly unchanged • Cl ~2 L/h

Enteral Administration and Nutrition Considerations

Compatibility, Stability, Bioavailability Considerations

- An aqueous solution of valsartan sodium (with solubility ~5 mg/mL) has a pH of ~5.5.[1]
- The solution formulation, as studied in a group of healthy subjects, exhibited greater oral bioavailability (1.74-fold) than the intact tablet.[2]

- An oral suspension (4 mg/mL) prepared from 80 mg tablets in OraPlus/ OraSweet SF (1:1) can be stored in amber glass bottles for 30 days at room temperature or 75 days at 2°C–8°C.[3]
- An extemporaneous oral suspension (4 mg/mL) exhibited greater oral bioavailability (1.56-fold) than the intact tablet in a study of healthy subjects.[2]
- An extemporaneously compounded oral suspension (4 mg/mL) prepared from drug powder in SyrSpend SF PH4, stored in low-actinic bottles at 2°C–8°C or 20°C–25°C, remained stable (HPLC analysis) for 90 days.[4]
- An extemporaneously compounded oral suspension (16 mg/mL) prepared from tablets (80 mg) in a complex aqueous vehicle, stored in opaque plastic containers at 23°C–27°C (60% relative humidity), remained stable (HPLC analysis) at 30 days.[5]
- One out of 27 tablet formulations in development for an orally disintegrating product exhibited a faster rate of absorption and greater oral bioavailability (1.35-fold) compared with the conventional oral tablet.[6]
- In an animal model, a solid dispersion formulation under evaluation exhibited less crystallinity, improved dissolution, and a 2-fold increase in oral bioavailability compared with pure drug.[7]
- Different solid dispersion formulations also exhibited improved dissolution (especially at pH 6.8) and bioavailability compared with pure drug in animal models.[8,9]
- Several solid dispersion formulations were developed for testing, with one exhibiting complete dissolution and higher bioavailability (2.65-fold) compared with the plain drug in an animal model.[10]
- Solid self-microemulsifying formulations under study exhibited rapid disintegration and dissolution, with an increased oral bioavailability (2.2-fold) in an animal model relative to pure drug powder.[11,12]
- A semisolid, self-microemulsifying formulation being evaluated exhibited an increased rate of dissolution and an increased oral bioavailability (~3-fold) in an animal model relative to oral solid formulation.[13]
- Tested nanoparticles performed better than microparticles in an animal model for oral bioavailability, although both exhibited improved dissolution compared with crude drug crystals across the pH range 1.2–6.8.[14]
- A nanoparticle formulation in development improved drug dissolution and increased oral bioavailability (1.8-fold) in an animal model compared with the commercial tablet.[15]
- Other nanoparticle formulations under study also demonstrated enhanced dissolution and oral bioavailability.[16,17]
- In research, several nanosuspension formulations have been prepared with adequate stability and improved dissolution.[18]

Drug-Nutrition Interactions
- Drug may influence nutrition status directly or indirectly:
  - CNS: fatigue, dizziness
  - GI: abdominal pain, diarrhea
  - Metabolic: angioedema, hyperkalemia
  - Other: arthralgia, back pain
- No data on the influence of malnutrition or obesity on drug disposition.
- Influence of food on oral absorption or bioavailability:
  - Food decreases the rate of drug absorption and reduces oral bioavailability by ~40% when using the tablet formulation.
  - The oral bioavailability is not influenced by a food effect when administered as part of a fixed combination tablet.[19]
  - In an animal model, a fructose-supplemented diet administered into the duodenum increased drug absorption compared with a control diet, at least in part by a reduction (~50%) in MRP2 expression.[20]

Recommendations

Gastric	• Dilute oral solution with water (at least 1:1) prior to administration. • No need to hold EN beyond the time required to flush-administer-flush, but administer medication consistently relative to EN administration.
Postpyloric	• As above. • Monitor for any unexpected change in effect.

References
1. Wang J, Chen L, Zhao Z, et al. Valsartan lowers brain beta-amyloid protein levels and improves spatial learning in a mouse model of Alzheimer disease. *J Clin Invest*. 2007;117: 3393–3402.
2. Sunkara G, Bende G, Mendonza AE, et al. Bioavailability of valsartan oral dosage forms. *Clin Pharmacol Drug Dev*. 2013;3:132–138.
3. Allen LV. Valsartan 4 mg/mL oral liquid. *Int J Pharm Compd*. 2008;12:269.
4. Polonini HC, Silva SL, Cunha CN, et al. Compatibility of cholecalciferol, haloperidol, imipramine hydrochloride, levodopa/carbidopa, lorazepam, minocycline hydrochloride, tacrolimus monohydrate, terbinafine, tramadol hydrochloride and valsartan in SyrSpend SF PH4 oral suspensions. *Pharmazie*. 2016;71:185–191.
5. Zaid AN, Assali M, Qaddomi A, et al. Preparation and stability evaluation of extemporaneous oral suspension of valsartan using commercially available tablets. *Int J Pharm Compd*. 2014;18:169–174.
6. Ibrahim HK, El-Setouhy DA. Valsartan orodispersible tablets: formulation, in vitro/in vivo characterization. *AAPS PharmSciTech*. 2010;11:189–196.
7. Chella N, Daravath B, Kumar D, Tadikonda RR. Formulation and pharmacokinetic evaluation of polymeric dispersions containing valsartan. *Eur J Drug Metab Pharmacokinet*. 2016;41:517–526.
8. Park YJ, Lee H-K, Im YB, Lee W, Han H-K. Improved pH-independent dissolution and oral absorption of valsartan via the preparation of solid dispersion. *Arch Pharm Res*. 2010;33:1235–1240.

9. Lee J-Y, Kang W-S, Piao J, et al. Soluplus®/TPGS-based solid dispersions prepared by holt-melt extrusion equipped with twin-screw systems for enhancing oral bioavailability of valsartan. *Drug Design Dev Ther.* 2015;9:2745–2756.
10. Chella N, Tadikonda R. Melt dispersion granules: formulation and evaluation to improve oral delivery of poorly soluble drugs: a case study with valsartan. *Drug Dev Ind Pharm.* 2015;41:888–897.
11. Yeom DW, Chae BR, Kim JH, et al. Solid formulation of a supersaturable self-microemulsifying drug delivery system for valsartan with improved dissolution and bioavailability. *Oncotarget.* 2017;8:94297–94316.
12. Yeom DW, Chae BR, Son HY, et al. Enhanced oral bioavailability of valsartan using a polymer-based supersaturable self-microemulsifying drug delivery system. *Int J Nanomedicine.* 2017;12:3533–3545.
13. Zhao K, Yuan Y, Wang H, et al. Preparation and evaluation of valsartan by a novel semi-solid self-microemulsifying delivery system using Gelucire 44/14. *Drug Dev Ind Pharm.* 2016;42:1545–1552.
14. Ma Q, Sun H, Che E, et al. Uniform nano-sized valsartan for dissolution and bioavailability enhancement: influence of particle size and crystalline state. *Int J Pharm.* 2013;441:75–81.
15. Biswas N. Modified mesoporous silica nanoparticles for enhancing oral bioavailability and antihypertensive activity of poorly water soluble valsartan. *Eur J Pharm Sci.* 2017;99: 152–160.
16. Kim M-S, Baek I-H. Fabrication and evaluation of valsartan-polymer-surfactant composite nanoparticles by using the supercritical antisolvent process. *Int J Nanomedicine.* 2014;9:5167–5176.
17. Gora S, Mustafa G, Sahni JK, Ali J, Baboota S. Nanosizing of valsartan by high pressure homogenization to produce dissolution enhanced nanosuspension: pharmacokinetics and pharmacodynamics study. *Drug Deliv.* 2016;23:940–950.
18. Vuppalapati L, Cherukuri S, Neeli V, Yeragamreddy PR, Kesavan BR. Application of central composite design in optimization of valsartan nanosuspension to enhance its solubility and stability. *Curr Drug Deliv.* 2016;13:143–157.
19. Sunkara G, Jiang X, Reynolds C, et al. Effect of food on the oral bioavailability of amlodipine/valsartan and amlodipine/valsartan/hydrochlorothiazide fixed dose combination tablets in healthy subjects. *Clin Pharmacol Drug Dev.* 2014;3:487–492.
20. Londero AS, Arana MR, Perdomo VG, et al. Intestinal multidrug resistance-associated protein 2 is down-regulated in fructose-fed rats. *J Nutr Biochem.* 2017;40:178–186.

Vardenafil Hydrochloride

Product Availability

Solid	• Tablet:
	    ○ Immediate-release: 2.5 mg, 5 mg, 10 mg, 20 mg (Levitra®
	       [Bayer]; others)
	    ○ Orally disintegrating: 10 mg (Staxyn® [Bayer]; others)

Physicochemical (drug)

Molecular weight: • 488.61 (salt 525.07)	Permeability: • LogP 2.23 (calc) • LogD n/a	Water solubility: • 0.11 mg/mL (salt)
pKa: • 4.7, 6.2	Classification: • BCS Class n/a; BDDCS Class 1	

Pharmaceutical (product)

Solid	• Immediate-release tablet products are film-coated. • Orally disintegrating tablet products can disperse in water, but they are not considered bioequivalent to immediate-release tablets. • Orally disintegrating tablet products may contain aspartame.

Pharmacokinetic (patient)

Absorption	• Specific site not known; t_{max} ~1 hour after an oral dose (fasted) • Bioavailability ~15% (immediate-release); ~21% (orally disintegrating)
Transport	• Substrate for P-glycoprotein, BCRP, and MRP2 efflux • Plasma protein binding ~95% • V_d ~208 liters
Metabolism	• Metabolized in part to an active metabolite ("M1") via CYP3A4, then excreted through bile • Cl ~56 L/h

Enteral Administration and Nutrition Considerations

Compatibility, Stability, and Bioavailability Considerations
- No data are available on the stability of tablets that are crushed and dispersed in water prior to administration.
- Administration of the 10 mg tablet (preparation step not described) via jejunal tube (size not reported) to a critically ill patient weaning off inhaled nitric oxide resulted in improvement in pulmonary artery pressures within 30 minutes, but the patient also experienced systemic hypotension; an attempt later in the hospital stay using 5 mg (2 or 3 times daily) was more successful.[1]

- The greater bioavailability (~21%) of the orally disintegrating tablet relative to the conventional tablet may be attributed to some oral mucosal absorption.[2]

Drug-Nutrition Interactions
- Drug may influence nutrition status directly or indirectly:
  - CNS: headache, dizziness, visual disturbances
  - GI: nausea, dyspepsia
  - Metabolic: elevated creatine kinase
  - Other: flu-like syndrome
- No data on the influence of malnutrition or obesity on drug disposition.
- Influence of food on oral absorption or bioavailability:
  - A high-fat meal (910 kcal, 58 g fat) reduced the rate of absorption, but with no influence on oral bioavailability.[3]
  - A moderate-fat meal (700 kcal, 23 g fat) has no influence on rate or extent of drug absorption.[3]
  - Grapefruit juice is likely to increase oral bioavailability.

Recommendations

Gastric	• If there is no therapeutic alternative (eg, sildenafil), disperse the orally disintegrating tablet in water just prior to administration. • No need to hold EN beyond the time required to flush-administer-flush.
Postpyloric	• As above. • Monitor for any unexpected change in effect.

References

1. Giacomini M, Borotto E, Bosotti L, et al. Vardenafil and weaning from inhaled nitric oxide: effect on pulmonary hypertension in ARDS. *Anaesth Intensive Care.* 2007;35: 91–93.
2. Heinig R, Weimann B, Dietrich H, Böttcher M-F. Pharmacokinetics of a new orodispersible tablet formulation of vardenafil. *Clin Drug Investig.* 2011;31:27–41.
3. Rajagopalan P, Mazzu A, Xia C, Dawkins R, Sundaresan P. Effect of high-fat breakfast and moderate-fate evening meal on the pharmacokinetics of vardenafil, an oral phosphodiesterase-5 inhibitor for the treatment of erectile dysfunction. *J Clin Pharmacol.* 2003;43:260–267.

Varenicline Tartrate

Product Availability

Solid	• Tablet: 0.5 mg, 1 mg (base) (Chantix® [Pfizer]; others)

Physicochemical (drug)

Molecular weight: • 211.27 (salt 361.35)	Permeability: • LogP 0.90 • LogD n/a	Water solubility: • 0.2 mg/mL
pKa: • 1.8, 9.7	Classification: • BCS Class 1; BDDCS Class 3	

Pharmaceutical (product)

Solid	• Tablet products have a thin film-coating. • Tablets can be crushed and dispersed in water.

Pharmacokinetic (patient)

Absorption	• Specific site not known; t_{max} ~3–4 hours after an oral dose • Bioavailability ~90%
Transport	• Possible substrate for OCT2 transport • Plasma protein binding ≤20% • V_d ~5.9 L/kg
Metabolism	• Eliminated primarily unchanged in urine • Cl ~100–150 mL/min

Enteral Administration and Nutrition Considerations

Compatibility, Stability, and Bioavailability Considerations
- No data are available on the efficacy or stability of tablets crushed and dispersed in water prior to administration.
- Tablet (1 mg) crushed and stored in sealed transparent glass bottles or light-shielded glass bottles at 30°C under diffuse light and 75% relative humidity remained stable (98.3%–99.4% content remained).[1]

Drug-Nutrition Interactions
- Drug may influence nutrition status directly or indirectly:
  - CNS: mood disorders (eg, depression, aggression), somnambulism
  - GI: nausea, vomiting, constipation
  - Metabolic: angioedema
- No data on the influence of malnutrition or obesity on drug disposition.
- Influence of food on oral absorption or bioavailability:
  - Food has no influence on the rate or extent of drug absorption.[2]

Recommendations

Gastric	• If there is no therapeutic alternative (eg, transdermal therapy), crush and disperse tablet in water just prior to administration. • No need to hold EN beyond the time required to flush-administer-flush.
Postpyloric	• As above. • Monitor for any unexpected change in effect.

References

1. Data on file (135) with Pfizer, Inc; 2016.
2. Faessel HM, Obach RS, Rollema H, et al. A review of the clinical pharmacokinetics and pharmacodynamics of varenicline for smoking cessation. *Clin Pharmacokinet*. 2010;49: 799–816.

Venlafaxine Hydrochloride

Product Availability

Solid	• Tablet:
	  ○ Immediate-release: 25 mg, 37.5 mg, 50 mg, 75 mg, 100 mg (base) (various)
	  ○ Extended-release: 37.5 mg, 75 mg, 150 mg, 225 mg (base) (various)
	• Capsule: Extended-release: 37.5 mg, 75 mg, 150 mg (base) (Effexor® XR [Wyeth Pharms]; others)

Physicochemical (drug)

Molecular weight: • 277.41 (salt 313.87)	Permeability: • LogP 2.74 • LogD n/a	Water solubility: • 572 mg/mL (salt)
pKa: • 9.4	Classification: • BCS Class 1; BDDCS Class 1	

Pharmaceutical (product)

Solid	• The immediate-release tablet disperses in water after crushing. • Do not crush extended-release tablet or capsule contents (coated granules) or place them in water.

Pharmacokinetic (patient)

Absorption	• Specific site not known; t_{max} ~2 hours after an oral dose • Bioavailability ~90%
Transport	• Plasma protein binding ~30% • V_d ~7.5 L/kg
Metabolism	• Extensively metabolized to an active metabolite O-desmethyl-venlafaxine by CYP2D6; excretion is primarily through the urine • Cl ~1.3 L/h/kg

Enteral Administration and Nutrition Considerations

Compatibility, Stability, and Bioavailability Considerations
- An oral liquid (5 mg/mL) prepared from tablets in OraSweet/OraPlus (1:1), stored in amber glass bottles, remained stable (HPLC analysis) for up to 10 days (at 22°C–28°C) or 15 days (4°C) and had a pH of ~4.[1]
- An extemporaneously compounded oral suspension (7.5 mg/mL) prepared from extended-release capsule contents in tragacanth mucilage, stored in amber glass bottles at 20°C–24°C, remained stable (HPLC analysis) with only 3%–6% drug loss within 30 days; the suspension had a pH of 3.2; viscosity was not reported, and there are no data on whether this suspension could be administered through an enteral access device.[2]

- An extemporaneous solution (7.5 mg/mL) made from extended-release capsule contents in sorbitol syrup and distilled water, stored in amber glass bottles at 20°C–24°C, remained stable (HPLC analysis) for 30 days; the solution had a pH of 3.4; osmolality and viscosity were not reported, and there are no data on whether this mixture could be administered through an enteral access device.[2]
- A extemporaneously compounded oral suspension (15 mg/mL) prepared from extended-release capsule contents in OraPlus/OraSweet (1:1) or simple syrup, stored in amber plastic bottles at 5°C and 23°C, remained stable (HPLC analysis) for 28 days, although higher losses (2%–7%) occurred in simple syrup; the initial drug concentration measured was actually ~12 mg/mL; osmolality and viscosity were not reported, and there are no data on whether this mixture could be administered through an enteral access device.[3]
- There were no differences in the oral bioavailability of venlafaxine or its active metabolite before and after gastric bypass when the extended-release capsule was used in patients serving as their own control.[4]
- Similar findings were reported previously.[5]

Drug-Nutrition Interactions
- Drug may influence nutrition status directly or indirectly:
  - Weight loss
  - CNS: somnolence or insomnia, headache, dizziness
  - GI: dry mouth, anorexia, nausea, constipation
  - Metabolic: hyponatremia, hypercholesterolemia
- No data on the influence of malnutrition or obesity on drug disposition.
- Influence of food on oral absorption or bioavailability:
  - Food may have a limited effect on the rate or extent of drug absorption without an influence on oral bioavailability, but food may reduce GI complaints.[6]

Recommendations

Gastric	• Crush and/or disperse tablet in water prior to administration. • No need to hold EN beyond the time required to flush-administer-flush.
Postpyloric	• As above. • Monitor for any unexpected change in effect.

References

1. Kervela JG, Castagnet S, Chiadmi F, et al. Assessment of stability in extemporaneously prepared venlafaxine solutions. *Eur J Hosp Pharm Pract*. 2009;15:30–32.
2. De Rosa NF, Sharley NA. Stability of venlafaxine hydrochloride liquid formulations suitable for administration via enteral feeding tubes. *J Pharm Pract Res*. 2008;38:212–215.
3. Donnelly RF, Wong K, Goddard R, et al. Stability of venlafaxine immediate-release suspensions. *Int J Pharm Compd*. 2011;15:81–84.

4. Krieger CA, Cunningham JL, Reid JM, et al. Comparison of bioavailability of single-dose extended-release venlafaxine capsules in obese patients before and after gastric bypass surgery. *Pharmacotherapy.* 2017;37:1374–1382.
5. Hamad GG, Helsel JC, Perel JM, et al. The effect of gastric bypass on the pharmacokinetics of serotonin reuptake inhibitors. *Am J Psychiatry.* 2012;169:256–263.
6. Troy SM, Parker VP, Hicks DR, Pollack GM, Chiang ST. Pharmacokinetics and effect of food on the bioavailability of orally administered venlafaxine. *J Clin Pharmacol.* 1997; 37:954–961.

Verapamil Hydrochloride

Product Availability

Solid	• Tablet:
	   ○ Immediate-release: 80 mg, 120 mg (Calan® [GD Searle]; others)
	   ○ Extended-release: 120 mg, 240 mg (Calan® SR [Pfizer]; others)
	• Capsule:
	   ○ Extended-release: 120 mg, 180 mg, 240 mg, 360 mg (Verelan®
	     [Recro]; others)
	   ○ Controlled-/extended-release: 100 mg, 200 mg, 300 mg
	     (Verelan® PM [Recro]; others)

Physicochemical (drug)

Molecular weight: • 454.61 (salt 491.07)	Permeability: • LogP 3.79 • LogD 3.12 (pH 7.4, calc), 2.24 (pH 6.5, calc)	Water solubility: • 0.005 mg/mL • 70–83 mg/mL (salt)
pKa: • 8.9	Classification: • BCS Class 1; BDDCS Class 1	

Pharmaceutical (product)

Solid	• Most tablet products are film-coated and do not disperse in water. • Do not crush extended-release tablets or capsule contents.

Pharmacokinetic (patient)

Absorption	• Specific site not known; t_{max} ~1–2 hours after an oral dose (immediate-release) • Bioavailability ~20%–35%
Transport	• Substrate for P-glycoprotein efflux • Plasma protein binding ~90% • V_d ~4.5–7 L/kg

Metabolism	• Significant first-pass effect
	• Metabolized to ≥12 metabolites via CYP3A4/CYP1A2
	  (major active metabolite is nor-verapamil) and excreted
	  renally
	• Cl ~15 mL/min/kg

Enteral Administration and Nutrition Considerations

Compatibility, Stability, and Bioavailability Considerations

- A 0.1% aqueous solution has a pH of 5.25, and a 5% aqueous solution
  has a pH of 4.5–6.5.
- Maximal drug stability occurs at pH 3.2–5.6; at pH >6, the drug
  decomposes and insoluble precipitate forms.[1]
- Verapamil does not interact with microcrystalline cellulose, magnesium
  stearate, hydroxyl-propyl-methyl cellulose, polyvinyl-pyrrolidone, or talc.[2]

- An extemporaneous suspension (10 mg/mL) prepared from 80 mg
  tablets in syrup, glycerin, and water with pH adjusted to 4–5 as needed
  to prevent precipitation had no reported stability data, but it was
  provided with BUD of 7 days under refrigeration.[3]
- The official USP oral solution and suspension (50 mg/mL) is expected
  to have pH 3.8–4.8 and has been provided a BUD of 60 days (at room
  temperature or refrigeration).
- An extemporaneous suspension (50 mg/mL) prepared from 80 mg
  tablets in one of several vehicles (OraSweet/OraPlus [1:1], OraSweet
  SF/OraPlus [1:1], or cherry syrup/simple syrup [1:4]), stored in amber
  polyethylene terephthalate plastic bottles at 5°C and 25°C, remained
  stable (HPLC analysis) at 60 days.[4]
- An extemporaneous suspension (50 mg/mL) prepared from tablets
  (80 mg) in simple syrup/methylcellulose 1% (1:1), stored in glass or
  plastic at 4°C and 25°C, remained stable (HPLC analysis) for 91 days.[5]
- An oral solution (50 mg/mL) prepared from drug powder in OraSweet
  SF/OraPlus (1:1) or in SyrSpend SF, stored in amber bottles at 2°C–8°C,
  exhibited no drug loss (HPLC analysis); however, a precipitate was noted
  in the OraSweet preparation.[6]
- When a dose (60 mg) of an oral, sugar-free solution available in the
  United Kingdom was administered (in error) via a subclavian central
  venous access device of similar size to the patient's nasogastric tube,
  the patient experienced rapid cognitive decline and respiratory arrest,
  requiring a difficult intubation; this outcome might have occurred
  because a Luer connector syringe compatible with both enteral and
  intravenous access devices was used.[7]

Drug-Nutrition Interactions
- Drug may influence nutrition status directly or indirectly:
  - CNS: dizziness, headache, lethargy, blurred vision
  - GI: dry mouth, nausea, dyspepsia, constipation, increased AST
    and ALT
  - Other: arthralgia
- Influence of malnutrition or obesity on drug disposition:
  - Although drug clearance is essentially unchanged in obesity, the
    volume of distribution (weight-normalized and absolute) is increased,
    suggesting the use of total body weight for the initial (loading) dose.[8]
- Influence of food on oral absorption or bioavailability:
  - Food has no known influence on oral bioavailability of immediate-
    release products, but food may decrease the oral bioavailability of
    extended-release products.
  - Anthocyanidins may compete with verapamil as a substrate for
    P-glycoprotein.[9]

o Grapefruit juice (either 200 mL once or larger, more-frequent volumes) may increase oral bioavailability from ~1.4-fold (immediate-release) to ~2.5-fold (extended-release) relative to orange juice or water; of note, there was significant interindividual variability.[10-12]

Recommendations

Gastric	• If there is no therapeutic alternative, use a stable, extemporaneously prepared liquid product and dilute with water just prior to administration. • No need to hold EN beyond the time required to flush-administer-flush.
Postpyloric	• As above. • Monitor for any unexpected change in effect.

References

1. Gupta VD. Quantitation and stability of verapamil hydrochloride using high-performance liquid chromatography. *Drug Dev Ind Pharm.* 1985;11:1497–1506.
2. Nunes RS, Semaan FS, Riga AT, et al. Thermal behavior of verapamil hydrochloride and its association with excipients. *J Therm Anal Calorim.* 2009;97:349–353.
3. Woods DJ. *Formulation in Pharmacy Practice.* Dunedin, New Zealand: Healthcare Otago, 1993.
4. Allen LV, Erickson MA. Stability of labetalol hydrochloride, metoprolol tartrate, verapamil hydrochloride, and spironolactone with hydrochlorothiazide in extemporaneously compounded oral liquids. *Am J Health-Syst Pharm.* 1996;53:2304–2309.
5. Nahata MC. Stability of verapamil in an extemporaneous liquid dosage form. *J Appl Ther.* 1997;1:271–273.
6. Voudrie MA, Alexander B, Allen DB. Stability of verapamil hydrochloride in SyrSpend SF compared to sorbitol containing syrup and suspending vehicles. *Int J Pharm Compd.* 2011;15:255–258.
7. Roberts TCN, Swart M. Enteral drugs given through a central venous catheter. *Anaesthesia.* 2007;62:624–626.
8. Abernethy DR, Schwartz JB, Verapamil pharmacodynamics and disposition in obese hypertensive patients. *J Cardiovasc Pharmacol.* 1988;11:209–215.
9. Vrzal R. Anthocyanidins but not anthocyanins inhibit P-glycoprotein-mediated calcein extrusion—possible implication for orally administered drugs. *Fundam Clin Pharmacol.* 2016;30:248–252.
10. Zaidenstein R, Dishi V, Gips M, et al. The effect of grapefruit juice on the pharmacokinetics of orally administered verapamil. *Eur J Clin Pharmacol.* 1998;54:337–340.
11. Ho PC, Ghose K, Saville D, Wanwimolruk S. Effect of grapefruit juice on pharmacokinetics and pharmacodynamics of verapamil enantiomers in healthy volunteers. *Eur J Clin Pharmacol.* 2000;56:693–698.
12. Fuhr U, Muller-Peltzer H, Kern R, et al. Effects of grapefruit juice and smoking on verapamil concentrations in steady state. *Eur J Clin Pharmacol.* 2002;58:45–53.

Warfarin

Product Availability

Solid	• Tablet: 1 mg, 2 mg, 2.5 mg, 3 mg, 4 mg, 5 mg, 6 mg, 7.5 mg, 10 mg (salt) (Coumadin® [Bristol Myers Squibb]; Jantoven® [USL Pharma]; others)

Physicochemical (drug)

Molecular weight: • 308.34	Permeability: • LogP 2.60 • LogD 1.12 (pH 7.4)	Water solubility: • 0.02 mg/mL
pKa: • 5	Classification: • BCS Class 2; BDDCS Class 2	

Pharmaceutical (product)

Solid	• Tablet products may disperse in water (20 mL) within 5 minutes. • Some products may be film-coated. • Bioequivalence between the innovator and generic product does not necessarily mean bioequivalence between one generic product and another.

Pharmacokinetic (patient)

Absorption	• Specific site not known; t_{max} ~3–6 hours after an oral dose • Bioavailability varies significantly between individuals.
Transport	• Plasma protein binding ~99%, mostly to albumin • V_d ~0.14 L/kg
Metabolism	• Metabolized to varying degrees by CYP2C9/19, CYP2C8/18, CYP1A2, and CYP3A4, with significant variability between individuals • Pharmacologic activity of the S-enantiomer is greater than the R-enantiomer • Cl can vary considerably; ~0.05 mL/min/kg

Enteral Administration and Nutrition Considerations

Compatibility, Stability, and Bioavailability Considerations
- An aqueous solution (1%) has a pH of 7.2–8.6; a precipitate is likely at pH <8.
- Different drug structure isomers may be present in aqueous solution, depending on pH; significant quantities of the cyclic hemiketal form at lower pH, which lowers drug solubility and can influence overall bioavailability.[1]
- Low drug solubility in acidic conditions improves in the presence of EN.[2]
- At lower pH (<7), warfarin can bind to polyvinyl chloride plastic but not to polypropylene.[3–5]

- Crushed tablet (5 mg) dispersed in water (10 mL) and administered through a nasogastric tube (12 Fr, 43 inches, polyurethane), with 5 mL water flush before and after, resulted in less drug being delivered and likely reflects drug binding to the feeding tube.[2]
- An extemporaneously compounded oral suspension (1 mg/mL) prepared from tablets (5 mg) or from drug powder in a vehicle containing tragacanth mucilage, sorbitol syrup, and distilled water, stored in amber glass bottles at 20°C–24°C, remained stable (HPLC analysis) for 28 days.[6]
- The admixture of drug to EN (Osmolite) at concentrations between 17 and 67 µg/mL results in loss of approximately one-third of drug (HPLC analysis) at each drug concentration, after ultrafiltration.[7]
- Holding EN for 1 hour before and after drug administration may improve therapeutic effect.[8,9]
- Crushing and mixing drug with thickened water (to aid swallowing) significantly delayed dissolution.[10]
- Crushing and mixing drug in yogurt (pH 4.5, viscosity 723 mPa·s) slowed dissolution compared with crushing/dispersing in water (pH 6.7, viscosity 0.8 mPa·s).[10]
- The oral warfarin dose required to maintain therapeutic INR may be decreased (by at least 25%) in the weeks/months following gastric bypass but eventually returns toward baseline.[11]
- The oral warfarin dose required to maintain therapeutic INR remains significantly lower (median 55% at 1 month, 39% at 12 months) following the less-common biliopancreatic diversion with duodenal switch procedure.[12]

Drug-Nutrition Interactions
- Drug may influence nutrition status directly or indirectly:
  - CNS: headache (related to intracranial bleed)
  - GI: anorexia, nausea, vomiting, abdominal cramps, paralytic ileus, intestinal obstruction (related to submucosal/intramucosal bleed)
- Influence of malnutrition or obesity on drug disposition:
  - Obesity is associated with higher dose requirements and longer time to achieve initial therapeutic INR compared with no obesity; however, no specific dosing recommendations other than close therapeutic monitoring are made for obese patients, given the many factors that play a role in drug disposition and effect.[13]
- Influence of food on oral absorption or bioavailability:
  - Food has no known influence on oral bioavailability, but drug should be taken consistently with respect to food.
  - Vitamin K content of EN <200 µg/d is not expected to interfere with drug action.
  - EN may contain other ingredients that interfere with warfarin absorption.[8,14]

- o Ascorbic acid supplementation (500 mg) interfered with oral drug bioavailability.[15]
- o Grapefruit juice is not expected to influence oral bioavailability.

Recommendations

Gastric	• If there is no therapeutic alternative, disperse tablet in water just prior to administration. • Consider holding EN for 1 hour before and at least 1 hour after drug administration.
Postpyloric	• As above. • Monitor for any unexpected change in effect.
Other	• Monitor patient INR as needed.

References

1. Rosengren AM, Karlsson BCG. Spectroscopic evidence for the presence of the cyclic hemiketal form of warfarin in aqueous solution: consequences for bioavailability. *Biochem Biophys Res Communic.* 2011;407:318–320.
2. Klang M, Graham D, McLymont V. Warfarin bioavailability with feeding tubes and enteral formula. *JPEN J Parenter Enteral Nutr.* 2010;34:300–304.
3. Kowaluk EA, Roberts MS, Polack AE. Interactions between drugs and intravenous delivery systems. *Am J Hosp Pharm.* 1982;39:460–467.
4. Ennis CE, Merritt RJ, Neff ON. In vitro study of inline filtration of medications commonly administered to pediatric cancer patients. *JPEN J Parenter Enteral Nutr.* 1983; 7:156–158.
5. Kane M, Jay M, DeLuca PP. Binding of insulin to a continuous ambulatory peritoneal dialysis system. *Am J Hosp Pharm.* 1986;43:81–88.
6. Sharley NA, Yu AMC, Williams DB. Stability of mixtures formulated from warfarin tablets or powder. *J Pharm Pract Res.* 2007;37:95–97.
7. Kuhn TA, Garnett WR, Wells BK, et al. Recovery of warfarin from an enteral nutrient formula. *Am J Hosp Pharm.* 1989;46:1395–1399.
8. Dickerson RN, Garmon WM, Kuhl DA, et al. Vitamin K-dependent warfarin resistance after concurrent administration of warfarin and continuous enteral nutrition. *Pharmacotherapy.* 2008;28:308–313.
9. Krajewski KC, Butterfoss K. Achievement of therapeutic international normalized ratio following adjustment of tube feeds. *J Clin Pharmacol.* 2011;51:440–443.
10. Manrique YJ, Lee DJ, Islam F, et al. Crushed tablets: does the administration of food vehicles and thickened fluids to aid medication swallowing alter drug release? *J Pharm Pharmaceut Sci.* 2014;17:207–219.
11. Martin KA, Lee CR, Farrell TM, Moll S. Oral anticoagulant use after bariatric surgery: a literature review and clinical guideline. *Am J Med.* 2017;130:517–524.
12. Bolduc C, Flamand-Villeneuve J, Giroux I, et al. Warfarin dose adjustment after biliopancreatic diversion/duodenal switch bariatric surgery. *Ann Pharmacother.* 2018;52: 425–430.
13. Wallace JL, Reaves AB, Tollex EA, et al. Comparison of initial warfarin response in obese patients versus non-obese patients. *J Thromb Thrombolysis.* 2013;36:96–101.
14. Dickerson RN. Warfarin resistance and enteral tube feeding: a vitamin K-independent interaction. *Nutrition.* 2008;24:1048–1052.
15. Sattar A, Willman JE, Kolluri R. Possible warfarin resistance due to interaction with ascorbic acid: case report and literature review. *Am J Health-Syst Pharm.* 2013;70:782–786.

Zolpidem Tartrate

Product Availability

Solid	• Tablet:
	  o Immediate-release: 5 mg, 10 mg (Ambien® [Sanofi Aventis]; others)
	  o Extended-release: 6.25 mg, 12.5 mg (Ambien® CR [Sanofi Aventis]; others)
	  o Sublingual: 1.75 mg, 3.5 mg (Intermezzo® [Purdue]; others); 5 mg, 10 mg (Edluar® [Mylan]; others)

Physicochemical (drug)

Molecular weight: • 307.40 (salt 764.88)	Permeability: • LogP 3.03 (calc) • LogD 2.35 (pH 7.4)	Water solubility: • 23 mg/mL
pKa: • 6.2	Classification: • BCS Class 1; BDDCS Class 1	

Pharmaceutical (product)

Solid	• Although often film-coated, immediate-release tablet products can be crushed and dispersed in water. • Do not crush extended-release or sublingual tablets. • Sublingual tablet may contain mannitol, sorbitol, saccharin, and/or sucralose. • Immediate-release and sublingual tablets are considered bioequivalent.

Pharmacokinetic (patient)

Absorption	• Specific site not known; t_{max} ~1–2 hours after an oral dose (immediate-release) • Bioavailability ~70%
Transport	• Plasma protein binding ~92%–93% • V_d ~0.54 L/kg
Metabolism	• Metabolized by CYP3A4 as well as CYP1A2 and CYP2D6 to inactive metabolites that are eliminated renally • Cl ~51 mL/min/kg

Enteral Administration and Nutrition Considerations

Compatibility, Stability, and Bioavailability Considerations
• No data are available.

Drug-Nutrition Interactions:
• Drug may influence nutrition status directly or indirectly:
  o CNS: drowsiness, dizziness, headache, amnesia, ataxia

- ○ GI: dry mouth, nausea, diarrhea
- ○ Metabolic: angioedema, increased BUN, polyuria
- ○ Other: myalgia, arthralgia
- No data on the influence of malnutrition or obesity on drug disposition.
- Influence of food on oral absorption or bioavailability:
  - ○ Food reduces the rate of drug absorption and reduces the oral bioavailability of immediate-release and sublingual tablets by ~15% and ~20%, respectively.
  - ○ Food effects may vary significantly between individuals for both immediate-release and modified-release formulations.[1]

Recommendations

Gastric	• Crush and/or disperse immediate-release tablet in water just prior to administration. • No need to hold EN beyond the time required to flush-administer-flush.
Postpyloric	• As above. • Monitor for any unexpected change in effect.

Reference

1. Andreas CJ, Pepin X, Markopoulos C, et al. Mechanistic investigation of the negative food effect of modified release zolpidem. *Eur J Pharm Sci.* 2017;102:284–298.

About the Editor

Joseph Boullata is a recognized expert in the field of nutrition support and nutritional pharmacotherapy. Dr. Boullata is a clinical professor in nutrition sciences at Drexel University and was previously professor of pharmacology and therapeutics at the University of Pennsylvania and professor of pharmacy practice at Temple University—all in Philadelphia, Pennsylvania. Dr. Boullata is also a clinician, most recently a pharmacy specialist with the clinical nutrition support services at the Hospital of the University of Pennsylvania.

He received his doctorate from the University of Maryland after completing undergraduate degrees in nutrition science (Penn State) and pharmacy (Philadelphia College of Pharmacy). He completed a postdoctoral fellowship in nutrition support at the University of Maryland Medical System, as well as a clinical residency at the Johns Hopkins Hospital.

Dr. Boullata has performed research and published in the areas of nutrition, gastroenterology, and critical care, authoring more than 70 chapters and papers in peer-reviewed journals. Furthermore, he has been an investigator on a number of grant-funded research projects. Dr. Boullata's teaching goal has always been to help develop clinicians who are well grounded in science and clinical evidence, who can use appropriate judgment in practice. It is hoped that this book will contribute toward that goal.

Index

Page numbers followed by *f* indicate a figure and page numbers followed by *t* indicate a table on the corresponding page.